DATE DUE

2/17/05			
4/3/05			

Osseointegration and Autogenous Onlay Bone Grafts

Osseointegration and Autogenous Onlay Bone Grafts:

Reconstruction of the Edentulous Atrophic Maxilla

Per-Ingvar Brånemark, MD, PhD
Professor
Institute for Applied Biotechnology
Brånemark Osseointegration Center
Göteborg, Sweden

Kerstin Gröndahl, DDS, PhD
Associate Professor
Department of Oral and Maxillofacial Radiology
Göteborg University
Göteborg, Sweden

Philip Worthington, MD, BSc, FDSRCS
Professor and Former Chairman
Department of Oral and Maxillofacial Surgery
University of Washington
Seattle, Washington

Christina Darle
Coordinating Editor

quintessence books

Quintessence Publishing Co, Inc
Chicago, Berlin, London, Tokyo, Paris, Barcelona,
São Paulo, Moscow, Prague, and Warsaw

Library of Congress Cataloging-in-Publication Data

Brånemark, Per-Ingvar.
Osseointegration and autogenous onlay bone grafts : reconstruction of the edentulous atrophic maxilla / Per-Ingvar Brånemark, Kerstin Gröndahl, Philip Worthington.
p. ; cm.
Includes bibliographical references.
ISBN 0-86715-398-9 (hardcover)
1. Maxilla–Surgery–Case studies. 2. Bone-grafting–Case studies.
[DNLM: 1. Maxilla–surgery–Case Report. 2. Bone Transplantation–methods–Case Report. 3. Dental Implantation, Endosseous–Case Report. WU 600 B821o 2001] I. Gröndahl, Kerstin. II. Worthington, Philip. III. Title.
RD526 .B66 2001
617.5'22059--dc21

2001000043

Quintessence Publishing Co, Inc
551 Kimberly Drive
Carol Stream, Illinois 60188
www.quintpub.com

Editor: Kathryn Funk
Production: Susan Robinson
Design: Michael Shanahan

Printed in Hong Kong

Contents

Preface vi

1 The Challenge of the Severely Resorbed Maxilla 1

2 Protocol for Long-Term Study of Autogenous Onlay Bone Grafting and Simultaneous Endosseous Fixture Placement 7

3 Routine Case Presentations 31

4 Compromised Case Presentations 65

5 Unusual Case Presentations 93

6 Appraisal of Restored Anatomy and Function 111

7 Patients with Discontinuous Maxillae 135

References 159

Preface

The term *osseointegration* was coined by P-I Brånemark to describe a direct and load-bearing union between a titanium fixture and vital bone without the ingrowth of fibrous tissue at the interface between the bone and the fixture. The concept is the direct result of Brånemark's research and clinical observations in the 1950s and early 1960s.[1,2] Based on these findings, Brånemark and coworkers developed predictable surgical techniques and biocompatible components for functional prosthetic rehabilitation of edentulous patients. The treatment became known as oral and maxillofacial rehabilitation ad modum Brånemark. Since the first patient was treated in 1965, applications of this concept have been documented in more than 100 doctoral theses and over 2,000 scientific publications. The first results were reported in 1969 in an article on the rehabilitation of completely edentulous patients with adequate bone height for grafting.[3] The 10-year results of the same patient population were published in 1977.[4]

During the following decades, the procedure was expanded to include the treatment of most types of edentulous patients.[5–8] Continued long-term follow-up of clinical results in patients with severe resorption of the maxilla initiated development of modified surgical procedures that included the transfer of autogenous bone and marrow grafts to the region of fixture anchorage. The motivation was twofold: to secure mechanical stability of the prosthesis and to restore the topography of the anterior maxillary bone, thereby providing support to the upper lip.

This book covers modifications in clinical procedures for treatment of patients with severely resorbed maxillae over a period of two decades, with an emphasis on problems, complications, solutions, results, and future developments. The resolution of early clinical and technical problems, which are described, resulted in a clinically predictable treatment modality based on 10-year follow-up rehabilitation data. Both typical clinical cases and some unusual cases with defect anatomies are reported, illustrating methodology and clinical features and emphasizing variations in healing patterns. In addition, a detailed description of observations of individual patients and their problems is included for the purpose of motivating maxillofacial surgeons to suggest future improvements and simplifications.

Finally, this text suggests that a considerable number of patients who were previously treated with bone grafting to provide osseointegrated prosthetic substitutes for teeth might benefit from fixture anchorage in os zygomaticum. Based on what was learned during this study and experience with reconstruction of major maxillofacial defects, it is evident that this technique can be a cost-effective adjunct or alternative to bone-grafting procedures.

This study could never have been completed without the devoted collaboration of Barbro Svensson, who participated in all the operative work and organized the clinical and computer records–a mammoth task. Also appreciated has been the skilled surgical assistance from Olle Hallén, Jörgen Lindström, Ragnar Adell, Ulf Lekholm, Arne Ridell, and Lars-Olof Öhrnell at the clinic in Göteborg, Sweden, as well as the excellent prosthetic work performed by a multitude of highly skilled prosthodontists around the world. The continuous work by Dan Tolman and Eugene Keller in the field of autogenous bone grafting has been both inspirational and informative. Dan's initial comments and encouraging advice after his review of the preliminary outline of this book were particularly appreciated.

Thanks are due to Nils-Gunnar Pehrson for his meticulous completion of all the statistical analyses, and to Kjell Hagberg and the staff at EXOPRO for the development and manufacturing of all the new fixtures and related components. Appreciation is extended to Johnny Lindquist for his assistance with computer programming and data administration, to Fredrik Persson for his illustrations, and to Ylwa Winsnes Johanson for excellent clinical photography. Thanks to Eva Lind for her administration of the donor site morbidity study, and Marianne Szabo and Rigmor Carlsson for their administrative assistance. Greatly appreciated was Richard Johns' contribution of reviewing the entire book before it was published. On the following page are the clinical centers that collaborated in the study.

Philip Worthington, MD, BSc, FDSRCS
University of Washington
Seattle, Washington

Collaborating Clinical Centers

The University Hospital
Department of Oral and Maxillofacial Surgery
Linköping, Sweden

Örebro Medical Center Hospital
Department of Oral and Maxillofacial Surgery
Örebro, Sweden

County Hospital
Department of Oral and Maxillofacial Surgery
Borås, Sweden

Karolinska Institute
Institute of Odontology
Department of Oral and Maxillofacial Surgery
Huddinge, Sweden

Stockholm Söder Hospital
Oral Maxillofacial Clinic
Stockholm, Sweden

Vancouver Hospital and Health Sciences Center
Department of Dentistry
Vancouver, Canada

Brånemark Osseointegration Center
Santiago, Chile

Argyle Professional Building
Oral and Maxillofacial Surgery
Ottawa, Ontario, Canada

University of Madrid
Faculty of Odontology
Madrid, Spain

Westmead Hospital
Department of Oral and Maxillofacial Surgery
Westmead, Australia

Ordre du Corps Dentaire du Liban
Beyoruth, Libanon

Queen Mary's University Hospital
London, England

University of Texas Health Science Center at San Antonio
Department of Oral and Maxillofacial Surgery
San Antonio, Texas, USA

McGill University Health Centre
Montreal General Hospital
Department of Dentistry
Montreal, Canada

Hospital de Lénfant-Jesus
Quebec City, Canada

Catholic University Leuven
Faculty of Medicine
Department of Periodontology
Leuven, Belgium

Brånemark Osseointegration Center
Madrid, Spain

Blackrock Clinic
Blackrock, Dublin, Ireland

Fundacao Antonio Prudente
Hospital AC Camargo
Departamento de Estomatologia
São Paulo, Brazil

Alfred Hospital
Plastic and Reconstructive Surgery Unit
Melbourne, Australia

Brånemark Osseointegration Center
School of Dentistry
Malmö, Sweden

Brånemark Osseointegration Center
Tokyo, Japan

Guy's and St Thomas's Medical and Dental School
Department of Oral and Maxillofacial Surgery
Guy's Hospital
London, England

Brånemark Osseointegration Center
Oderzo, Italy

The Mayo Clinic
Rochester, Minnesota, USA

Long Beach Memorial Hospital
Long Beach, California, USA

Spokane Center for Tissue Integrated Reconstruction
Spokane, Washington, USA

Universidade de São Paulo
Hospital de Pesquisa e Reabilitacao de Lesoes Lábio-Palatais
Bauru, São Paulo, Brazil

University of Washington
School of Dentistry
Department of Oral and Maxillofacial Surgery
Seattle, Washington, USA

CHAPTER 1

The Challenge of the Severely Resorbed Maxilla

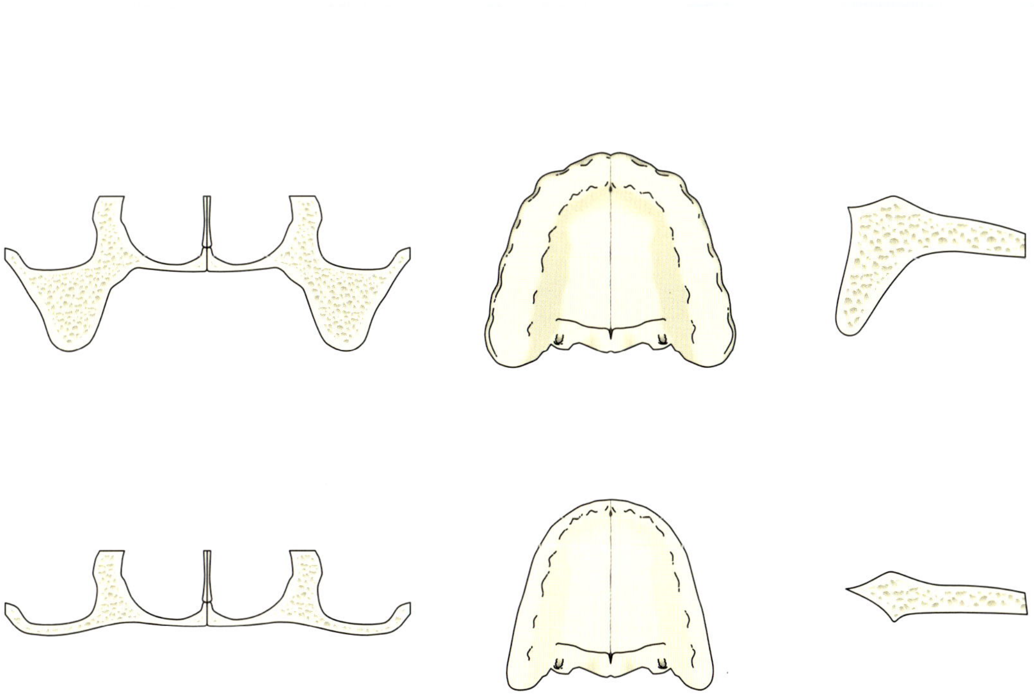

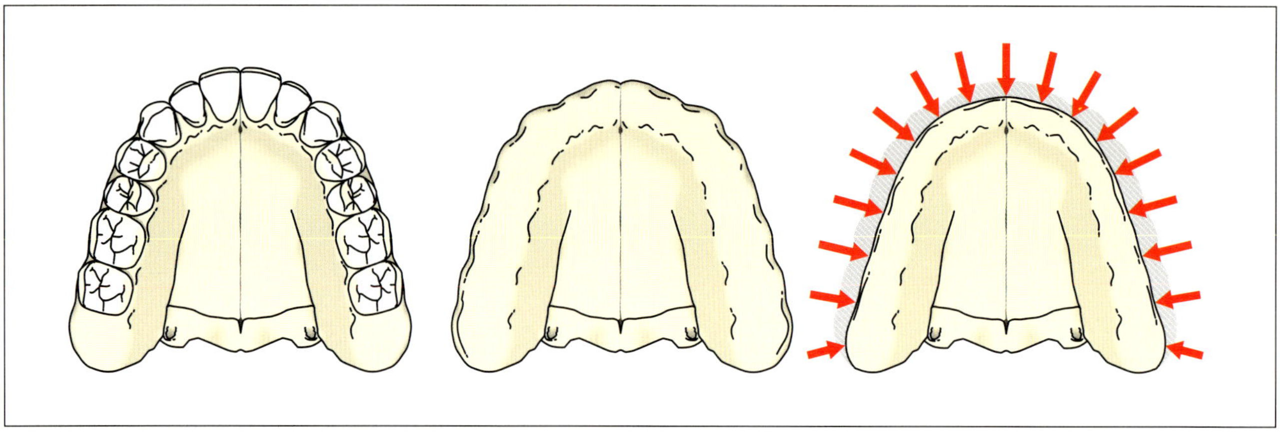

Fig 1-1 Typical resorption pattern in the edentulous maxilla with successive loss of bone.

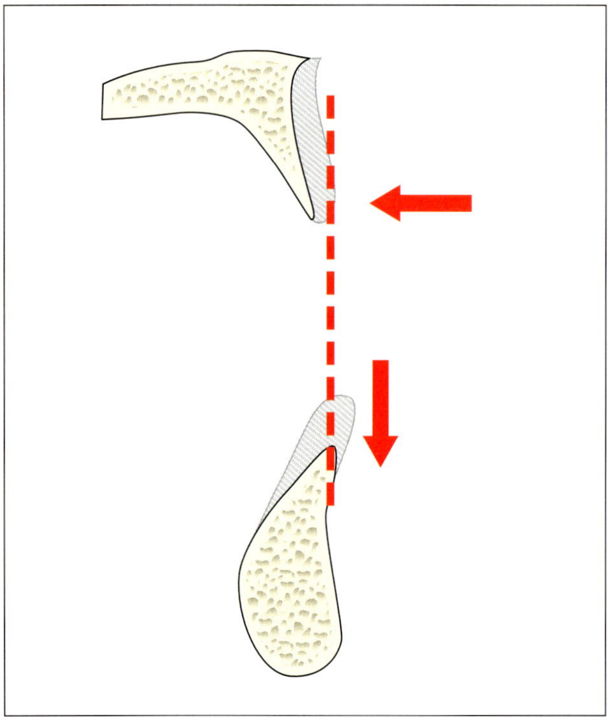

Fig 1-2 Effects of resorption. As the maxilla narrows, it appears to be more posterior in relation to the mandible.

In spite of refinements of the surgical technique and increased sophistication of prosthodontic reconstructions, there are limitations to what can be achieved with a prosthesis anchored in limited basal jawbone. The primary challenge involves treatment of the severely resorbed maxilla, where reduced bone volume and density often preclude predictable function of a bone-anchored prosthetic device.

Following the extraction of teeth, eg, because of periodontal disease, there is a loss of alveolar and basal bone. This resorption varies in degree from patient to patient. The pattern also differs in the maxilla when compared with the mandible.[9,10] There is usually a loss of bone height in the mandible, while the overall shape of the basal bone is preserved. In the maxilla, there is not only a loss of alveolar bone height, but also a loss of buccolabial width caused by bone resorption in the posterior direction (Fig 1-1). This causes a reduction of the maxilla and the interarch relationship progressively becomes one of skeletal class III.[11,12] The maxilla narrows and appears more posterior in relation to the mandible (Fig 1-2).

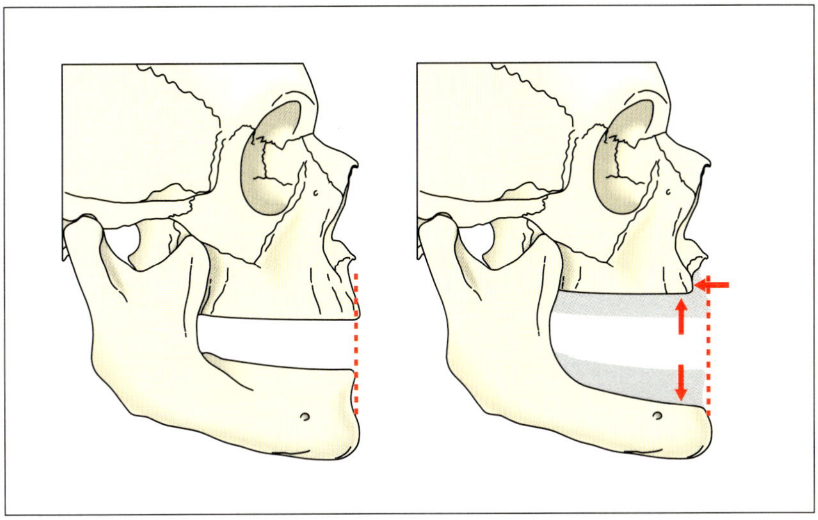

Fig 1-3 Increased interarch distance as a result of resorption.

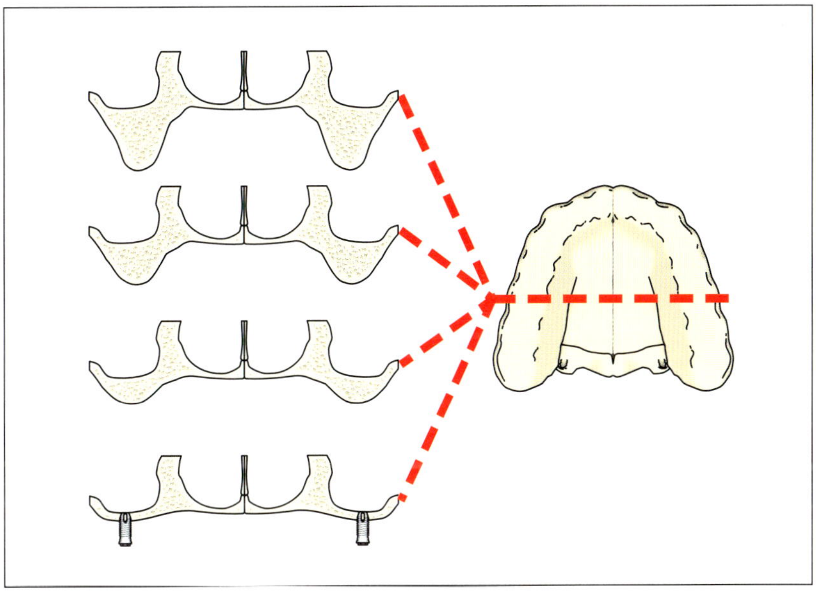

Fig 1-4 Reduced bone height as a result of resorption. Eventually the resorption process precludes or severely compromises optimal positioning and stable fixture placement.

As the interarch distance increases and the height of the available bone decreases, the ratio between the height of the prosthesis and the available bone for anchorage is increased (Fig 1-3). The reduced bone height can make fixture placement impossible or allow only for the use of short fixtures (Fig 1-4).

In cases where height is not lacking, extreme buccolabial resorption can compromise or even preclude fixture placement. In addition, a reduction in bone density frequently occurs. This increases the challenge associated with achieving adequate initial stability and/or stability in function. Both bone volume and bone density decrease once the functional stresses normally transmitted by natural teeth are lost. Different degrees of bone density are illustrated in Fig 1-5. The remodeling capacity is reduced in resorbed or insufficiently loaded bone tissue.

Resorption leaves the residual maxilla more retropositioned in relation to the mandible and the upper lip. Therefore, the prosthetic design must feature a greater anterior cantilever element. This, in turn, leads to progressively deteriorating retention capacity of a conventional maxillary denture. The problem is accentuated with age because deterioration of the neuromuscular system can lead to an inability to control the denture during function.

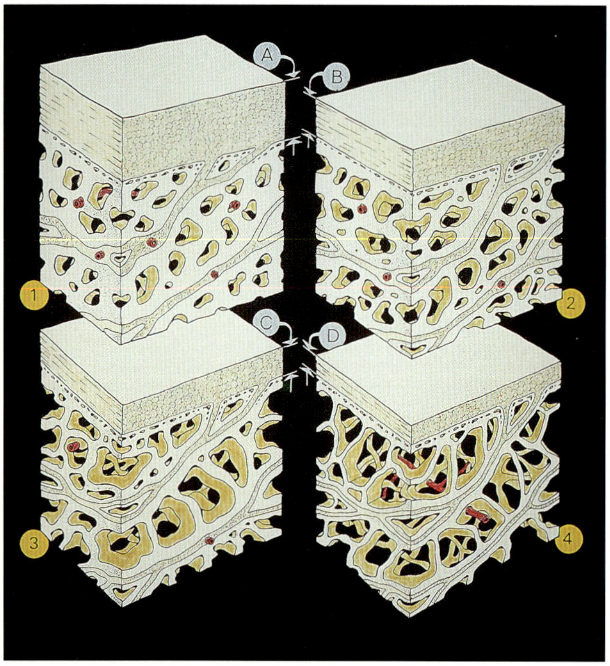

Fig 1-5 Differences in recipient and donor site bone density. Letters indicate reduction of cortical bone height; numbers indicate reduction of cancellous bone density.

Alternative Treatment Solutions

Various surgical remedies have been considered in the management of the severely resorbed maxilla. One example involves installing the fixture apex in the resorbed premaxilla and packing autogenous bone around the fixture in an effort to build an alveolar ridge. Experience has shown that this method is frequently followed by rapid bone loss.[13,14] The results improve when the bone grafts are allowed to incorporate prior to fixture placement.[15,16] The disadvantage with the latter method is that two surgical sessions, as well as an extended healing period, are required.

Grafting approaches can involve the use of particulate material or a corrective osteotomy together with an interpositional graft.[17] Many clinicians have attempted to augment the deficient bone of the maxillary sinus floor by grafting "upwards" into the lower part of the antrum (Fig 1-6).[18–23] These techniques are useful in certain circumstances, but when the grafting procedure is limited to the nasal and/or antral floors, the approach does not compensate for the anterior defect or the excessive interarch space resulting from alveolar atrophy.

A literature review conducted by Tolman in 1995 comprised 591 patients with 733 grafts and 2,315 fixtures.[24] The review included grafting procedures using blocks, autogenous bone (nonvascularized or vascularized), and a variety of particulate materials. Tolman concluded that "the fact that so many attempts have been made to find a solution to the problem is in itself an indication that no single solution has universal application."[24]

In a more recent study published in 1999, Keller, Tolman, and Eckert presented long-term (12-year) results on autogenous maxillary antral and nasal inlay grafts in the compromised maxilla.[25] The study included 118 inlay grafts and 248 Brånemark fixtures. The fixture survival rate was 87% and the prosthetic system survival rate was 95%.

A study from 1999 reported on 150 patients exposed to five different grafting techniques (local or full onlay graft, inlay, combination onlay/inlay, and LeFort I osteotomies).[15] A total of 781 Brånemark fixtures were placed. The majority of the patients were treated using a simultaneous approach and all received autogenous bone grafts. The overall fixture survival rate was approximately 80% after 3 years. Onlays, inlays, and LeFort I osteotomies showed almost the same success rates (76% to 84%), compared to 60% for the combined onlay/inlay technique. More implants were lost when they were placed simultaneously with grafting (23%) than when a delayed approach was used.

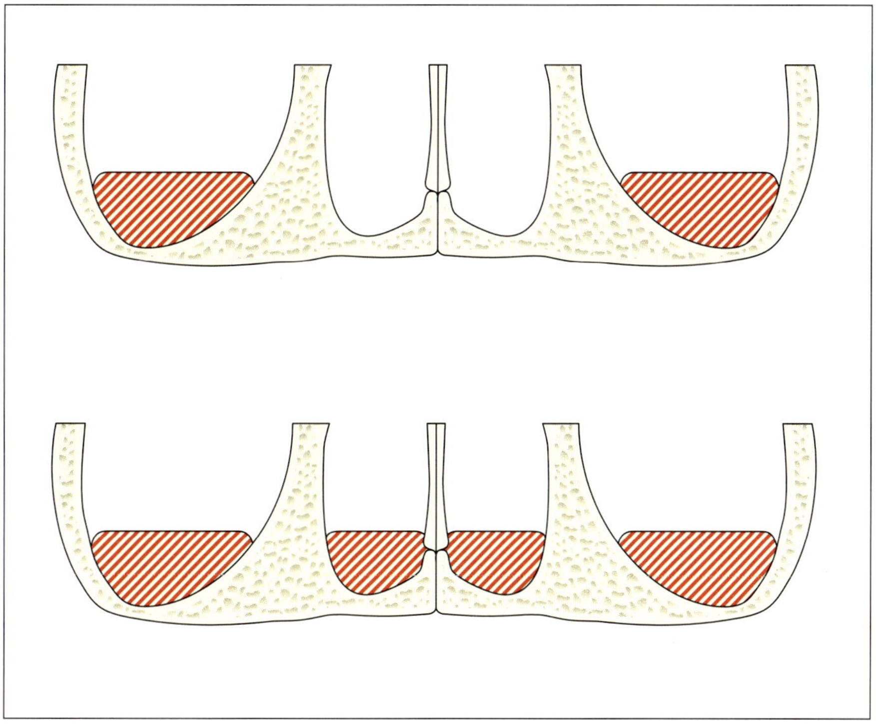

Fig 1-6 Sinus graft. Grafting the nasal and/or antral floors does not compensate for the anterior defect.

An interesting finding in this study was that the failure percentage for implants placed in nongrafted bone was comparatively lower (11%) than that of implants placed in grafted bone.

An ambitious attempt to evaluate the success of various aspects of sinus grafting was conducted in association with the Sinus Consensus Conference in 1996.[26] Yet the ultimate conclusion reached by the conference was essentially the same as Tolman's in 1995: the material was so "multivariate and multifactorial that it was difficult to draw definite conclusions; these must await controlled prospective studies."[26]

An alternative to grafting the atrophic maxilla is to place fixtures in nontraditional bone, eg, in the pterygoid plates (Fig 1-7). Another approach involves utilizing the relatively dense and mainly cortical bone of os zygomaticum[27] (Fig 1-8). Clinical results from these procedures indicate predictable and adequate long-term function. Yet the need remains for successful and predictable grafting procedures applicable to the severely resorbed maxilla.

Although valuable, many of the existing studies are characterized by small patient populations followed for short time periods. In addition, the surgeries of the limited observation groups were often conducted by different clinicians in a nonstandardized manner.

This book reports our long-term experiences with autogenous onlay bone grafting and simultaneous endosseous fixture placement. The patient population is sufficiently large for adequate statistical analyses. All patients were followed at least 2 years, and some up to 15 years. In addition, each surgery was performed by the same surgeon.

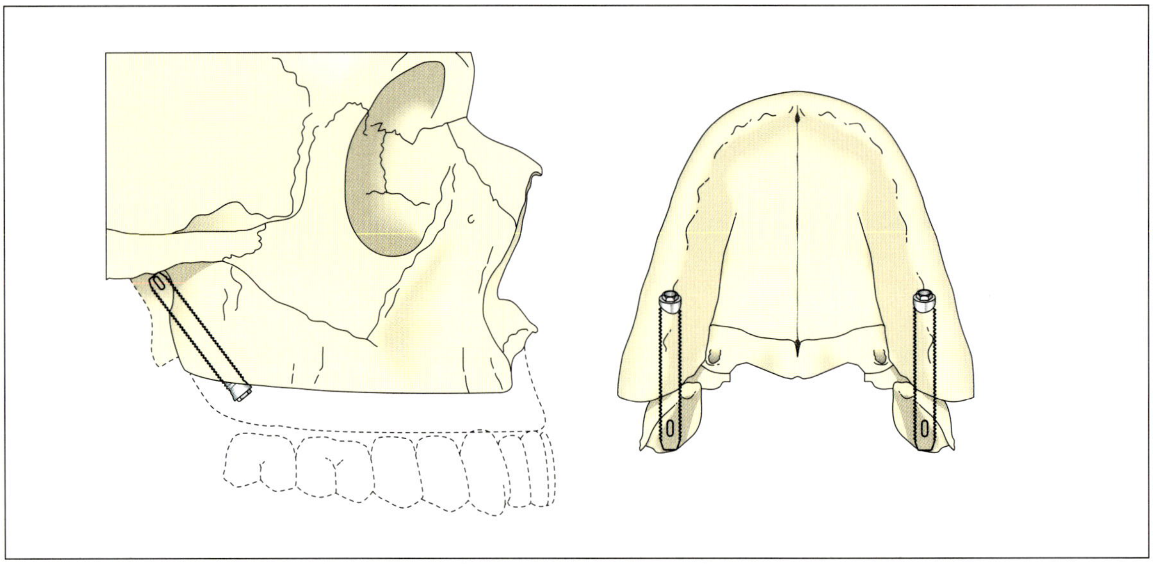

Fig 1-7 Anchorage of fixtures in the pterygoid plates as an adjunct to grafting.

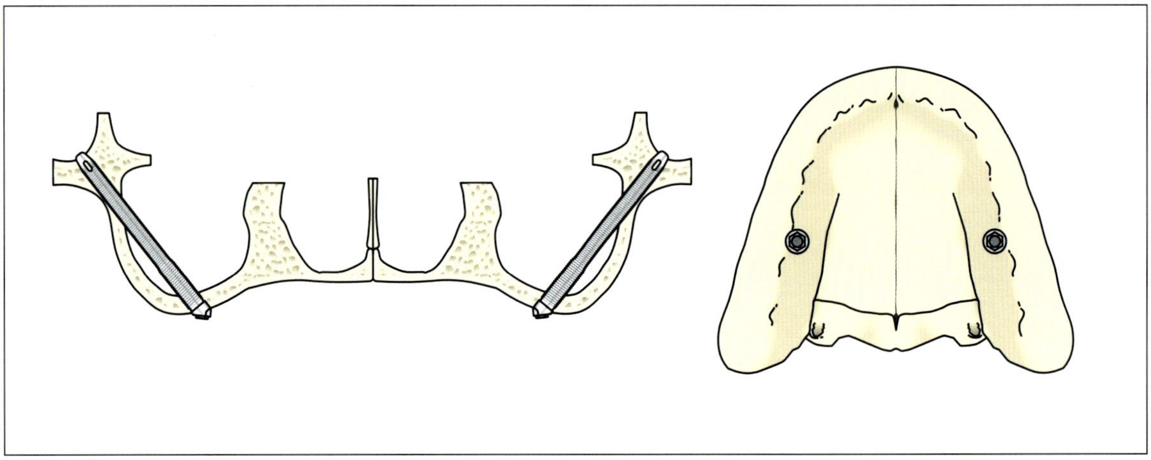

Fig 1-8 Placement of modified fixtures in the dense bone of os zygomaticum as another alternative to grafting.

CHAPTER 2

Protocol for Long-Term Study of Autogenous Onlay Bone Grafting and Simultaneous Endosseous Fixture Placement

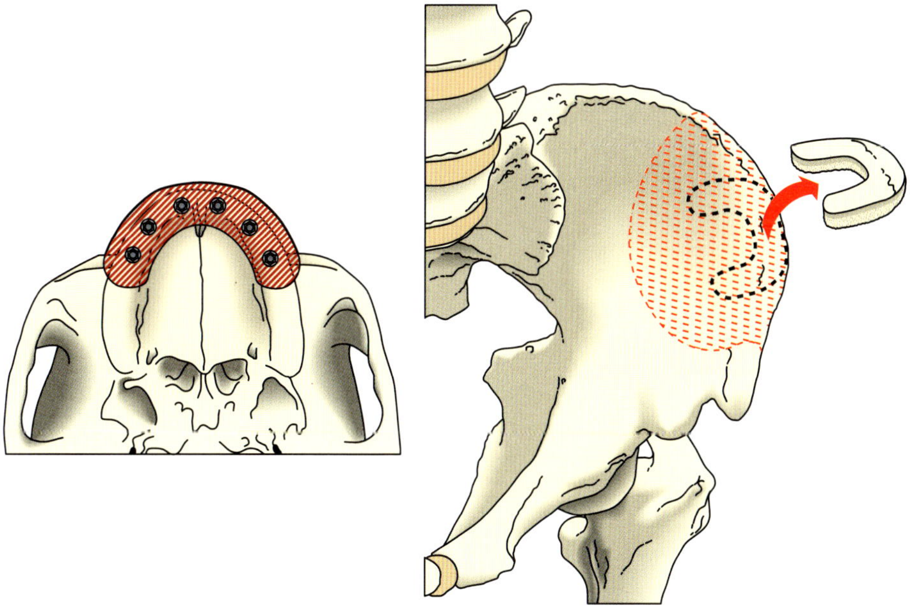

Study Objectives

The principal objective of this study was to evaluate the outcome of a surgical procedure in which severely resorbed maxillae were reconstructed with onlay block autogenous grafts and simultaneous fixture placement. The study intended to assess:

- The value of the maxillary augmentation procedure in combination with endosseous fixture installation
- The prosthetic long-term survival rates and the mechanical stability of the prostheses
- The condition of the peri-implant bone
- Potential complications, their causes, and preventive measures to avoid them

Study Design and Materials

The study ended in December 1998 when all patients had been followed for at least 2 years. All grafting and original fixture installation procedures were performed by P-I Brånemark.

Study population

The grafting procedure was initially developed during the years 1978 through 1985. During this developmental period, 27 patients underwent oral rehabilitation with autogenous onlay bone grafts and simultaneous fixture placement. An additional 138 patients were treated during the subsequent routine period, which took place during the years 1986 through 1996. In total, 165 patients with severe maxillary atrophy underwent autogenous onlay bone graft surgery. These defects were continuous; that is, they related to the entire maxilla. An additional 50 patients with discontinuous maxillary defects in the form of cleft (n = 25) or hemimaxillectomy (n = 25) were treated with onlay grafts during the study period. The data for the discontinuous defects are reported in chapter 7.

Jaw classifications

The majority of the patients demonstrated marked maxillary resorption and a cancellous bone quality of type 3 or 4 according to the index of Lekholm and Zarb.[28] In this study, however, the jaws were classified with respect to resorption pattern (Fig 2-1) and sinus configuration (Fig 2-2). Both indexes were constructed by P-I Brånemark in 1978.

Resorption pattern

The topographical pattern of the anterior frontal aspect of the maxilla was classified from I to V according to its degree of resorption in the anterior-posterior direction (see Fig 2-1).

Most patients (81%) exhibited a resorption pattern equivalent to type III or IV. In addition, 30 patients (18%) had extremely resorbed maxillae classified as type V. When a patient was classified with a type V resorption pattern, the thin ridge was used to stabilize the graft in the horizontal plane (Fig 2-3).

Determination of maxillary sinus shape

The thickness of the bony septum between the anterior border of the maxillary sinus and the lateral wall of the nasal cavity was classified from A to E (see Fig 2-2). In addition to the preoperative radiographic evaluation, the topography of the medial wall and the anterior floor of the sinus were explored during surgery, both from the nasal and from the sinus direction. The sinus was explored via a drilled hole using a special probe (Fig 2-4). The majority of the patients in the study (86%) exhibited sinus configurations of type A or B.

Baseline patient profile

The baseline patient profile is presented in Table 2-1. Most patients (61%) were treated in Göteborg, Sweden, while 64 (39%) of the 165 patients were treated elsewhere. The patients were of different ethnic backgrounds. Forty (24%) were men and 125 (76%) were women. Their mean age at the time of surgery was 55 (range, 17 to 81).

Retrospectively collected data on smoking and bruxing habits revealed that 18% of the patients for whom the information was available were bruxers, while 23% were smokers.

Type of grafting procedure

The preoperative anatomic conditions and the types of grafting procedures performed are shown in Table 2-2. The medial or lateral ilium constituted the donor site in 85% of the cases. In the remaining pro-

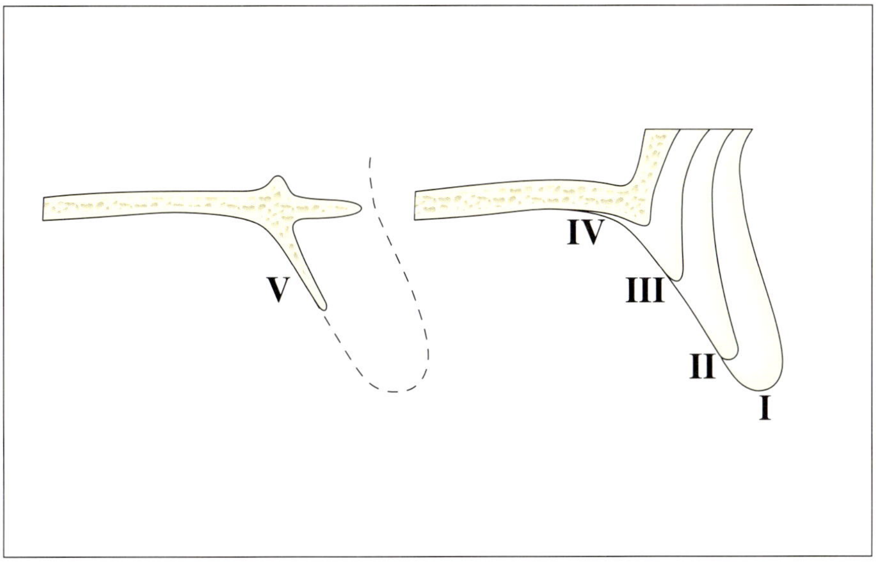

Fig 2-1 Pattern of resorption according to the index of P-I Brånemark 1978.

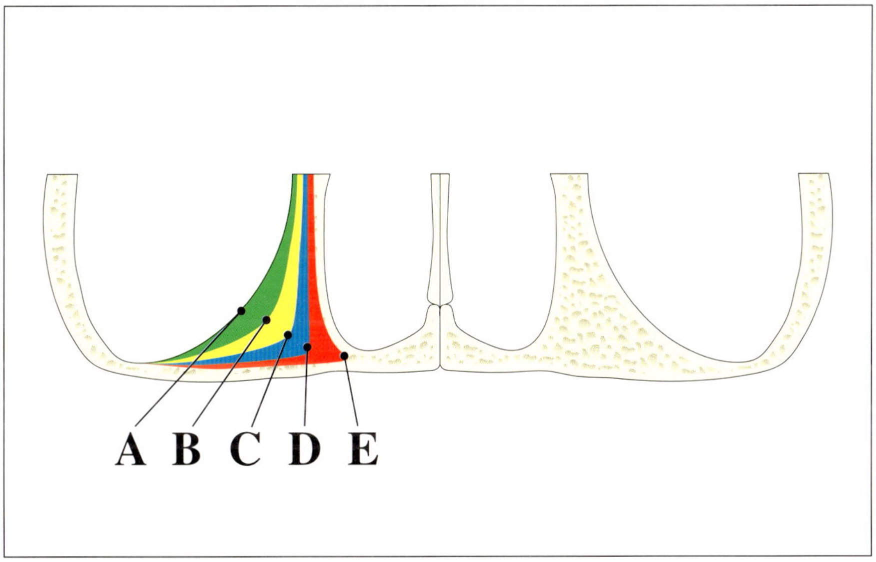

Fig 2-2 Determination of sinus anatomy according to the index of P-I Brånemark 1978.

cedures, the grafts were taken from the iliac crest or from both the lateral and medial aspects of the ilium (Figs 2-5 to 2-7).

Installed fixtures

In total, 929 fixtures were originally installed in association with the grafting procedure. Of these, 148 were placed during the development period and 781 during the routine period. An additional 118 fixtures were later placed in patients with complications and/or original fixture loss (Table 2-3).

The utilized fixture designs are described in Table 2-4. Those most frequently used are also illustrated in Fig 2-8, where the distance between the first thread and the reference point used for radiographic evaluation is indicated on each fixture.

The swan-neck fixture had a low conical profile. It was designed for tight adaptation of the graft to the recipient maxillary bone. It also helped avoid thread exposure to the mucosa or oral cavity in the event of bone resorption. In

Table 2-1 Baseline patient profiles

Baseline characteristics	Development group (n = 27)	Routine group (n = 138)	All patients (N = 165)
Age (y)			
< 50	9 (33.3%)	42 (30.4%)	51 (30.9%)
50–65	16 (59.3%)	61 (44.2%)	77 (46.7%)
> 65	2 (7.4%)	35 (25.4%)	37 (22.4%)
Mean age (range)	51.6 (30–66)	55.2 (17–81)	54.6 (17–81)
Sex			
Male	5 (18.5%)	35 (25.4%)	40 (24.2%)
Female	22 (81.5%)	103 (74.6%)	125 (75.8%)
Surgical clinic			
Göteborg	19 (70.4%)	82 (59.4%)	101 (61.2%)
Other	8 (29.6%)	56 (40.6%)	64 (38.8%)
Smoking*			
Yes	3 (33.3%)	25 (22.3%)	28 (23.1%)
No	6 (66.7%)	87 (77.7%)	93 (76.9%)
Bruxism*			
Yes	2 (28.6%)	11 (16.4%)	13 (17.6%)
No	5 (71.4%)	56 (83.6%)	61 (82.4%)
Opposing dentition			
Complete denture	1 (3.7%)	4 (2.9%)	5 (3.0%)
Natural teeth only	10 (37.0%)	42 (30.7%)	52 (31.7%)
Partial fixed prosthesis	1 (3.7%)	22 (16.1%)	23 (14.0%)
Removable partial denture	4 (14.8%)	27 (19.7%)	31 (18.9%)
Fixed prosthesis	11 (40.7%)	42 (30.7%)	53 (32.3%)
Time between fixture placement and delivery of fixed prosthesis			
< 9 mo	8 (32.0%)	82 (60.3%)	90 (55.9%)
9–12 mo	9 (36.0%)	35 (25.7%)	44 (27.3%)
> 1 y	8 (32.0%)	19 (14.0%)	27 (16.8%)
Time (d) between abutment connection and delivery of fixed prosthesis			
< 30	13 (52.0%)	36 (26.7%)	49 (30.6%)
30–60	9 (36.0%)	59 (43.7%)	68 (42.5%)
>60	3 (12.0%)	40 (29.6%)	43 (26.9%)

*Data on bruxing and smoking habits were collected retrospectively.

Table 2-4, the fixtures in the category "Other" under "Fixture design" were custom designed. Because the category includes the zygoma fixtures, the fixture lengths varied between 25 and 45 mm. The zygoma fixtures were developed during the study period. They were used with increased frequency to prevent or resolve complications. The mean number of original and additional (ie, total) fixtures installed per patient was 6.4; 61% of the patients received six original fixtures in association with the grafting procedure.

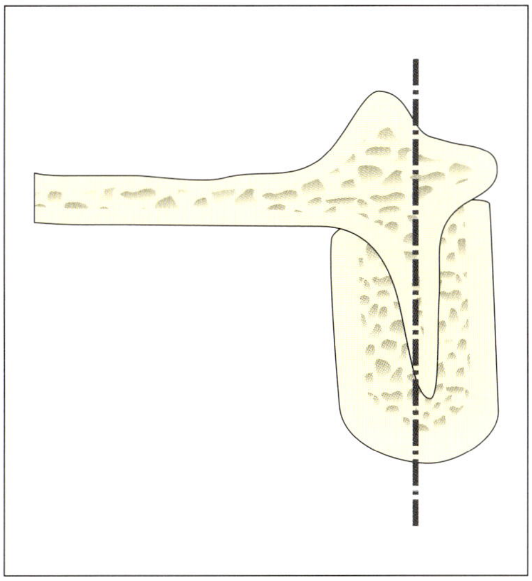

Fig 2-3 Maintenance of the thin bone crest to help stabilize the graft.

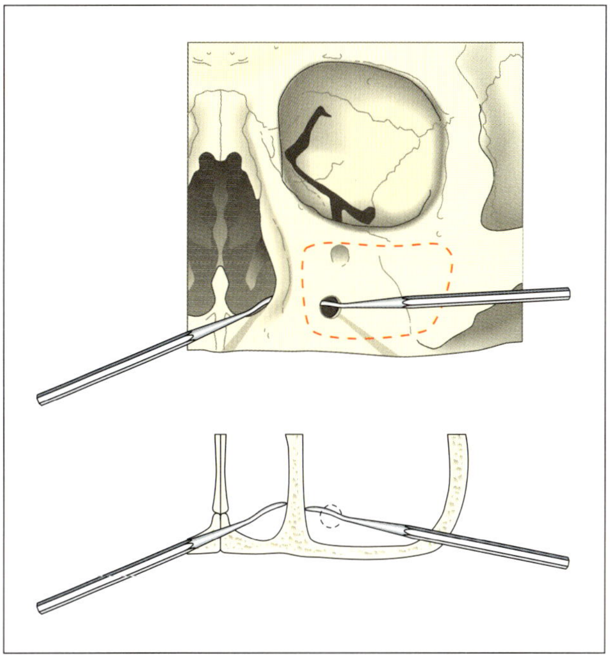

Fig 2-4 Drilling of an exploratory access hole to locate the bony septum between the maxillary sinus and the nasal cavity.

Table 2-2 Presurgical anatomical conditions and types of grafting procedures used by patient group

Anatomical conditions and types of grafting procedures	Development group (n = 27)	Routine group (n = 138)	All patients (N = 165)
Grade of resorption			
II	0	2 (1.4%)	2 (1.2%)
III	9 (33.3%)	44 (31.9%)	53 (32.1%)
IV	13 (48.1%)	67 (48.6%)	80 (48.5%)
V	5 (18.5%)	25 (18.1%)	30 (18.2%)
Sinus configuration			
A	7 (26.9%)	38 (32.8%)	45 (31.7%)
B	14 (53.8%)	63 (54.3%)	77 (54.2%)
C, D, or E	5 (19.2%)	15 (12.9%)	20 (14.1%)
Nasal floor bone graft			
Yes	0	45 (32.6%)	45 (27.3%)
No	27 (100%)	93 (67.4%)	120 (72.7%)
Onlay graft donor sites			
Medial ilium	0	83 (60.1%)	83 (50.3%)
Lateral ilium	27 (100%)	30 (21.7%)	57 (34.5%)
Medial and lateral ilium	0	8 (5.8%)	8 (4.8%)
Iliac crest only	0	17 (12.3%)	17 (10.3%)

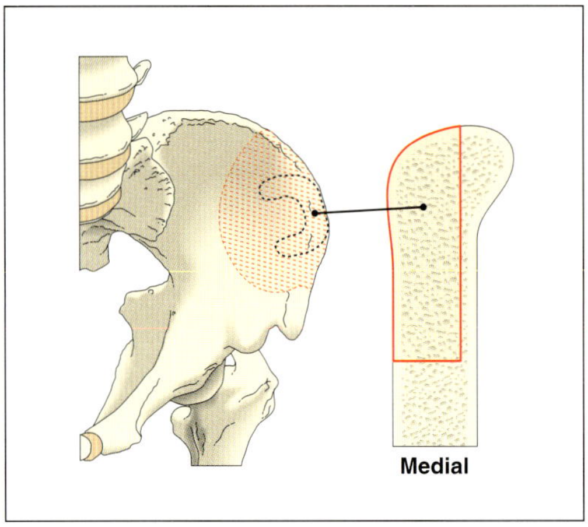

Fig 2-5 Graft taken from the medial ilium.

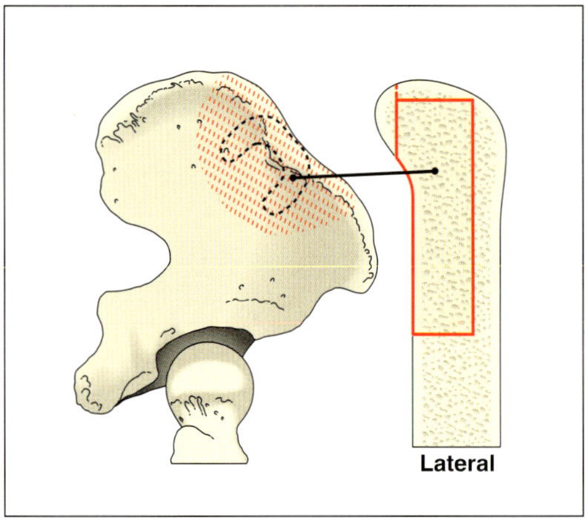

Fig 2-6 Graft taken from the lateral ilium.

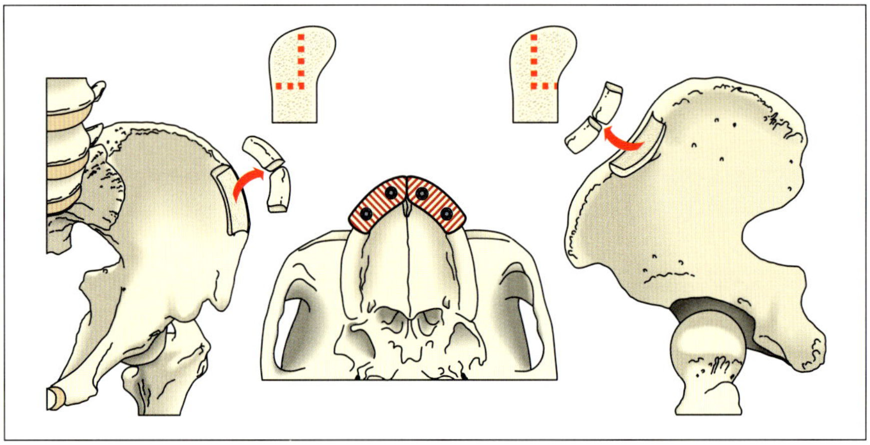

Fig 2-7 Grafts taken from the iliac crest.

Table 2-3 Placed fixtures by patient group

Patient group	Original fixtures	Additional fixtures	Total fixtures placed
Development	148	27	175
Routine	781	91	872
Total	929	118	1047

Table 2-4 Placed fixtures by fixture design

Fixture design	Original fixtures	Additional fixtures	Total fixtures placed
Standard	46	11	57
Self-tapping	139	4	143
Conical	137	0	137
Swan-neck	556	46	602
Other	51	57	108

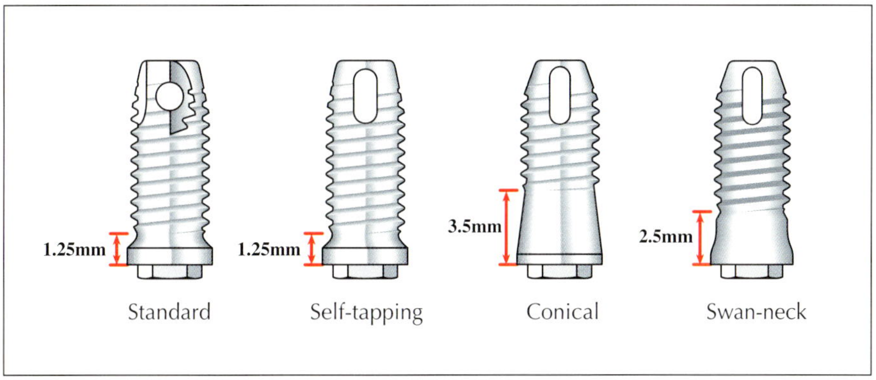

Fig 2-8 The most frequently used fixture designs. The distance between the reference point and the first thread is indicated on each fixture.

Table 2-5 Prosthetic reconstructions by patient group

Prosthesis	Development group (n=27)	Routine group (n=138)	All patients (N=165)
Bone-anchored fixed prosthesis	22 (81.5%)	119 (86.2%)	141 (85.5%)
Bone-anchored overdenture	3 (11.1%)	17 (12.3%)	20 (12.1%)
Early failure—no prosthesis	2 (7.4%)	2 (1.4%)	4 (2.4%)

Prosthetic design

The objective was to allow all patients the option of a fixed prosthesis, except in a few instances at clinics where the prosthodontist preferred to deliver an overdenture to the patient. As reported elsewhere,[29] four to six fixtures are usually sufficient to support a fixed prosthesis and therefore constituted the treatment plan for the majority of the patients.

A fixed prosthesis was delivered to 86% of the patients and an overdenture to 12%. The treatment failed in 4 patients who were unable to be fitted with an initial prosthesis (Table 2-5). In the overdenture group, 11 of the 20 patients had four or more fixtures and therefore could have carried a fixed prosthesis if desired.

Treatment and follow-up time

The mean follow-up time in the development group was 15 years (median, 15; maximum, 20). The same figure for the routine group was 8 years (median, 8; maximum, 13). The mean follow-up time was 8.7 years (median, 8.8), and the whole study comprised 1,444 patient years.

The time between fixture placement and connection of the fixed prosthesis was less than 1 year in 83% of the cases and less than 9 months for 56% of the patients (see Table 2-1).

Multidisciplinary study of donor site morbidity

Donor site morbidity in terms of pain was assessed through interviews with 61 patients in the routine group who underwent consecutive operations. As described elsewhere,[30] a protocol involving a multidisciplinary approach was used to complete the sequence of examinations and questionnaires. The study was carried out in collaboration with orthopedic experts and physiotherapists. The protocol was divided into three evaluation periods:

1. The initial postoperative period
2. Three to four weeks later
3. At the last scheduled follow-up visit

The donor site morbidity was rated in the questionnaires on a scale from 0 to 10. Physiotherapeutic tests were employed to detect sensorial and motor alterations.

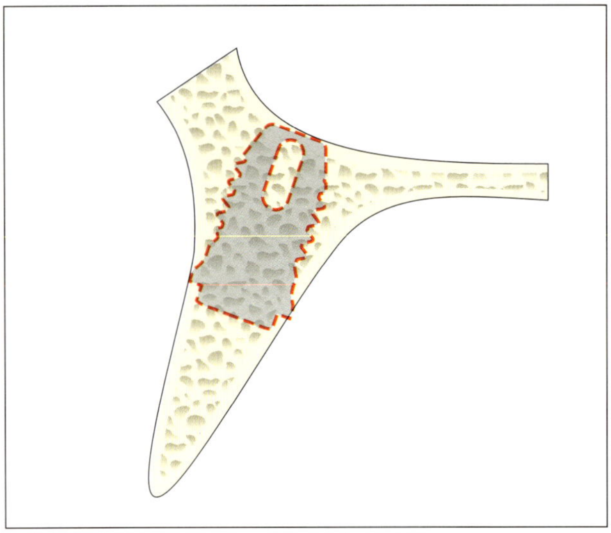

Fig 2-9 Total versus available bone height.

Radiographic aspects

The radiographic evaluation was based on 77 patients (19 men and 58 women) on whom postoperative radiographic examinations had been performed at Göteborg University, Sweden. The mean age of these patients was 56 (range, 30 to 79) at the time of fixture placement.

Radiographs for several patients who underwent surgery abroad or at distant clinics were not available for follow-up measurements. The postoperative radiographic material included 19 (70%) of the 27 patients in the development group and 58 (42%) of the 138 patients in the routine group.

The 77 patients had received 421 fixtures of different designs: 58 conical, 262 swan-neck, 40 standard, 44 self-tapping, and 17 fixtures of other designs; 8 of the fixtures remained unloaded. Only originally placed fixtures were included in the analyses. One observer (Gröndahl) performed all evaluations.

The preoperative radiographic examinations were performed according to the same principles as those applicable to ordinary fixture treatment. The preoperative lateral cephalograms and, when present, tomographic images were evaluated with respect to total bone height and available bone height. The available height was calculated based on the fixture dimension versus the height between the nasal floor and the bone level, ie, the required buccolingual width of 4 mm adjacent to the fixture (Fig 2-9). The radiographic magnification was taken into account. The measurements were performed to the closest millimeter.

The postoperative radiographs were used to measure the distance between a reference point on the fixture and the most apical marginal bone level on the mesial and distal surfaces of each fixture. The uppermost cervical part was chosen as the reference point on all fixture types (see Fig 2-8). The linear measurements were performed to the closest 0.1 mm when assessing the intraoral radiographs (first choice) and to the nearest 0.5 mm for images obtained with an extraoral technique. The radiographs were also evaluated with respect to the presence of peri-implant radiolucency or other signs of lost osseointegration.

Surgical and Prosthetic Procedures

Treatment planning

The fixture positions were planned in conjunction with the preoperative determination of facial profile and contours, existing parafunctional habits, horizontal and vertical jaw relations and occlusal plane level and angulation. Preoperative or intraoperative prosthetic reinforcement of the mandible was carried out when needed to minimize bending forces and assure optimal occlusion and loading conditions. When the prosthetic requirements had been fully considered, a surgical stent was manufactured. Considering that the graft would alter the topography of the alveolar crest, the palatal portion of the replica was cut off so that only the buccal contours of the teeth and a posterior supporting connection remained.

Figs 2-10 to 2-70 Clinical and radiographic views of surgical and prosthetic procedures in a typical patient.

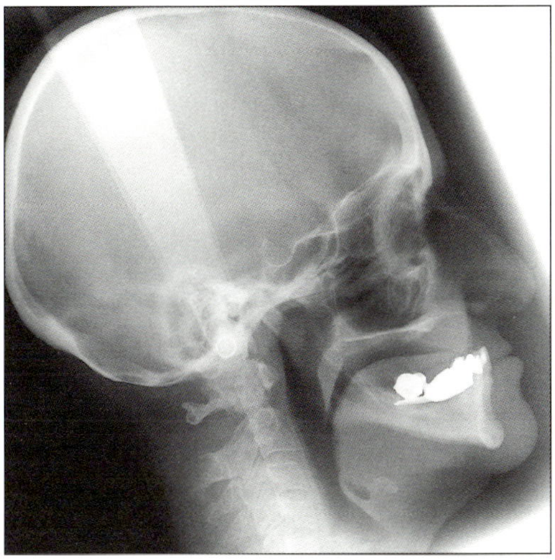

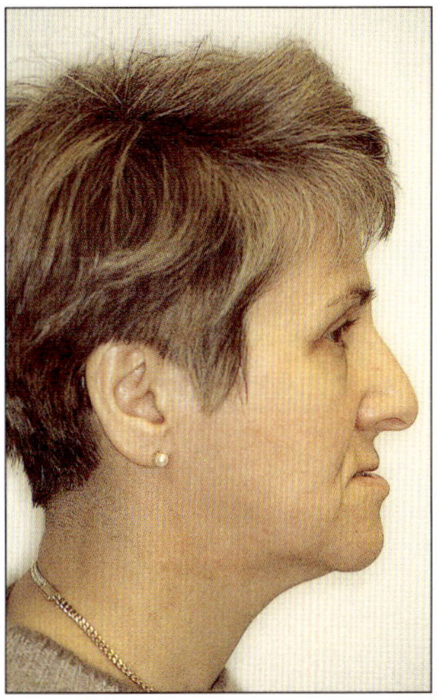

Figs 2-10 and 2-11 Preoperative status.

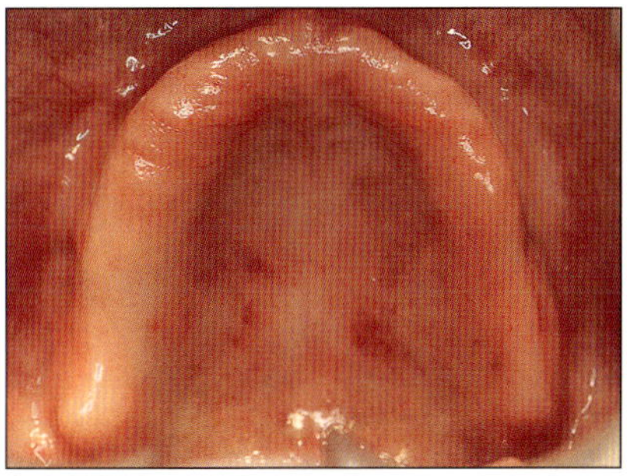

Fig 2-12 Preoperative clinical view of the maxilla.

Surgical procedure

The surgical method is presented as a summary of a typical case. The original scenario is illustrated in Figs 2-10 to 2-12. The treatment is further exemplified in the additional 24 case presentations.

The surgical procedure was conducted under general anesthesia. Antibiotics were administered intravenously 1 hour prior to surgery. The patient was positioned supine on the operating table with a large pad (a rolled towel or equivalent) placed under the donor hip to elevate the iliac crest region. A pillow was also placed under the knees of the patient, with the leg on the donor side slightly flexed and drawn partly across the other leg. Adhesive tape was then drawn from table edge to table edge over the elevated leg. An indwelling, self-retaining urinary catheter was used if needed, depending on the anticipated duration of the surgery.

Preparation of the recipient site

The recipient site was infiltrated with a local anesthetic solution (lidocaine 1% with epinephrine .001%) to elevate the mucoperiosteal flap and to assist hemostasis. The intended incision line was marked on the oral mucosa by scratching lightly with a dissector (Fig 2-13). It extended in a curved line from a point near the orifice of one parotid duct to the other and followed the inner surface of the upper lip (Fig 2-14).

Dissection and elevation of the mucoperiosteal flap aimed at developing a large, thick flap rather than a thin mucosal flap (Fig 2-15). Because of the extremely shallow premaxilla, the dissection started at the anterior and lateral segments of the incision. Direct dissection near the midline posed the risk of inadvertently entering the nasal cavity.

As the thick mucosal flap was elevated, the periosteum of the residual alveolar ridge was incised as high up as possible (Fig 2-16). On the labial aspect of the premaxilla, the periosteal dissection proceeded in a superior direction to allow exposure of the lower part of the piriform aperture and resection of the anterior bony wall of the nasal aperture (Fig 2-17).

Next, the palatally pedicled mucoperiosteal flap was elevated almost to the greater palatine foramina. This required section of the neurovascular contents of the incisive canal and careful curettage of the soft tissue remnants within the canal (Fig 2-18). This step not only minimized the risk of incorporating soft and possibly epithelial tissue elements into the paramedian fixture sites, but also allowed the surgeon to later plug the canal with densely

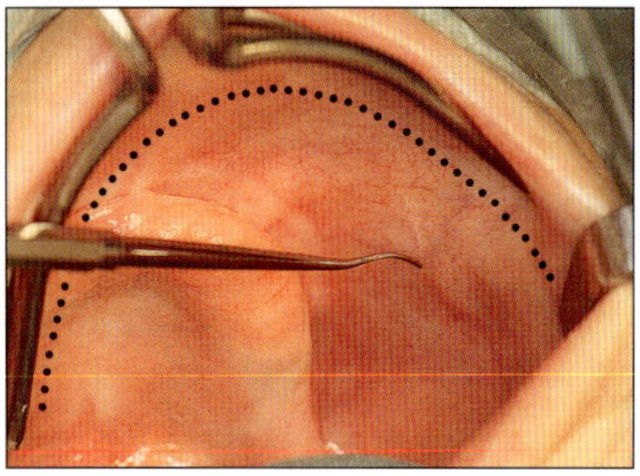

Fig 2-13 Intended incision line. The incision was to extend from a point near the orifice of the parotid duct.

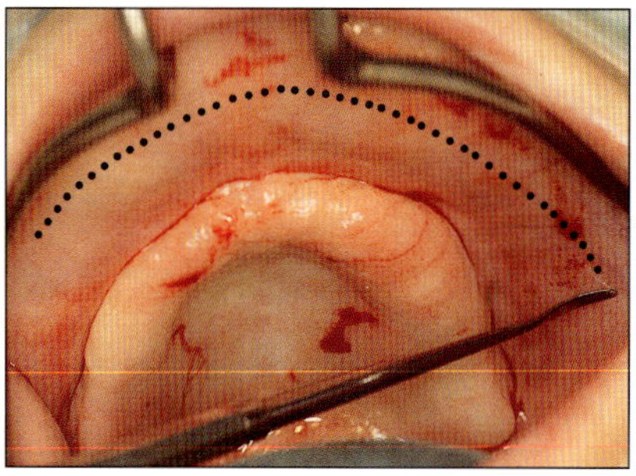

Fig 2-14 Intended incision line. The incision was to follow the inner surface of the upper lip.

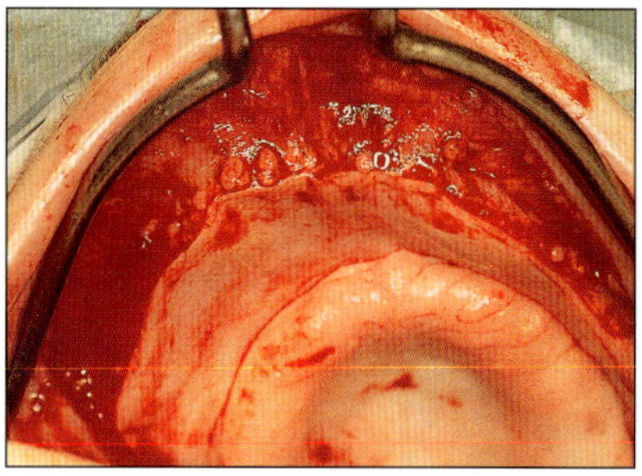

Fig 2-15 Dissection and elevation of the mucoperiosteal flap.

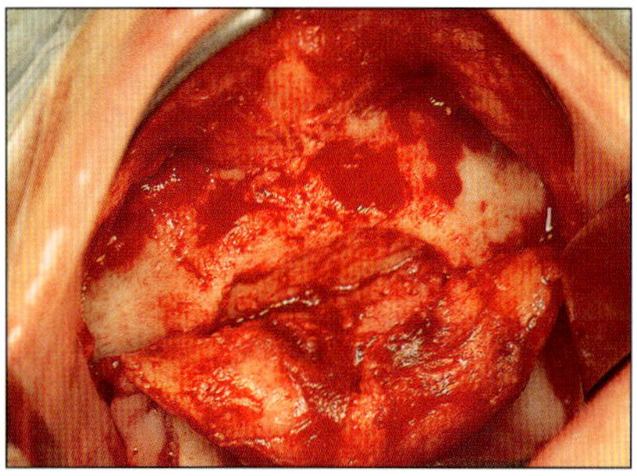

Fig 2-16 Incision of the periosteum of the residual alveolar ridge.

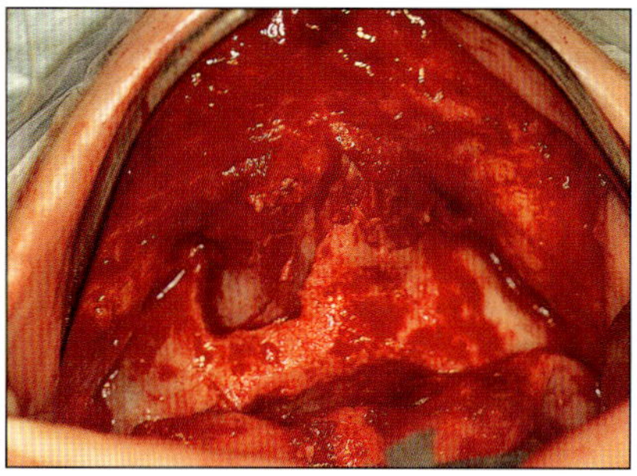

Fig 2-17 Resection of the bony wall of the nasal aperture.

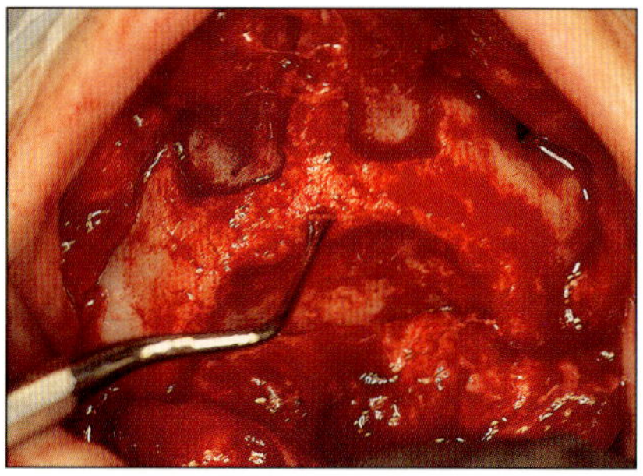

Fig 2-18 Section of the contents of the incisive canal and removal of any soft tissue remnants.

compacted cancellous bone to further extend the area available for fixture placement.

An exploratory access hole was drilled with a small round bur to penetrate the anterior lateral wall of the sinus and locate the bony septum between the maxillary sinus and the nasal cavity (see Fig 2-4). The mucoperiosteum of the nasal floor was elevated on each side (similar to a Le Fort I osteotomy procedure), and the anterior lower and mesial part of the nasal floor was removed by a conchotome while the anterior lower part of the septum cartilage was cut away.

At this stage, the elevated mucoperiosteum could be compressed and the bleeding reduced by placing narrow strips of gauze soaked in an epinephrine solution into the nasal floor beneath the elevated mucosa (Fig 2-19). The rough edges of the alveolar crest were then smoothed.

An aluminum foil sheet was pressed against the premaxillary ridge to produce a template of the bony area that could act as a guide when trimming and carving the bone graft (Fig 2-20).

A metal semicircular template (Fig 2-21) was used to gauge the size and curvature of the maxillary arch. A corresponding template was used to transfer this information to the hip donor site (Fig 2-22). Small, occasional perforations were then made in the cortex of the premaxilla to facilitate vascular connections between the mucoperiosteum and the original and grafted bone (Figs 2-23 to 2-25). The site was then protected with a moist pack while the graft donor site was accessed.

Graft retrieval

Following infiltration of epinephrine at the iliac crest area, an approximately 10-cm long linear in-

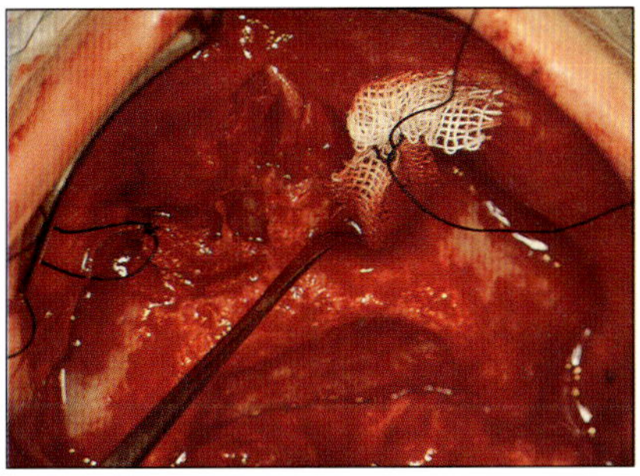

Fig 2-19 Placement of gauze soaked in epinephrine in the nasal floor to compress the elevated mucoperiosteum.

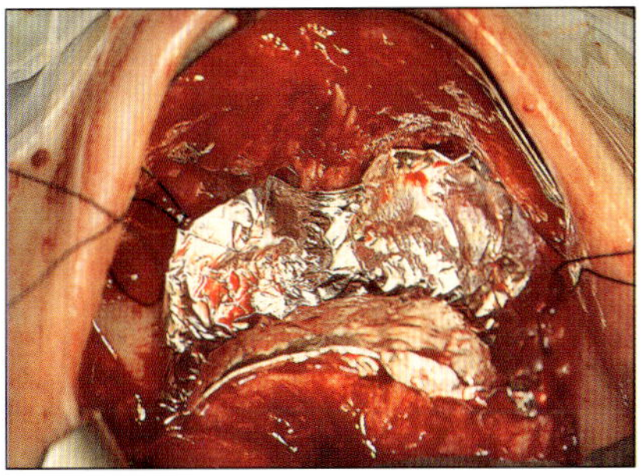

Fig 2-20 Formation of a template of the anatomy of the graft donor site using aluminum foil.

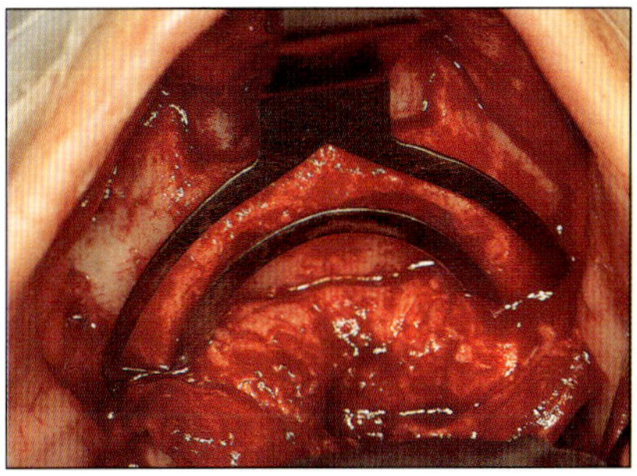

Fig 2-21 Metal template used to gauge the size and curvature of the maxillary arch.

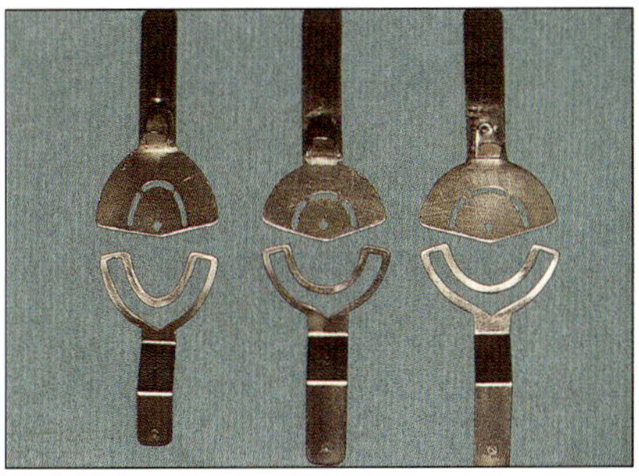

Fig 2-22 Paired metal templates used to determine the size of the needed graft and to transfer the information to the hip.

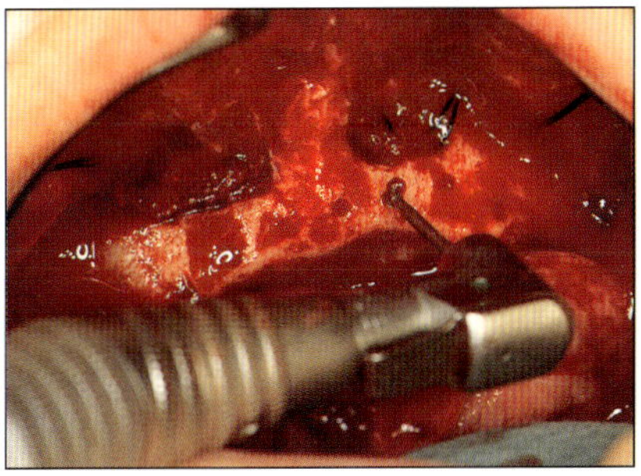

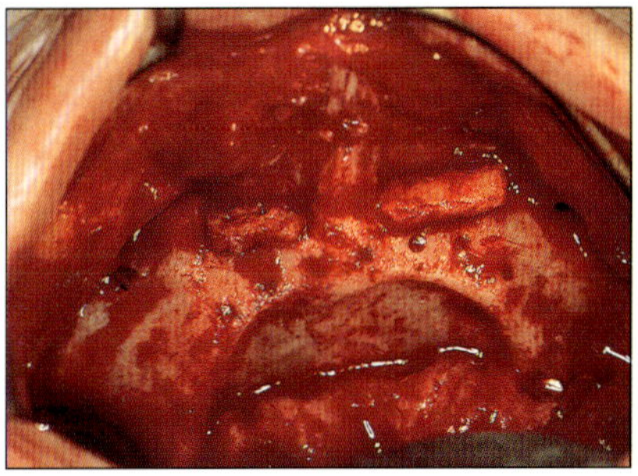

Figs 2-23 and 2-24 Drilling of small perforations in the premaxilla to facilitate vascular connections between the mucoperiosteum, the premaxilla, and the grafted bone.

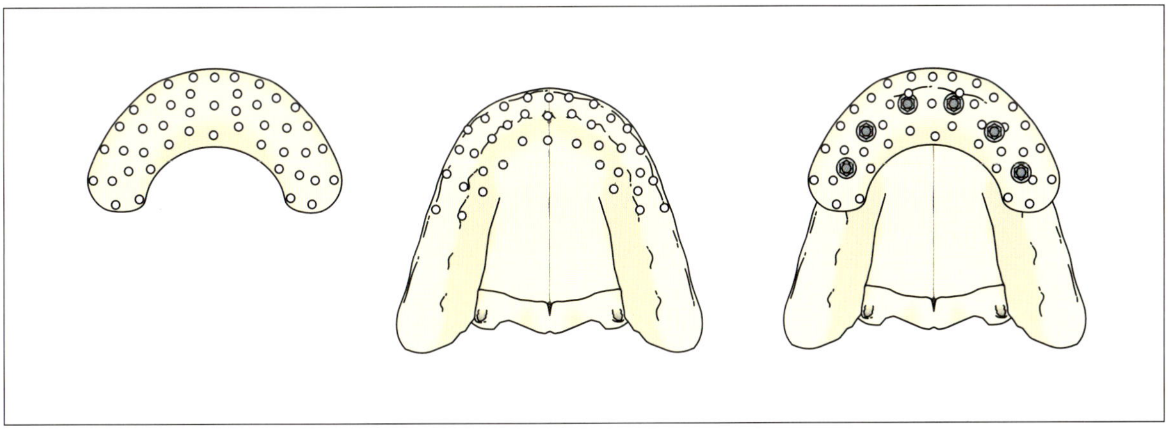

Fig 2-25 Holes prepared for vascular connections.

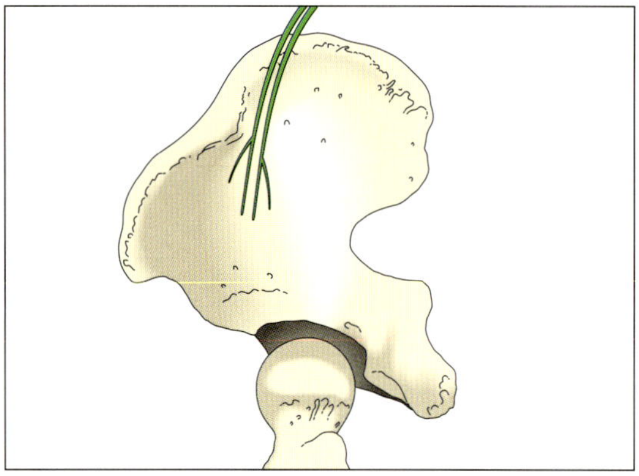

Fig 2-26 Incision for graft removal. The incision passes through the skin lateral to the crest to avoid injury to the lateral cutaneous nerves.

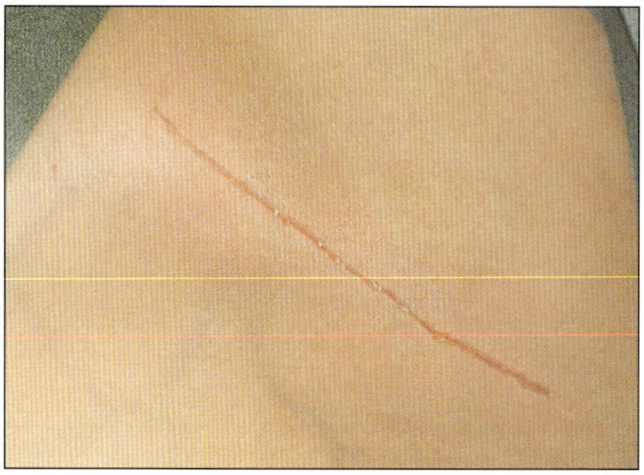

Fig 2-27 First incision at the anterior superior iliac crest.

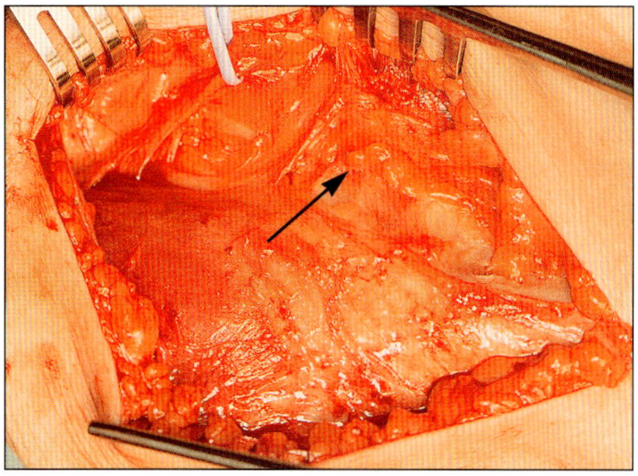

Fig 2-28 The lateral cutaneous nerve.

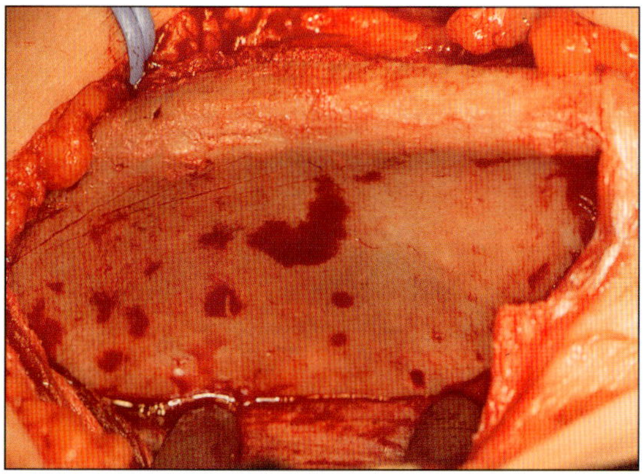

Fig 2-29 Exposure of the medial iliac crest.

cision was made about one finger's width lateral to the bony crest, starting at the anterior superior iliac crest (Figs 2-26 and 2-27). To facilitate this, the assistant would "roll up" the skin from the upper thigh over the iliac crest. This allowed the incision to pass through the skin lateral to the crest. A sharp dissection through the dermis and fascial layers to the periosteum followed, with care taken to avoid injury to the lateral cutaneous nerves (Rr laterales, N subcostales, and iliohypogastricus [Th12 + L1]) (Fig 2-28) in the thigh at the iliac crest.

The periosteum of the crest was incised as far posterior as possible along the exposed length of the crest, starting from a point about 1 cm behind the superior anterior iliac crest. Then the periosteum was elevated and the crest of the ilium was exposed (Fig 2-29).

During the initial study period, the graft was taken from the lateral aspect of the ilium because that was the routine approach to reconstruction of discontinuous mandibular defects at the time.[31] When the graft was taken from the lateral side, a subperiosteal dissection of the gluteal muscle was necessary to provide access to the donor area. We soon learned that taking the graft from the medial ilium resulted in easier access and decreased morbidity.

When the lateral ilium was to be the donor site (Fig 2-30), it was exposed after cutting off the superolateral margin of the crest with saws and osteotomes. The periosteal flap and gluteal muscle were then reflected from the lateral surface of the ilium. The flap was held in position with broad retractors. The bony rim within the upper part of the flap facilitated closure and repositioning of the musculoperiosteal flap.

When the medial ilium was to be the donor site (Fig 2-31), the medial periosteum and musculus iliacus were reflected medially from the bone as a

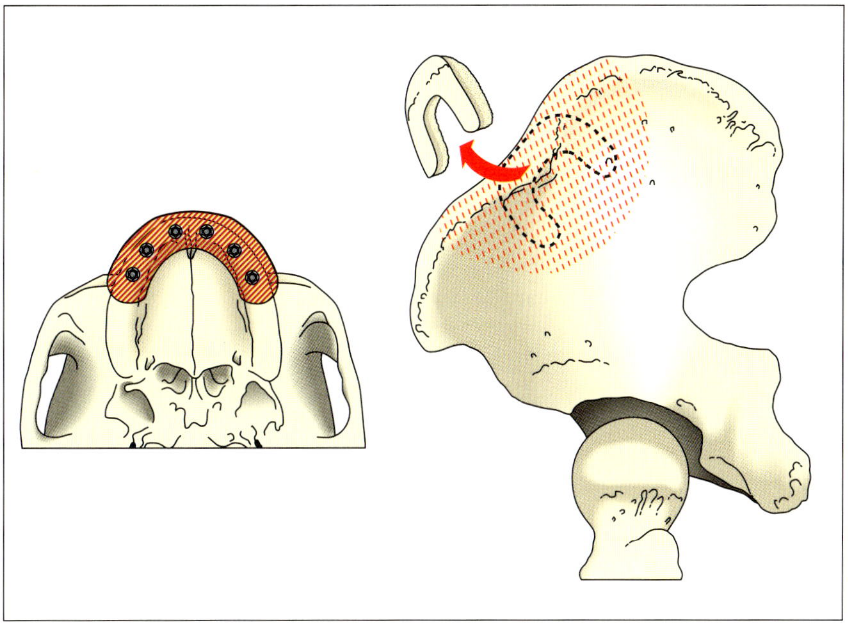

Fig 2-30 Removal of the graft from the lateral ilium. This was the procedure followed in the beginning of the study.

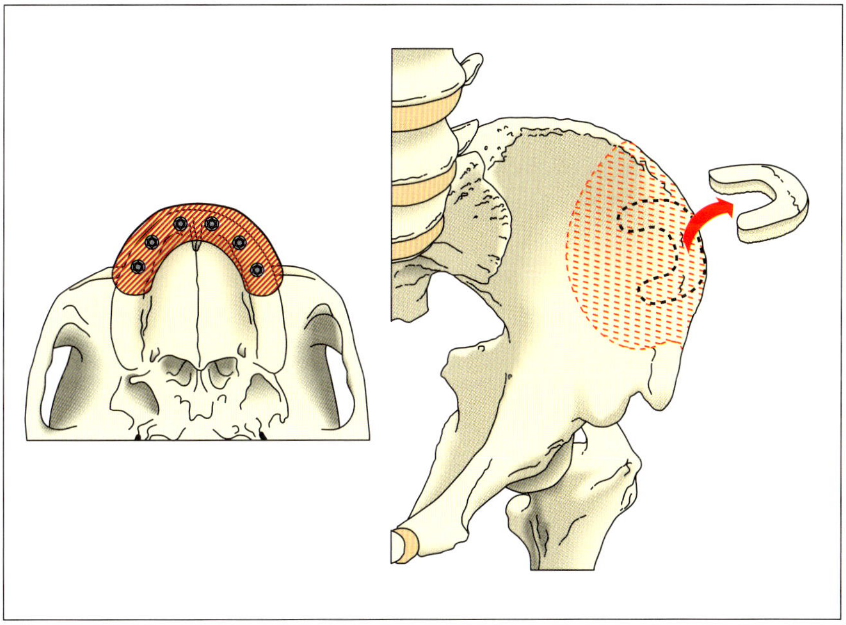

Fig 2-31 Removal of the graft from the medial ilium. The medial ilium eventually became the preferred donor site because it simplified harvesting of the graft and reduced postoperative pain.

combined musculoperiosteal flap. With the ilium exposed, lateral or medial, a semicircular template matching that chosen to fit the maxilla was held against the bone, with the handle at the center of the curve located near the tubercle of the crest. The template was temporarily stabilized with a direction indicator placed into a 3-mm–diameter hole drilled in the bony cortex (Fig 2-32). The template could then be outlined with a series of small perforations using a round bur (Fig 2-33). The iliac graft, shaped like a horseshoe, was delineated, and the template and direction indicator could be removed. Reciprocating cuts joining the peripheral perforations were made through the cortex and the cancellous bone with saw blades (Fig 2-34).

To free the graft, an osteotomy had to be made parallel to and just within the opposite margin of the iliac crest using a circular or oscillating saw (Fig 2-35). It was sequentially deepened in an immediate subcortical plane with thin-bladed osteotomes

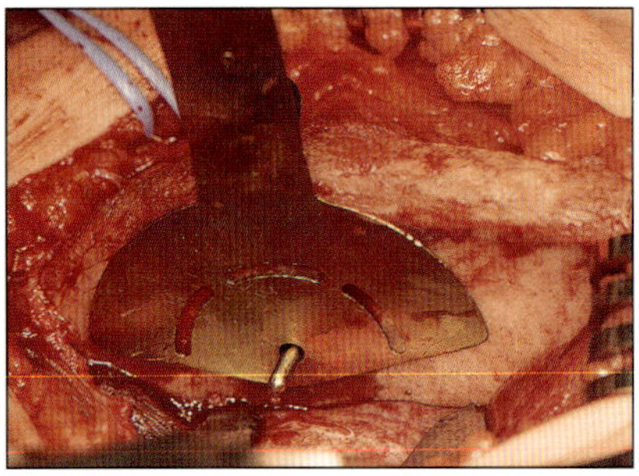

Fig 2-32 Placement of the template matched to the maxilla on direction indicator at the donor site.

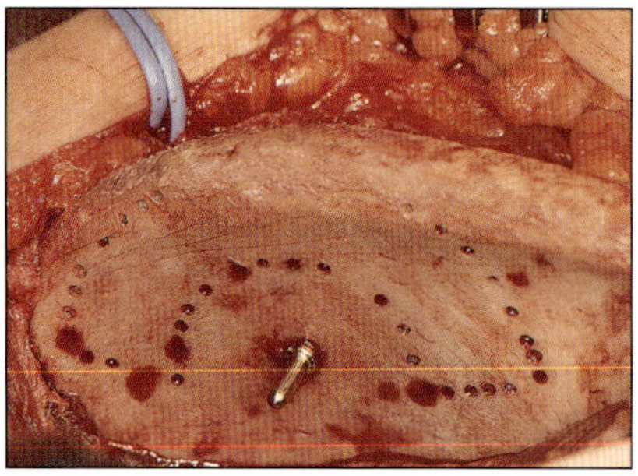

Fig 2-33 Outline of template with small bur.

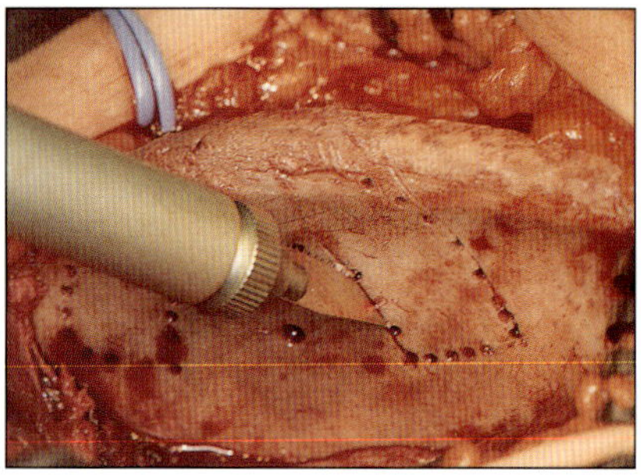

Fig 2-34 Perforations joined by reciprocating cuts made by a saw blade.

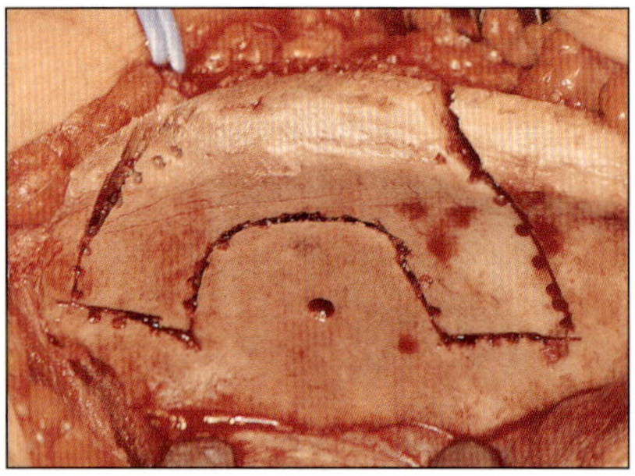

Fig 2-35 After osteotomy.

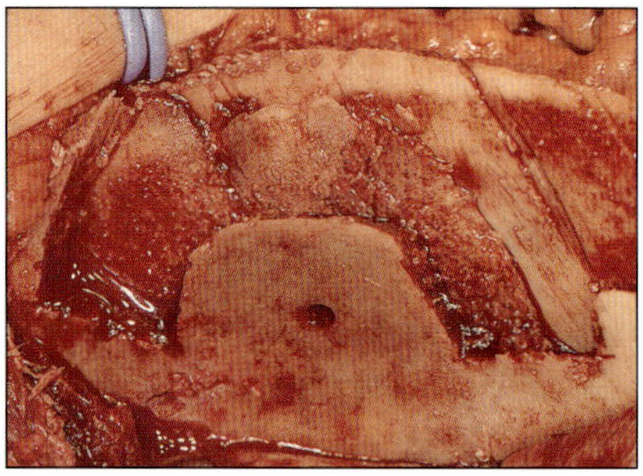

Fig 2-36 Sequential deepening of the osteotomy.

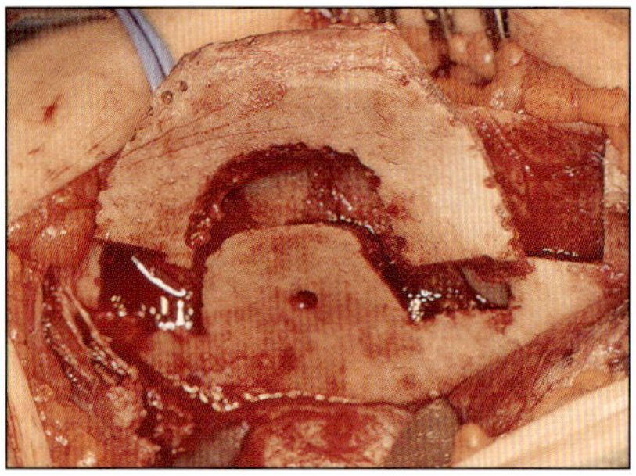

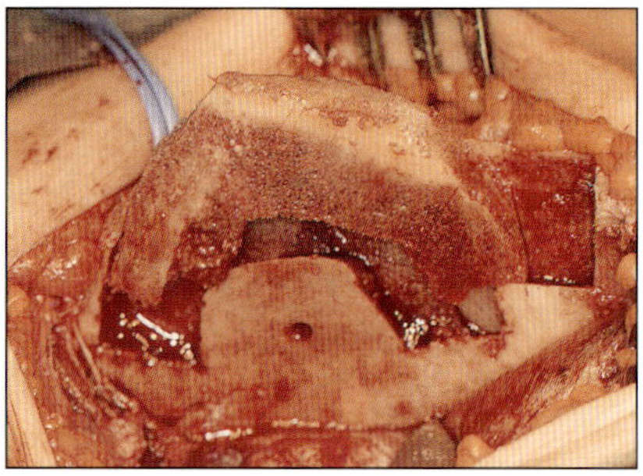

Figs 2-37 and 2-38 Graft retrieval.

(Fig 2-36). Before the graft was completely detached, the edges of the cortical bone usually required trimming to eliminate sharp angles. The graft was then removed (Figs 2-37 and 2-38).

Before the hip wound was closed, additional cancellous and marrow bone was collected between the cortical plates of the ilium using large curettes and gouges. A syringe of marrow-rich blood was collected and stored at room temperature.

When hemostasis of the hip had been achieved, the wound was closed in layers (Fig 2-39). The periosteal, subcutaneous, and skin incisions were closed using individual sutures (Fig 2-40). A series of towel clips helped close the edges of the periosteal incisions during suturing. A hip drain was usually not required. A circumferential pressure pad was tightly applied to the hip wound postoperatively to prevent hematoma formation and reduce pain (Fig 2-41). While the hip wound was closed, the graft was preserved in marrow-rich blood.

The detached graft (Figs 2-42 and 2-43) was placed in a special titanium tray holder to facilitate further carving and trimming until the graft adequately corresponded with the template of the maxillary recipient bone (Figs 2-44 to 2-46). Rongeurs were used to make a channel in the cancellous aspects of the graft to make it fit the residual maxillary ridge (Figs 2-47 and 2-48). The graft topography was then once again verified against the foil impression of the premaxillary ridge (Fig 2-49).

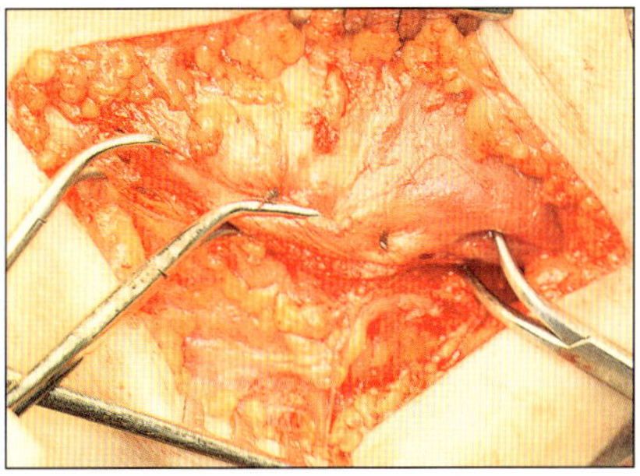

Fig 2-39 Closure of the site in layers.

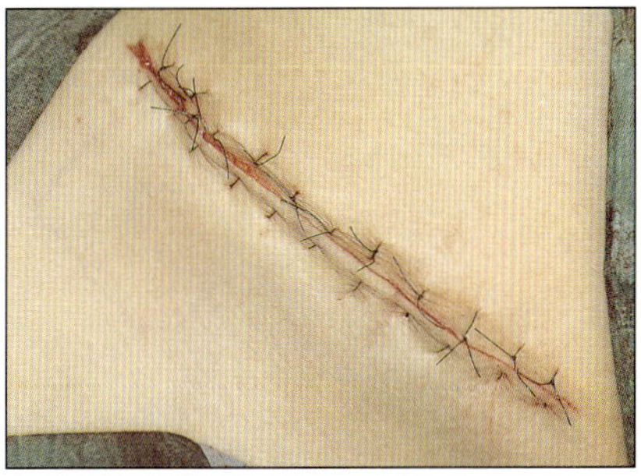

Fig 2-40 After closure of wound by individual sutures.

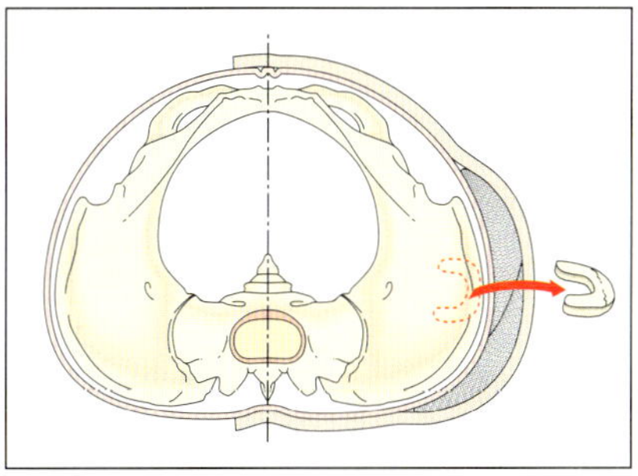

Fig 2-41 Cross-section illustrating placement of pressure pad against the hip wound.

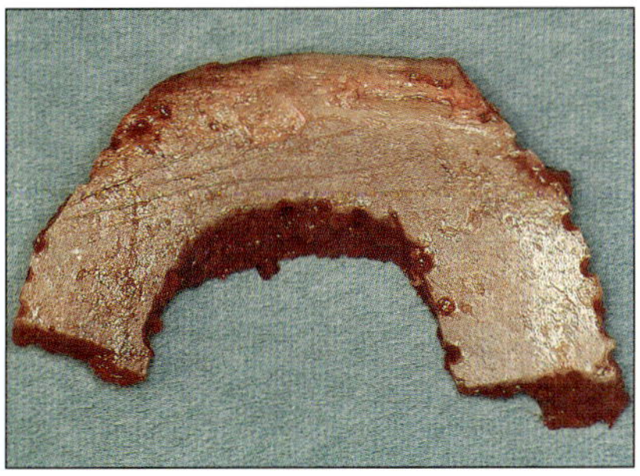

Fig 2-42 The cortical bone of the graft.

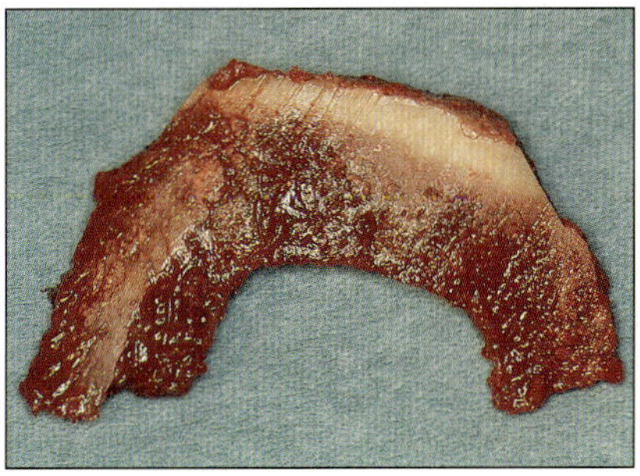

Fig 2-43 The side of the graft that is to be adapted to the premaxilla.

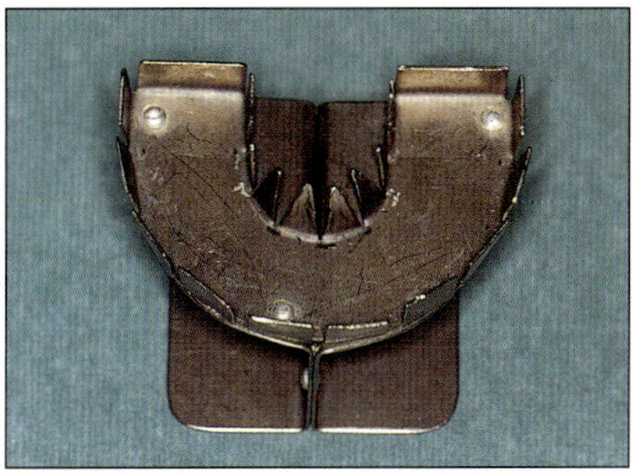

Fig 2-44 Titanium tray holder used when trimming the graft.

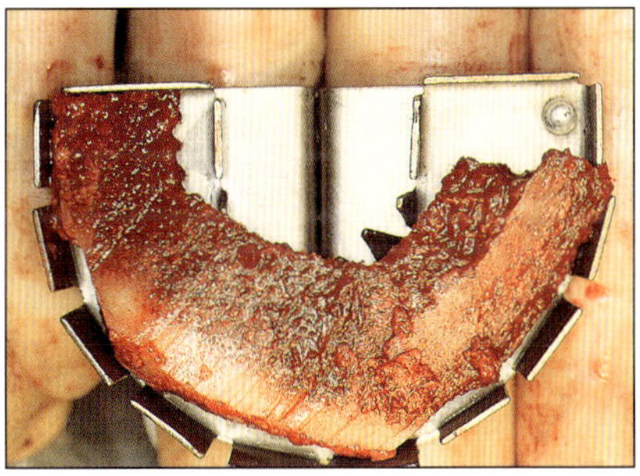

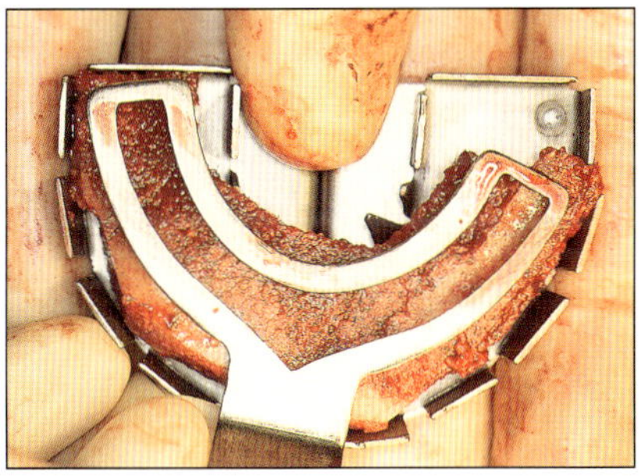

Figs 2-45 and 2-46 Trimming and carving of the graft.

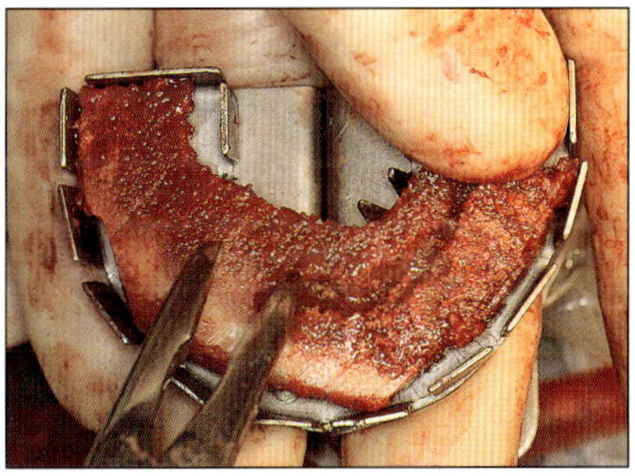

Fig 2-47 Formation of a channel in the cancellous aspect of the graft using rongeurs.

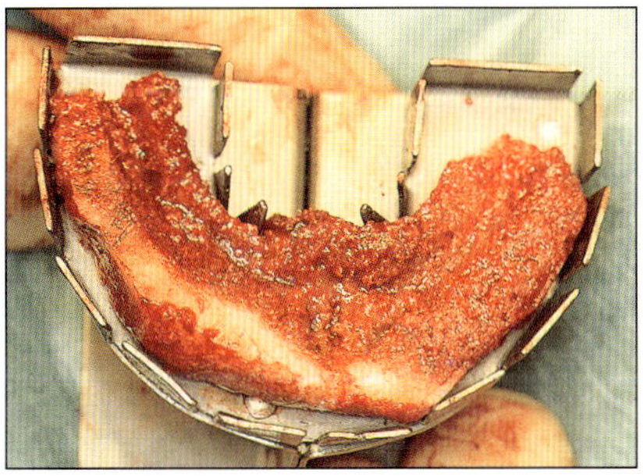

Fig 2-48 Adapted graft topography.

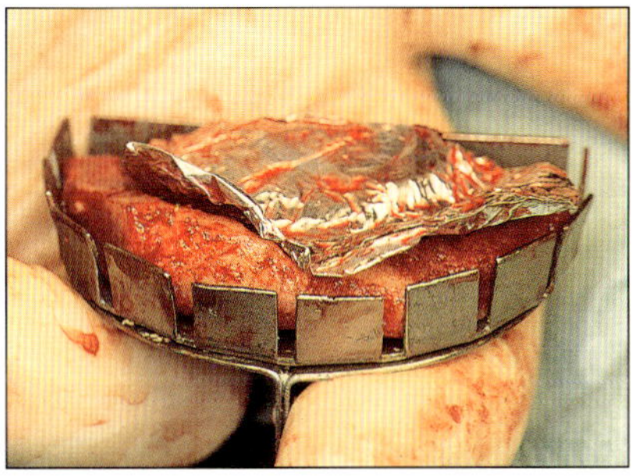

Fig 2-49 Verification of graft topography against the foil model.

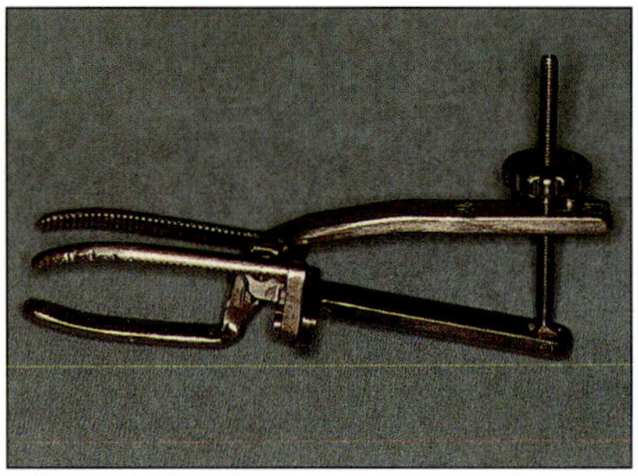

Fig 2-50 Clamp used to secure the graft to the recipient site.

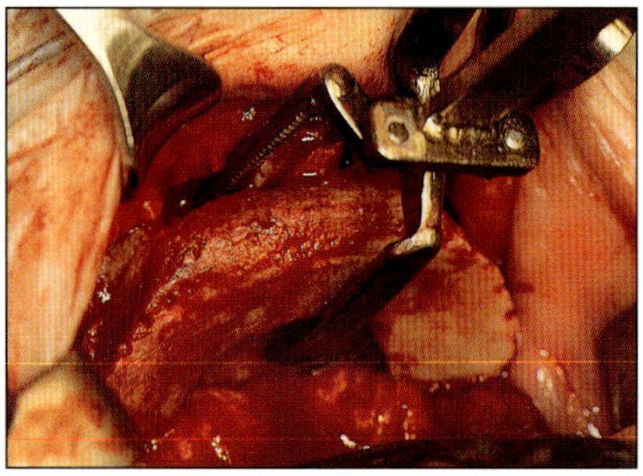

Fig 2-51 Securing of graft with three-pronged clamp.

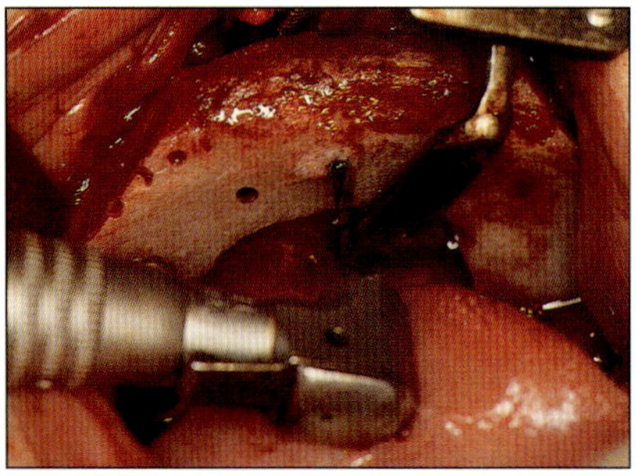

Fig 2-52 Location of initial fixture sites.

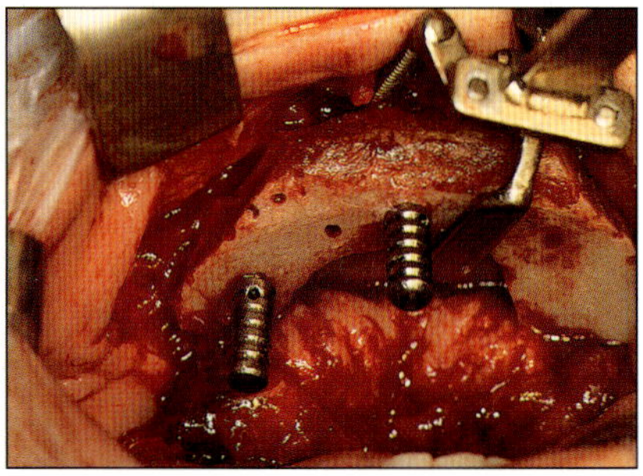

Fig 2-53 Direct indicators are used to support final positioning of fixtures.

Graft adaptation

As stated, the trimming of the graft was performed with utmost care to obtain a precise fit. Closely adapting the graft to the premaxilla prevented ingrowth of soft tissue at the interface. After adaptation, the graft was securely attached to the premaxilla using a special clamp with three prongs (Fig 2-50). Two prongs fit into the previously dissected and exposed nasal floor, one on each side of the nasal septum, and the third was placed underneath the cortical layer of the graft (Fig 2-51). To facilitate the fitting of the clamp without any rocking motion, it was helpful to remove any bone irregularities at the lower margins of the piriform aperture (see Figs 2-17 and 2-18).

With the graft firmly clamped in place, the surgeon tried to locate two sites–one on each side of the former canine areas–where fixtures could be placed to transfix the graft and penetrate the residual basal bone of the maxilla (Fig 2-52). This was carried out with careful consideration of the topographical requirements of the final prosthesis.

Simultaneous fixture placement

It was often possible to find suitable basal bone in the area between the anterior border of the maxillary sinus and the lateral wall of the nasal cavity by probing with a curved dissector through the exploratory access hole (see Fig 2-4). A special direction indicator was placed in the first fixture site, while the second site was identified and prepared on the opposite side. Another direction indicator was then placed in the second site (Fig 2-53).

Cancellous bone was ground using a special mortar and pestle into a soft, particulated, pastelike consistency (Fig 2-54). Using a custom-made titanium instrument, particulated bone was packed into each site prior to fixture placement. Bone marrow and spongious bone were also introduced into each site before the fixtures were placed (Fig 2-55). In addition, the marrow-rich blood retrieved from the donor site was gently applied to each fixture prior to placement.

With the clamp still in situ, the fixture sites were prepared (Figs 2-56 to 2-58). It was common to use

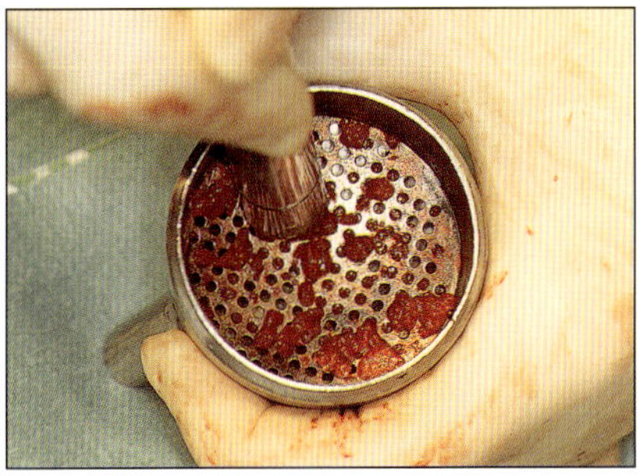

Fig 2-54 Grinding of cancellous bone.

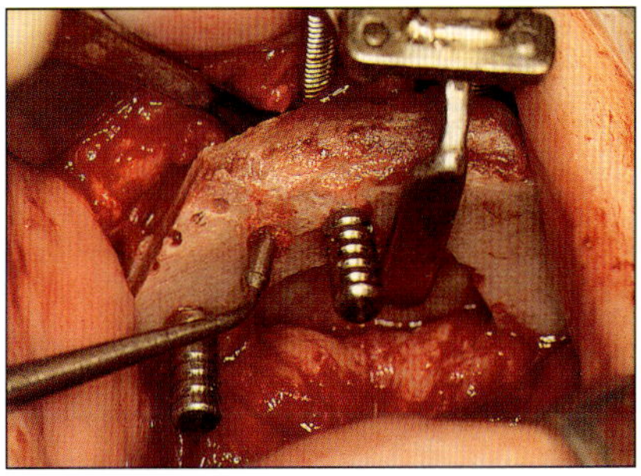

Fig 2-55 Addition of bone marrow and particulated spongious bone to each site using a custom-designed titanium instrument.

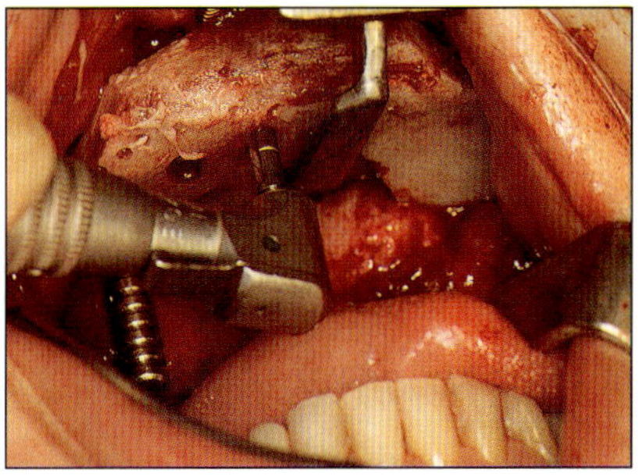

Fig 2-56 Preparation of the second site using a pilot drill.

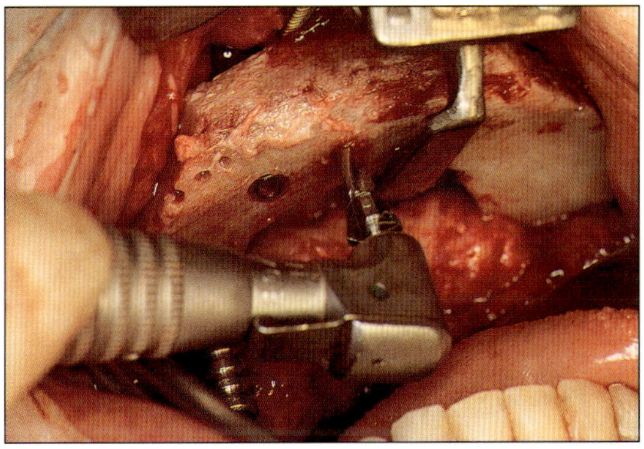

Fig 2-57 The 2.85-mm drill countersink in use.

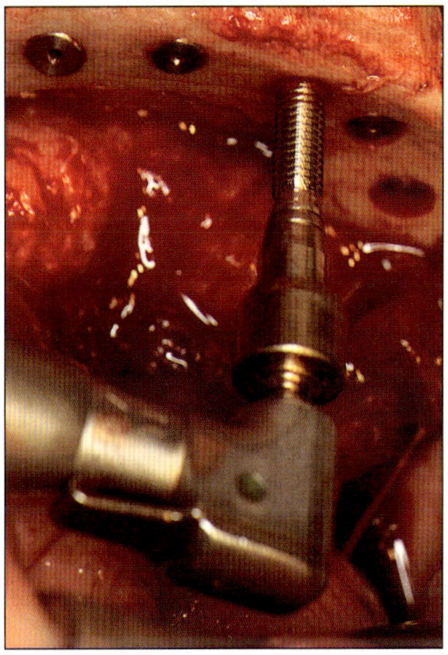

Fig 2-58 Fixture insertion.

the 2-mm twist drill, the pilot drill, and the 3-mm drill, or–if the bone was cancellous–the 2.85-mm drill countersink. Judicious countersinking was prescribed, in contrast to tapping, which was avoided to the extent possible.

Self-tapping fixtures with a low conical profile (swan-neck) were commonly used to avoid thread exposure to the mucosa or the oral cavity in the event of bone resorption (see Fig 2-8). The conical shoulder was also expected to exert some compressive influence and help stabilize the graft. The fixtures were tightened using a manual wrench in cross-ordered sequences.

Usually four to six fixtures were installed (Fig 2-59), although the number varied depending on the position of the fixtures, their angulation, and the mechanical properties of available basal and grafted bone. An attempt was always made to place a minimum of four fixtures to support a fixed prosthesis and to engage available cortical basal bone (eg, in the nasal floor, the maxillary sinus, or the nasal cavity walls).

Once the graft was secured with fixtures, the margins were trimmed again with particular focus on smoothing sharp edges, corners, and the heels of the horseshoe graft (Fig 2-60). Cortical areas of the graft were perforated with a small round bur to allow for vascular connections between the premaxilla, the grafted bone, and the mucoperiosteum (Figs 2-61 and 2-62). This step was important because it optimized revascularization of all affected tissues. Moreover, in all of the graft reconstructions

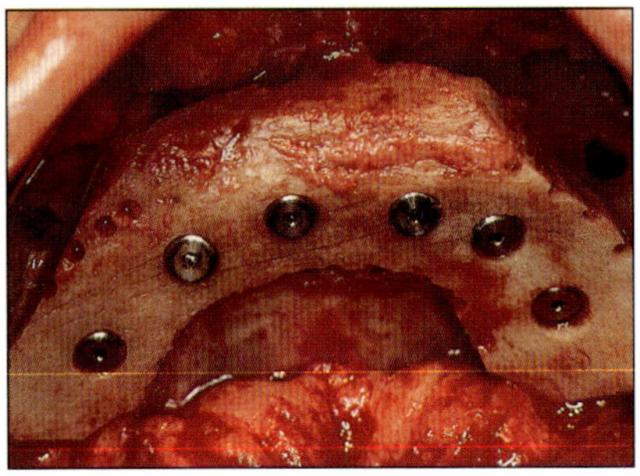

Fig 2-59 Six fixtures in place.

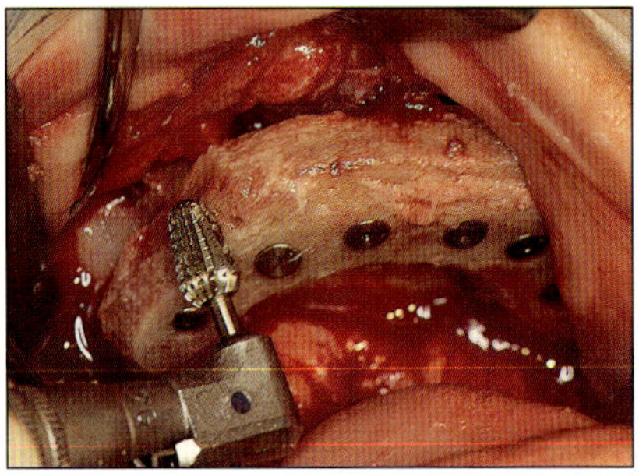

Fig 2-60 Smoothing of sharp edges.

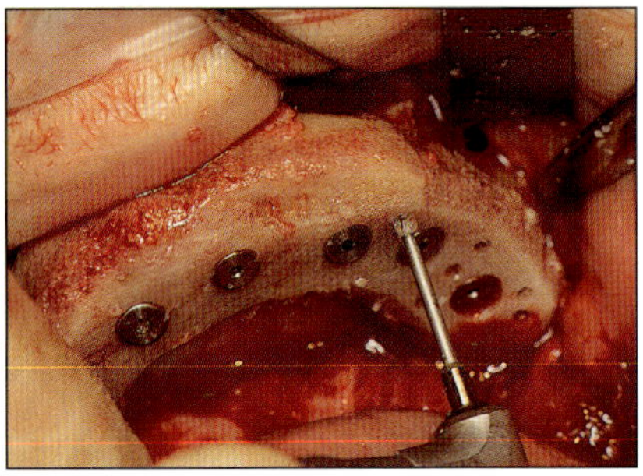

Fig 2-61 Perforation of cortical areas of the graft to allow for vascular connections.

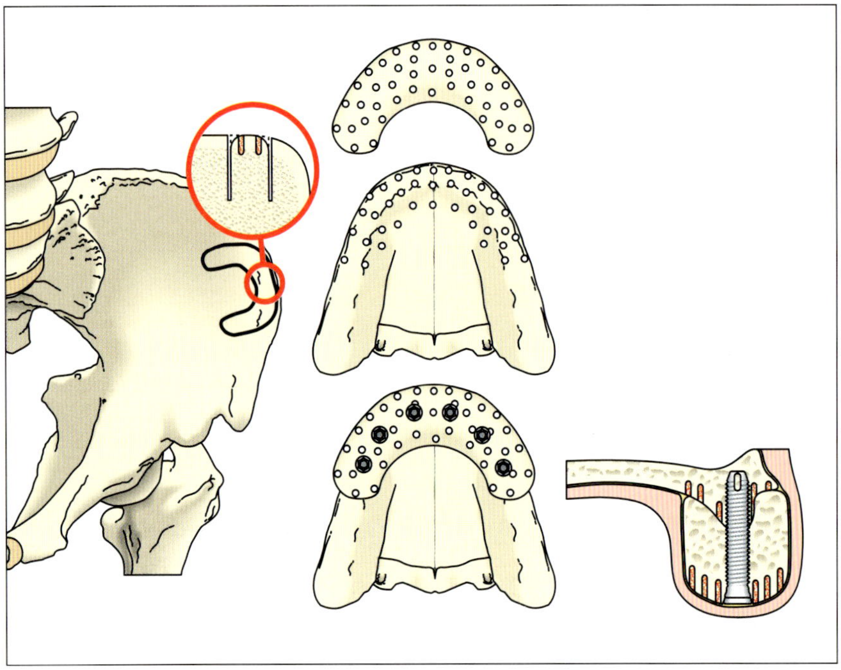

Fig 2-62 Schematic of revascularization principles.

it was absolutely essential to minimize the risk of thermal injury in the bone, both original and grafted, by profused irrigation of room-temperature saline.

The particulated bone (see Fig 2-54) was packed into any space remaining between the graft and the maxilla on both the buccolabial and palatal sides (Fig 2-63). If voids were allowed to persist between the graft and the recipient maxilla, bone was less likely to form and the discrepancies could become occupied by granulating soft tissue. It was therefore essential to pack the particulated bone into all such peripheral spaces.

A low-profile, soft-edge cover screw (or space screw) was used on each fixture to close the internal threaded cavity. It was important that the fixtures were positioned deep enough for the cover screws to be placed flush with the bony surface (Fig 2-64). This was done to avoid undue pressure on the mucoperiosteum. Such pressure could otherwise cause ulceration when the adjusted denture was delivered 6 to 8 weeks later.

Immediately before closure, marrow-rich blood was gently injected into the recipient site. The palatally pedicled mucoperiosteal flap was then repositioned (Fig 2-65). The incision was closed without tension in two layers: first the periosteum with individual resorbable sutures, then the submucosa and mucosa with individual nonresorbable sutures (Figs 2-66 and 2-67). Complete closure was important for success and could be obtained with vertical mattress polyamide monofilament sutures. The initial patient status can be compared with the 5-year follow-up results in Figs 2-68 to 2-70.

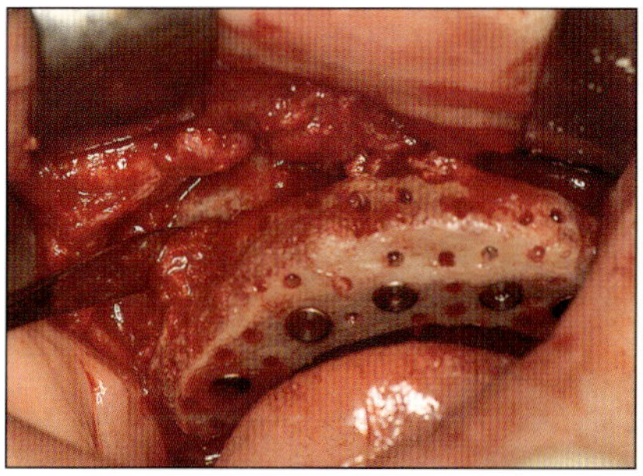

Fig 2-63 Filling of space between the graft and the premaxilla with particulated bone.

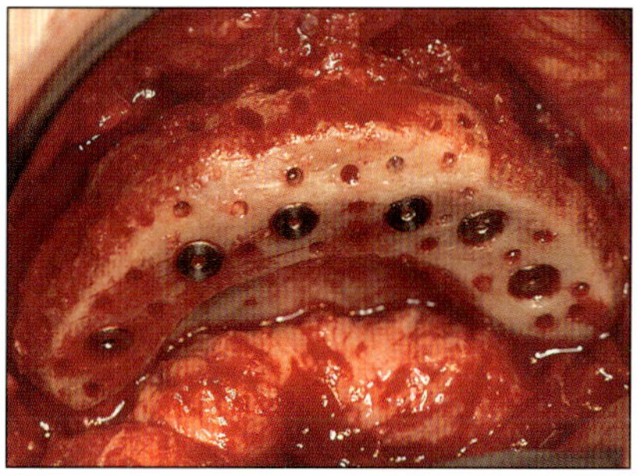

Fig 2-64 The cover screws placed flush with the bony surface.

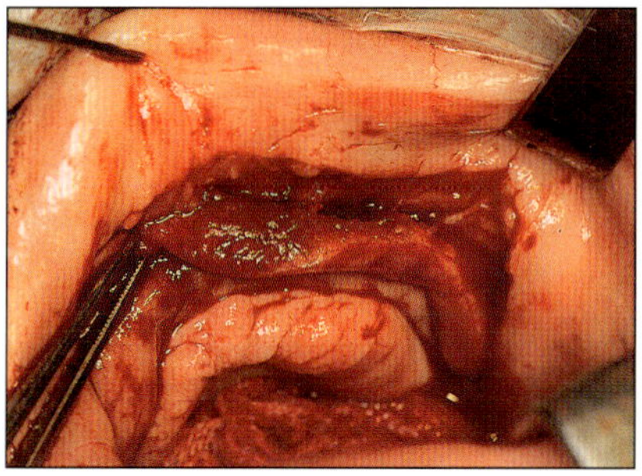

Fig 2-65 Repositioning of the mucoperiosteal flap.

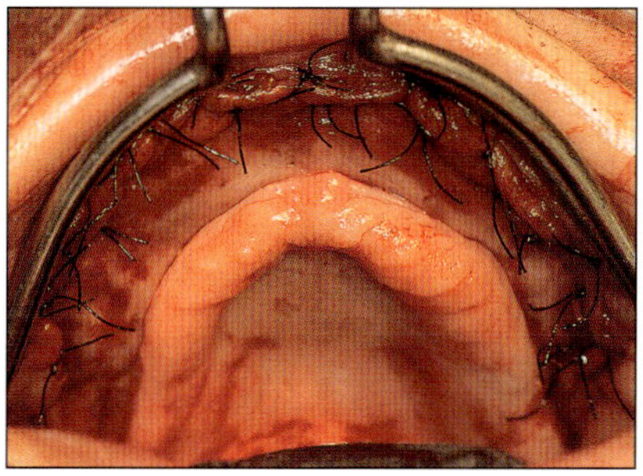

Fig 2-66 Closure of the periosteum with individual sutures.

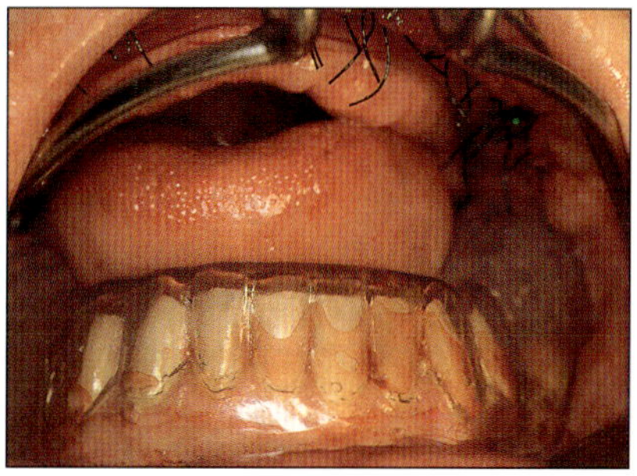

Fig 2-67 Closure of the submucosa and mucosa with nonresorbable sutures. A soft occlusal splint covered the mandibular dentition.

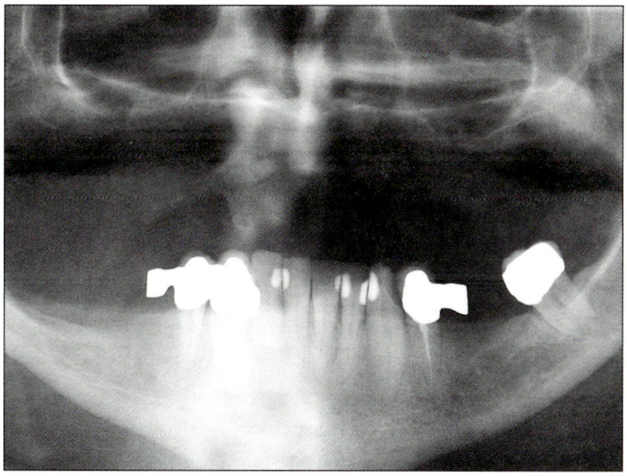

Fig 2-68a Preoperative view.

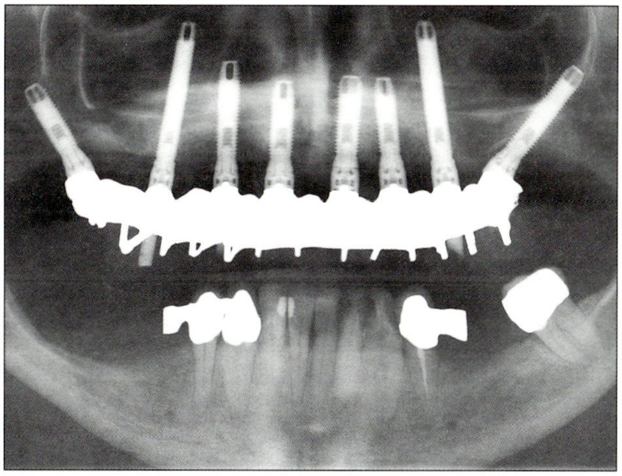

Fig 2-68b Five years after surgery.

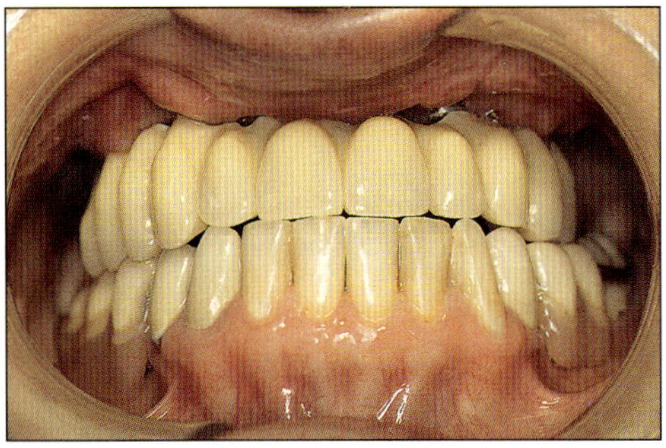

Fig 2-69 Five years after delivery of fixed prosthesis.

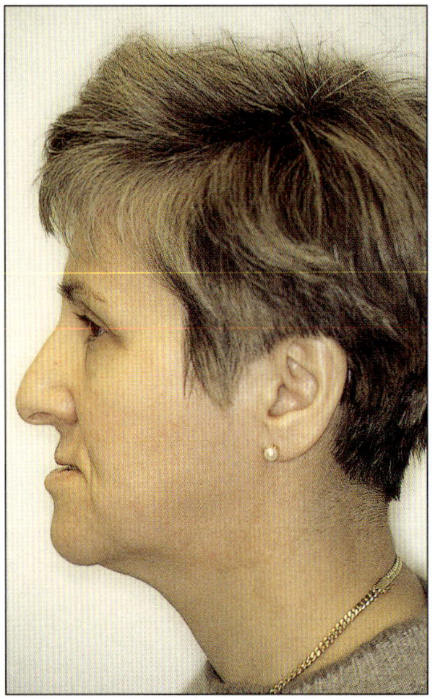

Fig 2-70a Initial clinical profile.

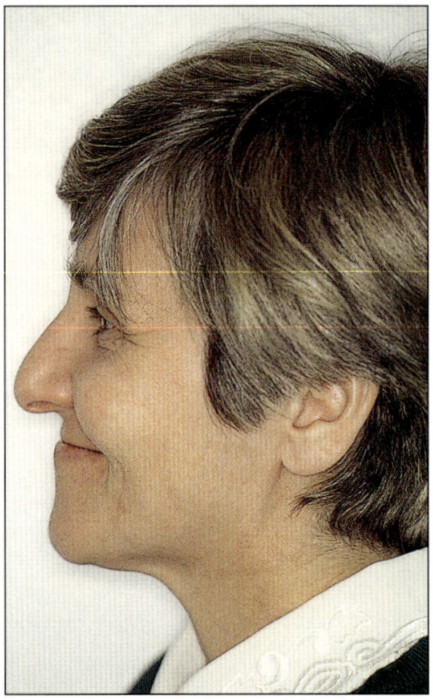

Fig 2-70b Five-year postoperative result.

Postoperative care

A gauze roll soaked in saline solution was placed into the vault of the palate on the grafted area after completion of the surgery (Fig 2-71). This was done to compress the mucoperiosteum and diminish the risk of developing a palatal hematoma or seroma. If a hematoma formed, it was aspirated under appropriate sterile conditions. A prophylactic antibiotic (two 2-g doses of penicillin V) was administered for 10 days postoperatively.

Normally there was no need to apply a drain to the hip. When there was, the drain was usually removed within 48 hours. The patient was advised to move the legs in a pedaling exercise to ensure adequate circulation and to avoid venous stasis of blood.

On a few occasions, a narrow (20-gauge) indwelling catheter was left in the depths of the wound and sutured to the skin at a separate exit point prior to closure of the hip wound. Periodically during the first 2 to 3 days postoperatively, a long-acting local anesthetic solution (eg, 3 mL 0.5% bupivacaine hydrochloride every 6 hours) was injected via the catheter to minimize postoperative donor site pain. This offered the patient increased comfort, simplified movement, facilitated early ambulation, and decreased the need for narcotic analgesics.

The patient initially required assistance during movement, and then used a walking frame or cane until the initial soreness and stiffness had subsided from the hip region. The period of hospitalization varied with age, general health, and resilience of each patient, but generally lasted 5 to 7 days.

The hip sutures were removed in two stages: every other suture after 10 days and the remaining ones after 2 weeks. The oral sutures were removed in a similar fashion: every other suture after 1 week and the remaining sutures after 10 days. No maxillary prosthesis was worn for at least 6 weeks postoperatively. The initial prosthesis (usually the patient's old denture) was then carefully adapted to avoid undue pressure on the tissue above the cover screws.

Prosthetic procedures

General

The prosthetic clinical procedure mainly followed the same sequence as the classic Brånemark system approach with the addition of rigid splinting of the abutments immediately after second-stage surgery.

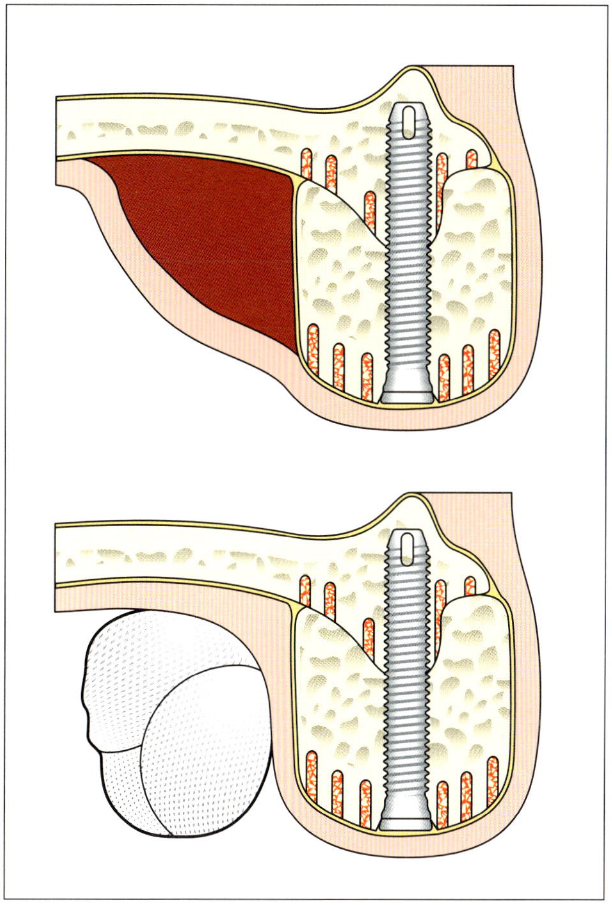

Fig 2-71 Placement of a gauze roll to prevent hematoma formation.

Biomechanical considerations

Torque can cause deformation and deflection of the supporting bone, which in turn can result in fixture mobility. Unfavorable bending forces were minimized by decreasing buccal lever arms and cantilevers (mesiodistal and anteroposterior) to the extent possible. Cross-arch stabilization, controlled occlusion, and decreased cuspal inclination also helped decrease bending moments (Fig 2-72).

Prosthetic impressions, laboratory work, and patient discussions

The prosthetic procedure began with an impression taken immediately following abutment connection, after proper seating of the abutments had been verified radiographically. Abutment screw stability was also checked. A rigid impression material (eg, impression plaster) and squared two-piece impression copings were used in most cases. A rubber dam was used to cover the surgical incisions and sutures as needed. When used, the abutments and impression copings penetrated the dam. An impression of the mandible and a preliminary registration of the jaw relations were also recorded.

A laboratory working cast was poured and gold cylinders were attached to the abutment replicas. A gold bar was adjusted to fit and was then soldered to the gold cylinders. The rigid bar was attached to the abutments and secured with the connecting screws. The patient's removable denture was carefully adjusted and relined with a soft material.

A second rigid impression was taken after suture removal and soft tissue healing. The impression was taken to the dental laboratory where a master cast was produced. An acrylic record base with a wax occlusal rim was made on the cast. The record base was attached to the abutments and the occlusal rim was adjusted to the correct vertical height and occlusal plane orientation. Adequate lip support and facial contours were also evaluated. Tooth shape and shade were selected in consultation with the patient.

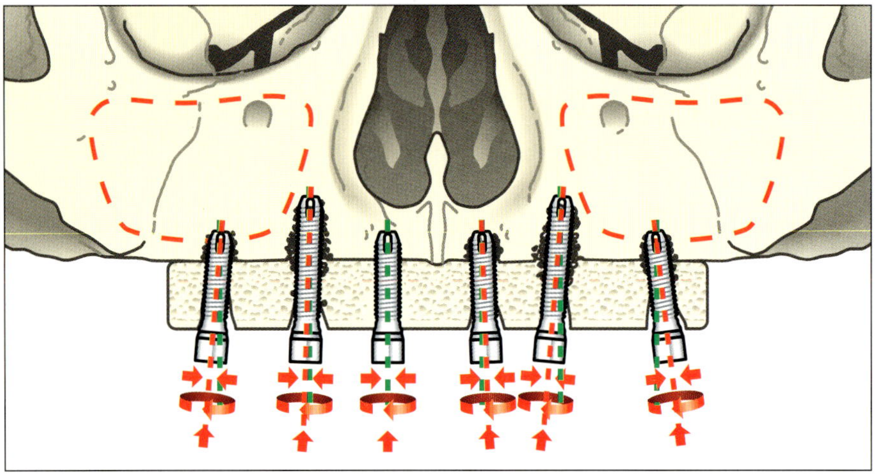

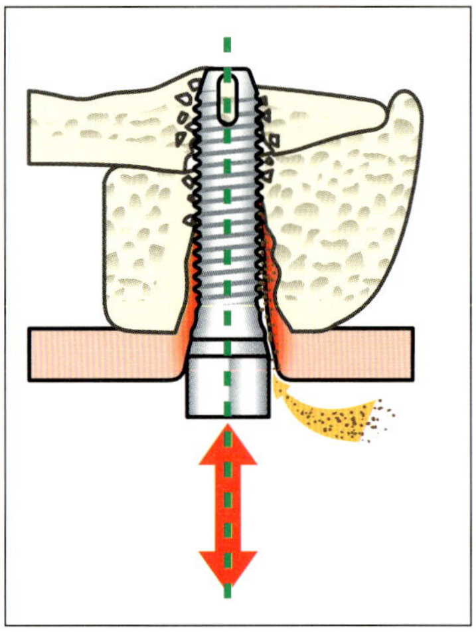

Figs 2-72a and 2-72b *(a)* Damage caused by torque and bending forces on individual fixtures after abutment connection. *(b)* Damage to the anchoring bone caused by relative motion resulting from individual fixture loading.

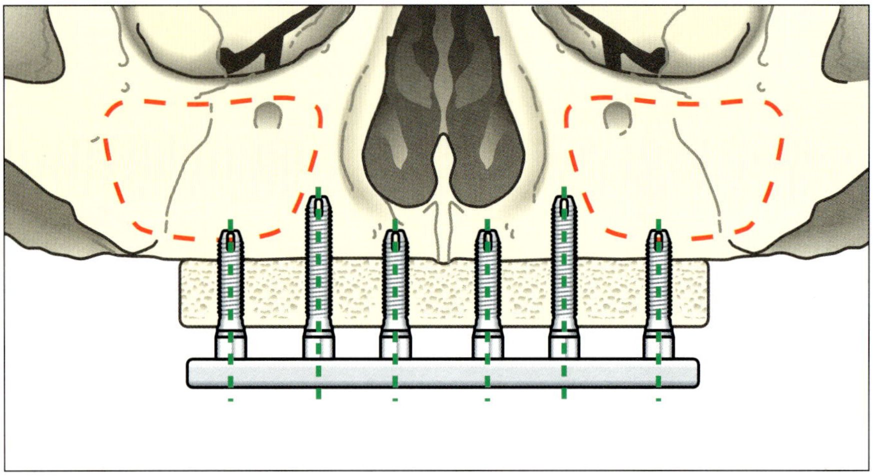

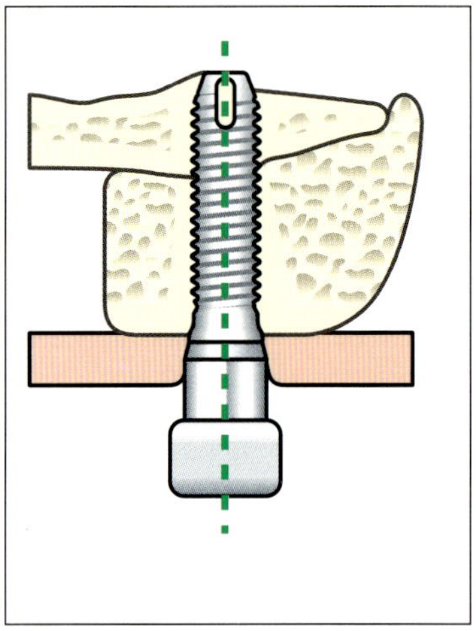

Figs 2-72c and 2-72d Cross-arch stabilization achieved through the placement of a rigid bar.

A preliminary tooth set-up then was made according to conventional principles. The wax set-up was tried in the patient so that vertical dimensions, occlusion, cantilevers, cuspal inclination, shade, shape, hygiene accessibility, lip support, and facial contours could be evaluated and approved by the patient.

A rigid framework with adequate dimensions and precision was then fabricated using cast gold alloy or a precision-milled titanium beam. It was carefully assured that the framework fit passively on the laboratory abutment replicas. The passive fit of the framework was verified intraorally and the use of magnifying loupes facilitated the procedure. The final restoration was then produced.

Delivery of the fixed prosthesis

At delivery of the fixed prosthesis, passive fit of the final restoration was once again verified. The gold retaining screws were then tightened to 10 Ncm. The occlusion was carefully checked, and primary occlusal contacts on the distal cantilevers were eliminated. The screw access holes were temporarily sealed, and oral hygiene requirements were discussed with the patient. Finally, intraoral radiographs were taken to verify component fit and to record the baseline marginal bone levels.

Typical case results are shown in Figs 2-73 to 2-80.

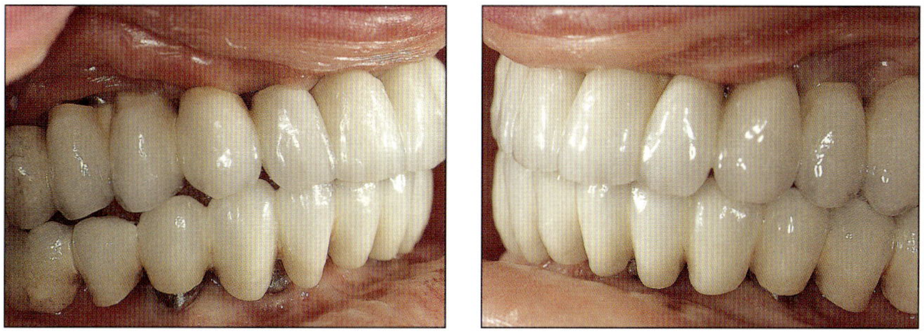

Figs 2-73 and 2-74 Ceramo-metal constructions in the maxilla and mandible of a patient with multiple agenesia of her permanent teeth.

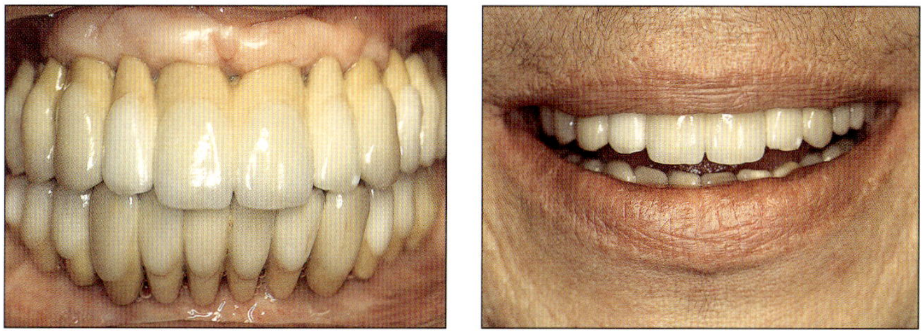

Figs 2-75 and 2-76 Ceramo-metal restorations in the maxilla and mandible after 4 years of function.

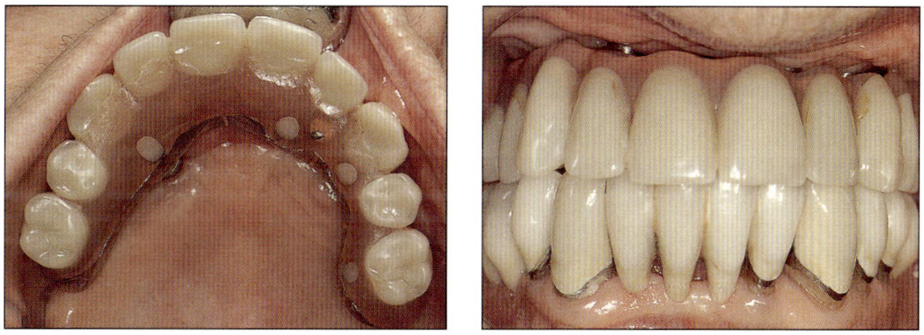

Figs 2-77 and 2-78 Conventional gold-acrylic fixture-supported maxillary fixed prosthesis after 10 years of function.

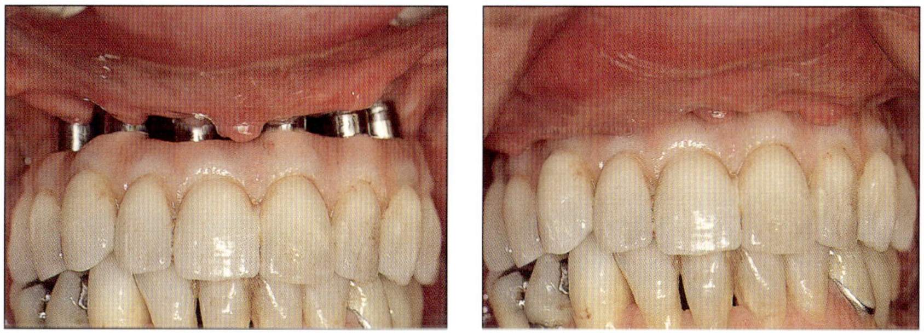

Figs 2-79 and 2-80 Ceramo-metal construction with stainings and characterizations of teeth and soft tissue imitations. Note how the suturing technique results in hygiene accessibility around the abutments. The adaptation of the soft tissue is demonstrated when the upper lip is retracted and the sealing of the interabutment spaces when the lip is folded down.

Follow-up

The patient returned after 1 or 2 weeks for an evaluation of the stability, function, phonetics, and esthetics of the fixed prosthesis. The connecting screws were retightened if necessary, and the screw access holes were permanently sealed. A soft and easily removable material was used near the screw head, while composite resin or another hard filling material was used on top to completely seal the access holes.

The healing time to abutment connection was usually about 6 months. The subsequent follow-up protocol was similar to that used for routine fixture placement, ie, the patient was placed on an annual clinical recall schedule that included regular radiographic examinations.

Statistical Methods

System survival curves were calculated by the product-limit estimate, ie, the Kaplan-Meier survival curve.[32] The log rank test[33] was used to analyze prognostic factors related to system survival. The Cox proportional hazard regression model[34] was used for calculation of the hazard ratios and the 95% confidence intervals for the hazard ratios. The Pitman nonparametric permutation test was used for all correlation analyses.[35] In addition, the Pearson correlation coefficient was calculated for descriptive purposes. For comparison between groups, the Fisher nonparametric permutation test was used.[36] Comparison of proportions between groups was analyzed by the Fisher exact test. Changes over time in mean bone loss were analyzed with the Fisher nonparametric permutation test for matched pairs.[37] All statistical tests were based on patients rather than fixtures. The significant tests were two-tailed and conducted at the 5% significance level.

Patient Withdrawals

Seven patients died during the course of the study. Of these, four were treated during the routine period and three during the development period. One of the patients who died during the study was a heavy smoker with an extremely resorbed maxilla. She died from the progression of a preexisting disease shortly after losing her fixed prosthesis. At the time of her death at the age of 69, she had worn the fixture-supported prosthesis for almost 3 years. The six other patients died with a functioning bone-anchored fixed prosthesis in situ. Three of these patients had worn their fixed prostheses for more than 5 years at the time of death. The other three patients had carried their bone-anchored prostheses for 8, 18, and 42 months.

CHAPTER 3

Routine Case Presentations

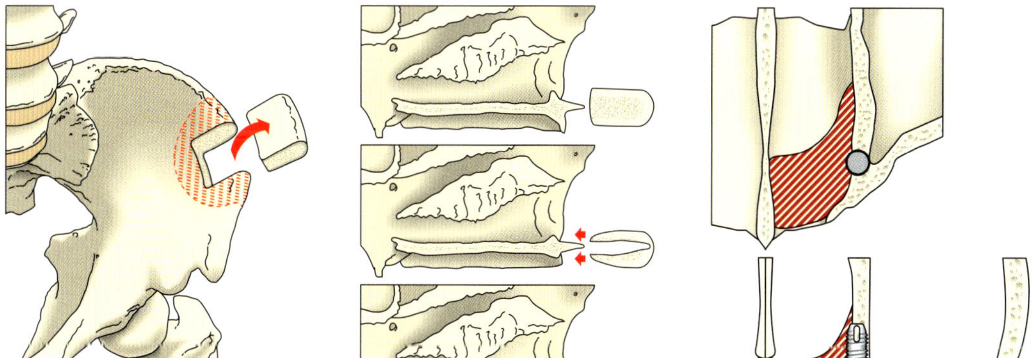

The following overview of our most important findings serves as an introduction to the routine case presentations. These 13 clinical presentations summarize the scenarios most frequently encountered during the autogenous onlay bone grafting study.

Summary of Important Clinical Findings

- Proper preoperative or intraoperative treatment of a dysfunctional or partial mandibular dentition was essential in the minimization of bending forces and the assurance of optimal occlusion.
- When grafts were taken from the medial ilium graft harvesting was simplified and postoperative pain reduced.
- Small holes were randomly drilled in the mucoperiosteum, the premaxilla, and the grafted bone before graft attachment to enable revascularization.
- The mucoperiosteal flap was carefully sutured in two layers. A compromised closure might allow communication between the oral cavity and the sinus and/or the nasal cavity. Such connections inevitably caused severe complications unless they were remedied immediately.
- Four fixtures were frequently sufficient for adequate support of the fixed prosthesis in the grafted maxilla. Short fixtures could also function well when indicated.
- The grafted bone could remineralize if the dynamic functional load was optimal during the remodeling process.
- Both clinical and radiographic evaluations verified that the bone responded favorably to controlled early prosthetic loading. The reduced bone resorption associated with early loading required all fixtures to be rigidly connected with a bar, thus avoiding torque and early loading of individual fixtures.

Patient 1 (Routine Group)

Background

This male patient was born in 1931. He had been edentulous in the maxilla since he was 28 years old (1959). He had a dysfunctional maxillary prosthesis; however, his mandibular dentition was viewed as acceptable.

Preoperative comments

Nutrient canals and few bone trabeculae indicated a thin alveolar crest in the frontal jaw region. The patient exhibited a resorption pattern equivalent to type III and a sinus configuration equivalent to type D (see Figs 2-1 and 2-2).

Surgical procedure

Surgery was conducted in May 1985, when the patient was 54 years old. The graft was taken from the left lateral ilium and attached with five 15-mm conical self-tapping fixtures and one self-tapping standard 10-mm fixture in the right distal site.

Postoperative comments

The total bone loss between connection of the fixed prosthesis and the 10-year follow-up visit was 0.4 mm (Figs 3-5 to 3-8). At the latest examination, the marginal bone was still located above the first thread of each fixture. The functional loading of the grafted bone was sufficient to preserve its degree of mineralization throughout the 10-year follow-up. As exemplified in the enlargements from 1986 and 1996 of the second fixture on the right side (R2) (Figs 3-6 and 3-8), the marginal bone level remained in contact with the conical portion of the fixtures throughout the follow-up period.

Today a patient under similar circumstances would be treated with a smaller graft to restore the anterior maxillary topography and four standard and two zygoma fixtures to anchor the prosthesis.

Patient 1 (Routine Group)

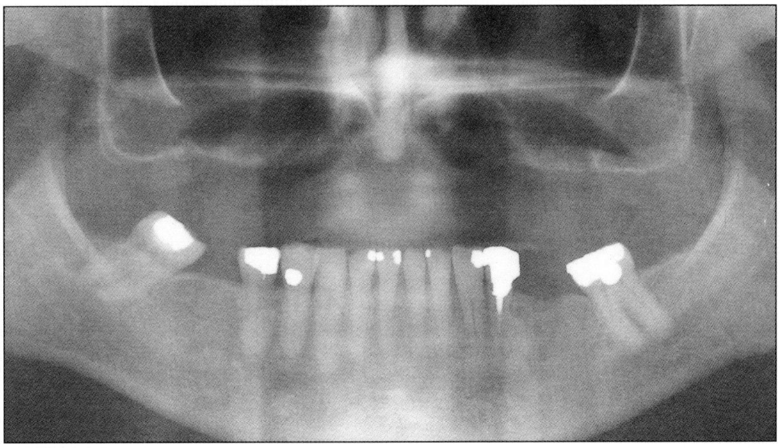

Fig 3-1 Preoperative panoramic view.

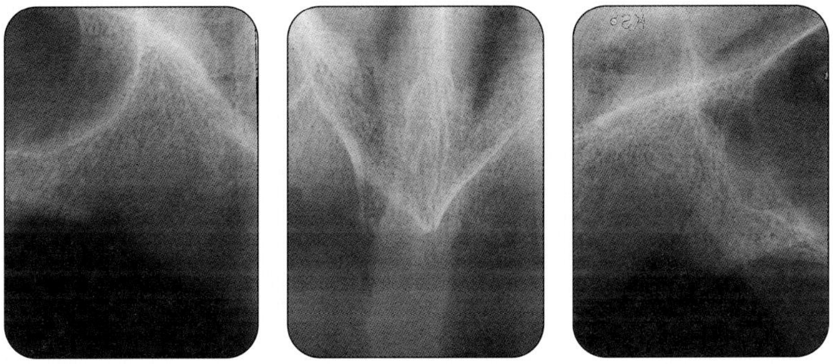

Fig 3-2 Preoperative intraoral radiographs.

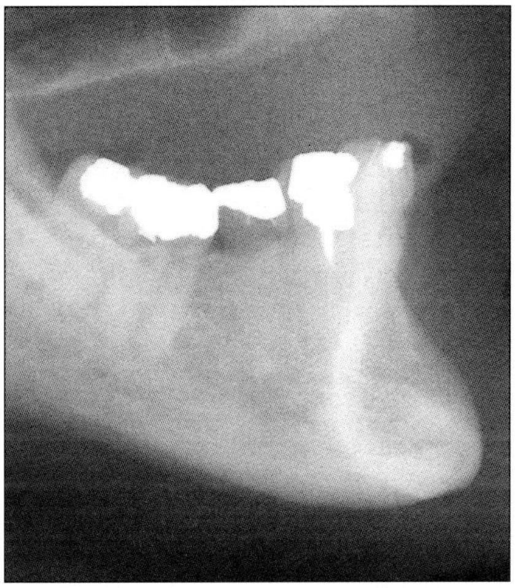

Fig 3-3 Preoperative profile.

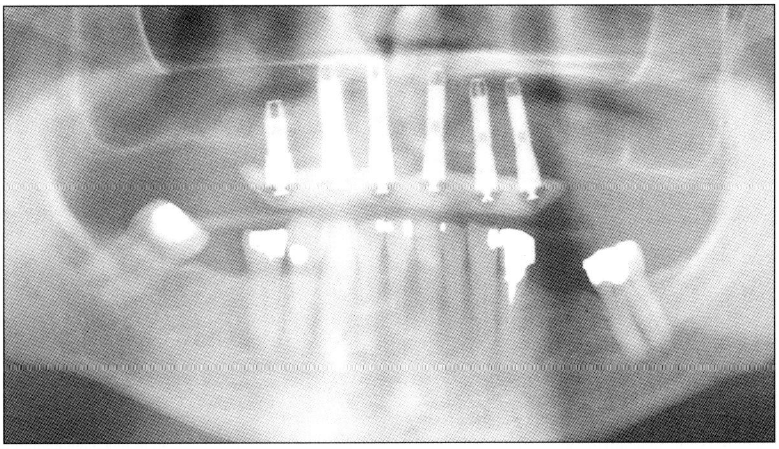

Fig 3-4 Abutment connection (1986).

Patient 1 (Routine Group) continued

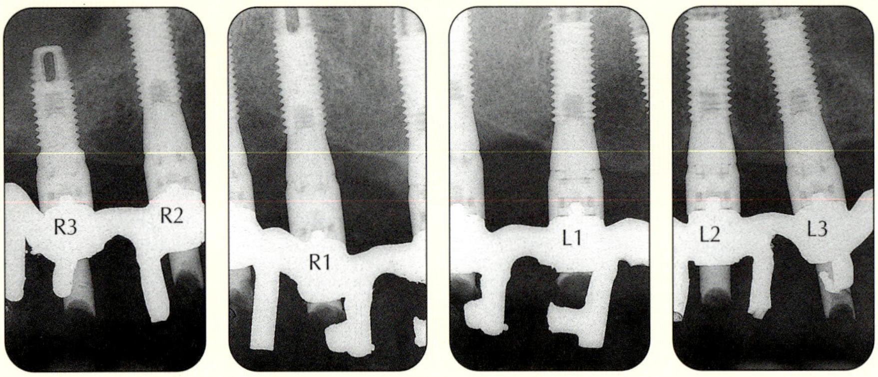

Fig 3-5 Connection of the fixed prosthesis (1986).

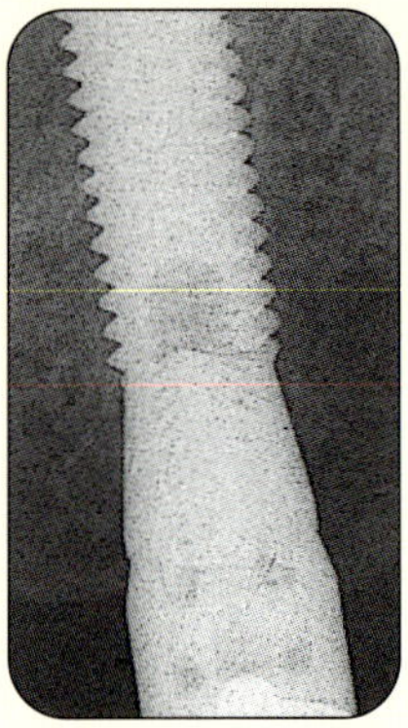

Fig 3-6 Enlargement of R2 from Fig 3-5.

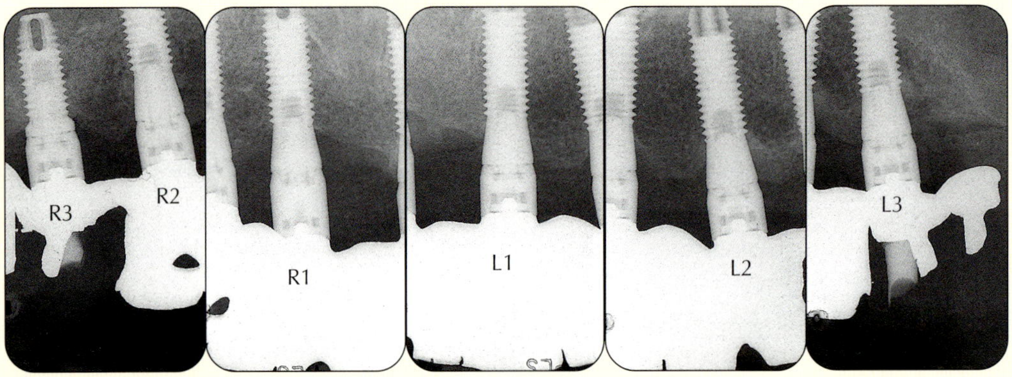

Fig 3-7 Fixed prosthesis at the 10-year follow-up (1996).

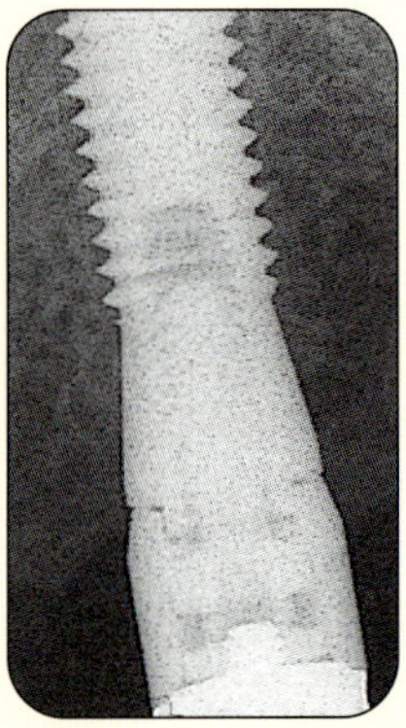

Fig 3-8 Enlargement of R2 from Fig 3-7.

Patient 2 (Routine Group)

Background

This male patient, born in 1951, had aplasia but was otherwise healthy. He never had any permanent teeth in the maxilla and had only five primary teeth remaining in the mandible. These teeth were replaced with fixtures prior to the grafting procedure to optimize occlusion and loading conditions.

Preoperative comments

The maxillary sinus expanded in an anterior direction. The radiographic distance between the anterior border of the maxillary sinus and the incisive canal was approximately 10 mm bilaterally. The available bone height for fixture anchorage was only 4 mm. The patient exhibited a resorption pattern equivalent to type III and a sinus configuration equivalent to type D (see Figs 2-1 and 2-2).

Surgical procedure

The surgery was performed in September 1984, when the patient was 33 years old. The graft was taken from the left lateral ilium and was stabilized with three 15-mm standard fixtures. One of the three fixtures was placed in the midline after the incisive canal had been cleaned out and filled with particulated bone and marrow. In addition, two 7-mm fixtures (R2 and L2) were placed in the distal areas where the anterior expansion of the sinus only allowed for fixture placement through the graft and in 1 mm of the basal bone.

Postoperative comments

The mean bone loss between connection of the fixed prosthesis and the 10-year follow-up visit was 1.4 mm (Figs 3-13 and 3-14). Note the distinctly increased corticalization of the bone crest, which can be seen, for example, around the midline fixture (M). The bone adjacent to the 7-mm fixtures also retained its degree of mineralization. New bone was formed in the maxillary sinus (Fig 3-14).

Had this patient been treated as a child, small-diameter provisional fixtures would have been placed in preparation for adult treatment with a graft and regular fixtures. Placement of the two 7-mm fixtures could then have been avoided.

Patient 2 (Routine Group)

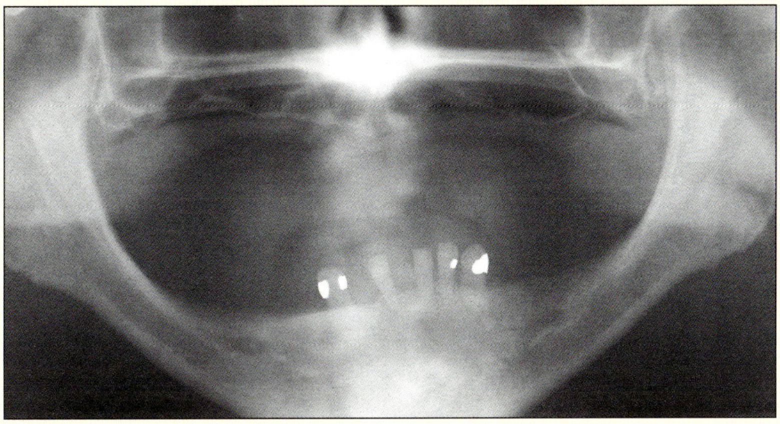

Fig 3-9 Preoperative panoramic view.

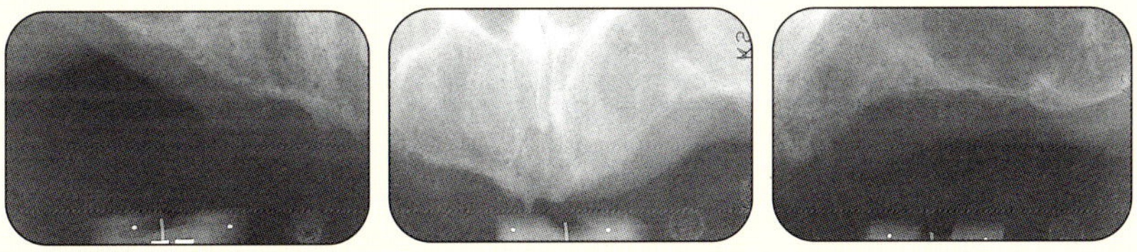

Fig 3-10 Preoperative intraoral radiographs.

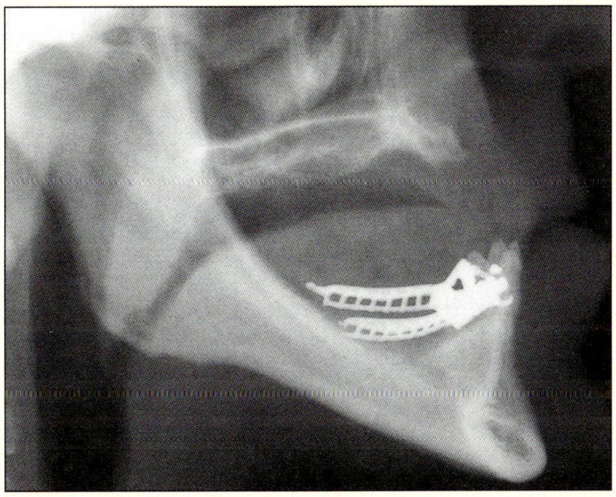

Fig 3-11 Preoperative profile.

Patient 2 (Routine Group) continued

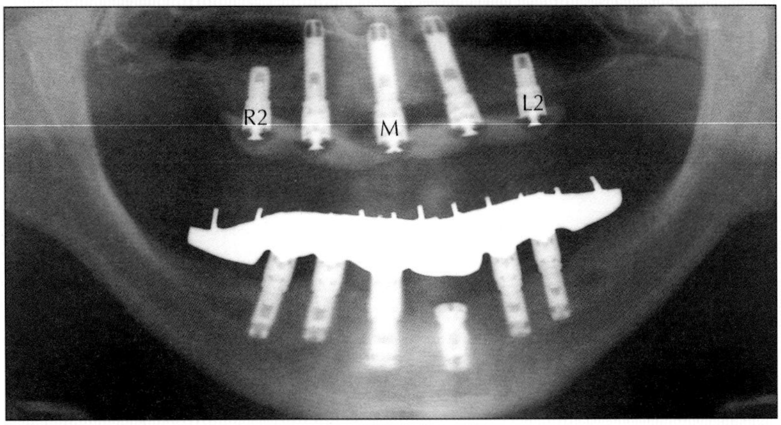

Fig 3-12 Abutment connection (1985).

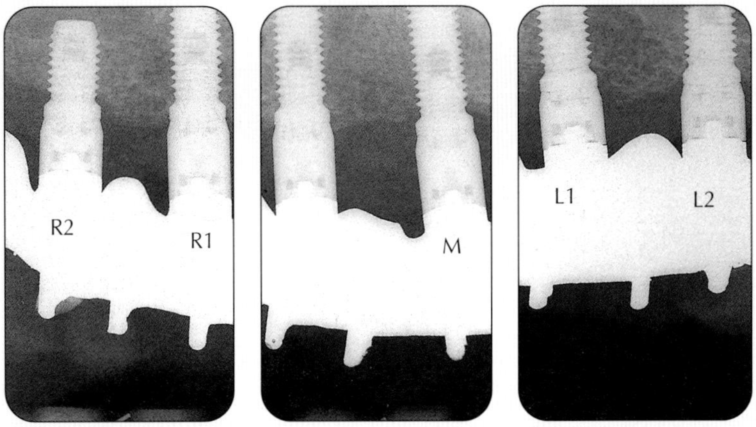

Fig 3-13 Connection of the fixed prosthesis (1985).

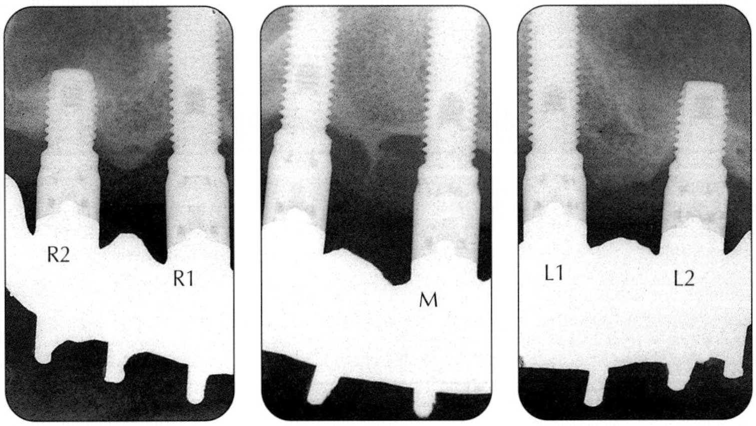

Fig 3-14 Fixed prosthesis at the 10-year follow-up (1995).

Patient 3 (Routine Group)

Background

This female patient was born in 1925. She had asthma and was retired because of disability. The partial dentition in the mandible required reinforcement.

Preoperative comments

The total height of the alveolar crest was 15 mm, but the low bone density indicated a thin crest, which was verified in tomographic radiographs. The available bone height for fixture anchorage in the maxilla was only 4 mm. The patient exhibited a resorption pattern equivalent to type III and a sinus configuration equivalent to type B (see Figs 2-1 and 2-2).

Surgical procedure

Surgery was performed in September 1987 when the patient was 62 years old. The graft was taken from the left lateral and medial ilium. It was attached to the maxillary base with five conical fixtures (10, 12, and 15 mm). In the mandible, two standard fixtures (10 and 13 mm) were placed bilaterally after nerve transposition.[37]

Postoperative comments

The most distal maxillary fixture on the right side (R3) perforated the maxillary sinus. The stability of this fixture was questioned at the last follow-up visit in 1998 (Fig 3-21). A 2-mm loss of bone support, possibly caused by insufficient functional loading of the fixture, had occurred during the past 2 years. In addition, the graft was particularly thin in this area. The mean bone loss for all fixtures was 2.8 mm between connection of the fixed prosthesis and the 10-year follow-up examination.

In the mandible, only minor bone loss was noted on the right side in spite of a long anterior cantilever. The fixtures on the left side lost approximately 2 to 3 mm of bone support during the follow-up period (Fig 3-22).

Today, a patient under similar circumstances would receive two zygoma and four standard fixtures. This would allow for a longer construction of the fixed prosthesis with reduced cantilevers as well as adequate functional loading of all fixtures–without fixture placement in the R3 position.

Patient 3 (Routine Group)

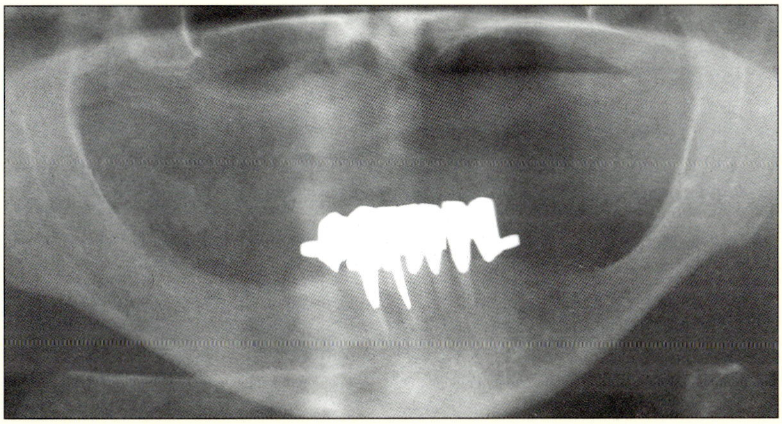

Fig 3-15 Preoperative panoramic view.

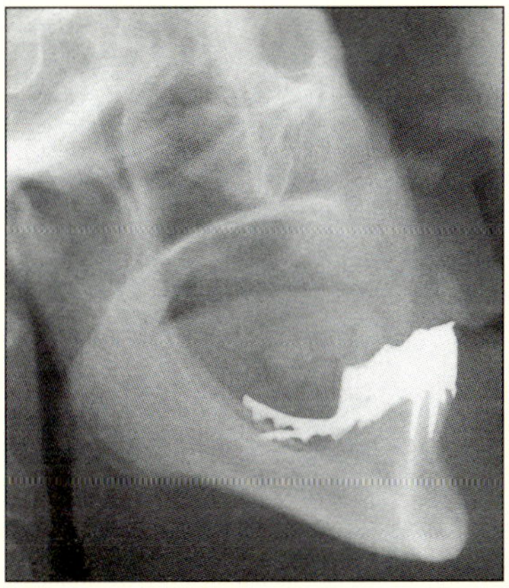

Fig 3-16 Preoperative profile.

Patient 3 (Routine Group) continued

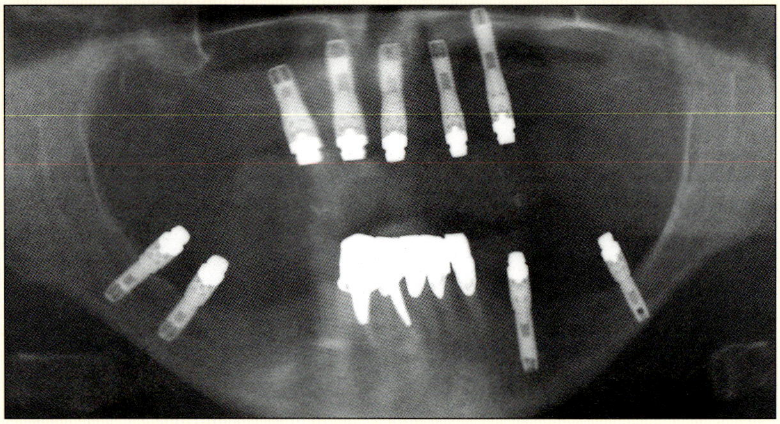

Fig 3-17 Connection of the provisional fixed prosthesis (1988).

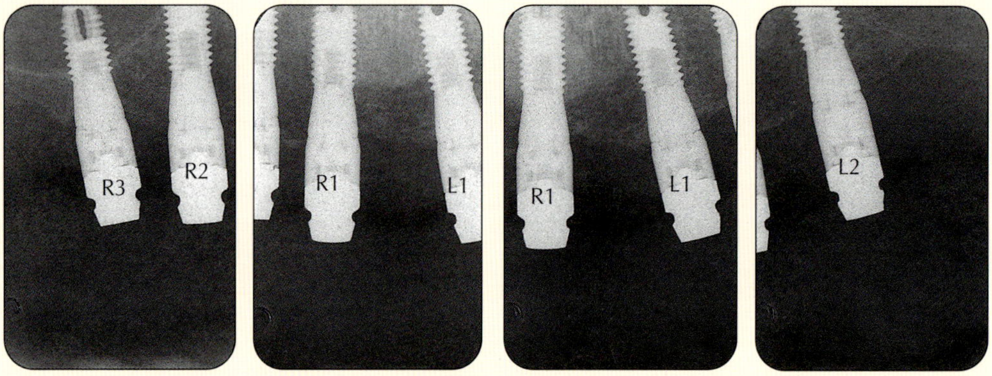

Fig 3-18 Connection of the provisional fixed prosthesis (1988).

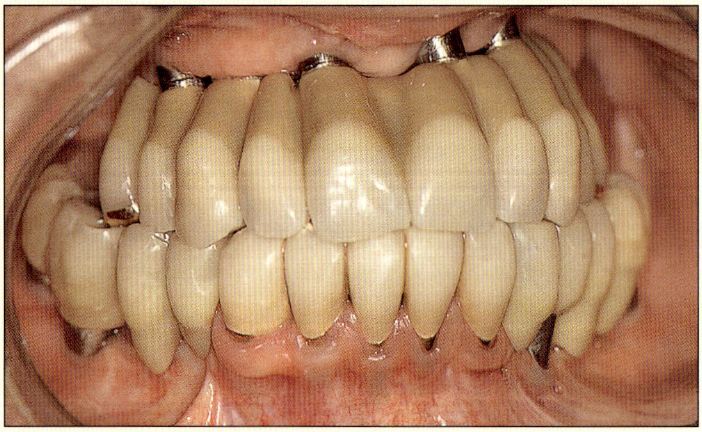

Fig 3-19 Intraoral view (1988).

Patient 3 (Routine Group) continued

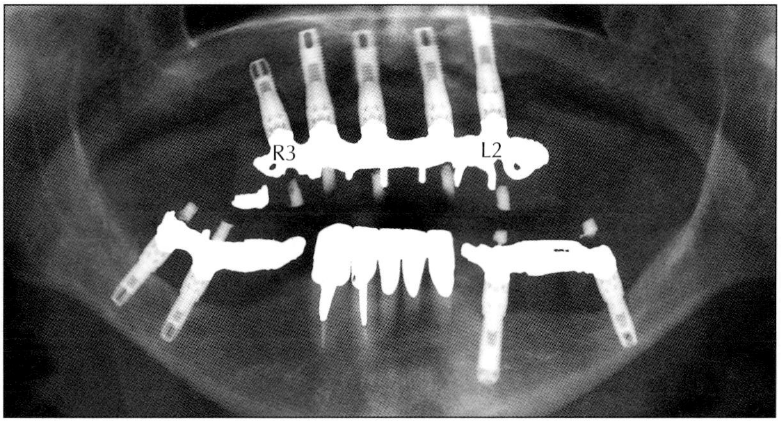

Fig 3-20 Fixed prosthesis at the 10-year follow-up (1998).

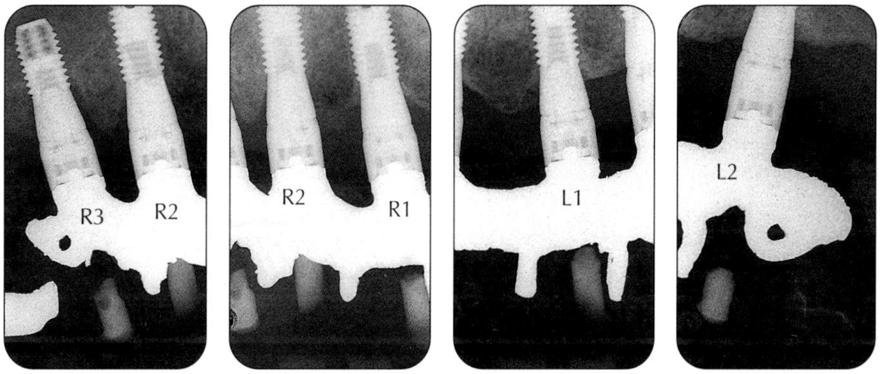

Fig 3-21 Fixed prosthesis at the 10-year follow-up (1998).

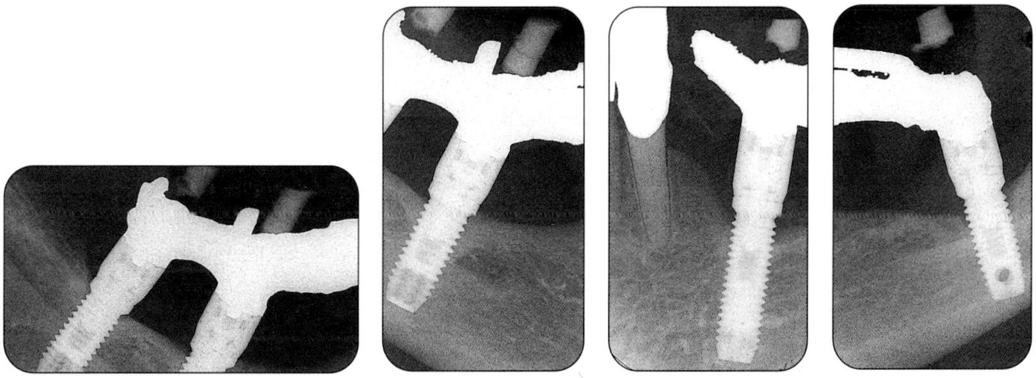

Fig 3-22 Fixed prosthesis in the mandible at the 10-year follow-up (1998).

Patient 4 (Routine Group)

Background

This female patient was born in 1936. She had been edentulous in the maxilla since the age of 25 (1961). She was neither a bruxist nor a smoker.

Preoperative comments

The available bone for fixture anchorage was only 2 mm in the patient's extremely resorbed maxillary base. The partial dentition in the mandible was severely deteriorated and required substitution with fixtures at the time of maxillary reconstruction (Figs 3-23 and 3-24). The patient exhibited a resorption pattern equivalent to type IV and a sinus configuration equivalent to type D (see Figs 2-1 and 2-2).

Surgical procedure

Surgery was performed in March 1991, when the patient was 55 years old. The grafted bone was taken from the left lateral ilium. Bilateral nasal inlay grafts were performed. In addition, a special grafting procedure called the "sandwich" procedure was conducted in the frontal region to compensate for the highly resorbed alveolar crest (Fig 3-25). Five swan-neck fixtures (15 and 18 mm) penetrated the grafts, going through the exterior aspect, the thin nasal floor, and the internal part of the graft. After extraction of the partial dentition, five standard fixtures (10 and 13 mm) were placed in the mandible.

Postoperative comments

Significant bone loss was noted around several fixtures at the time of connection of the fixed prosthesis (Figs 3-26 and 3-27). This particularly applied to the most distal fixture on the left (L2). The average distance between the reference point and the bone crest was 3.5 mm at the time of connection of the fixed prosthesis.

At the 5-year follow-up in 1997, the mean bone loss was 1.5 mm. The initial bone loss may have resulted from the fact that vascular connections were not made in the grafts. As can be noted in the intraoral radiographs from the examination in 1999 (Fig 3-30), the bone loss continued around the two distal fixtures on the left. Two zygoma fixtures may be indicated if the problems persist.

Patient 4 (Routine Group)

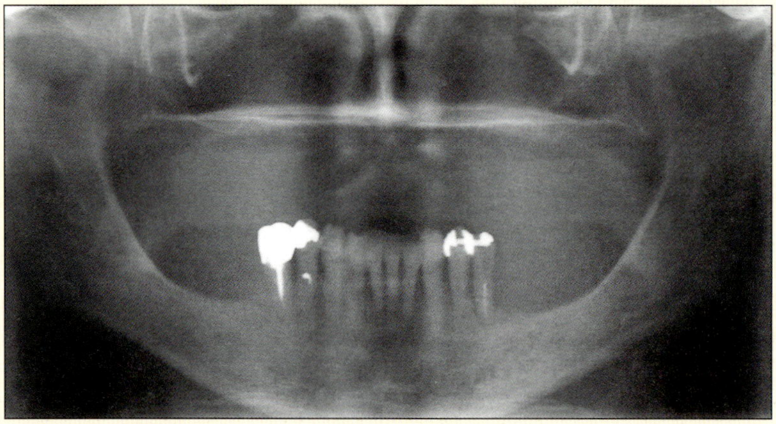

Fig 3-23 Preoperative panoramic view.

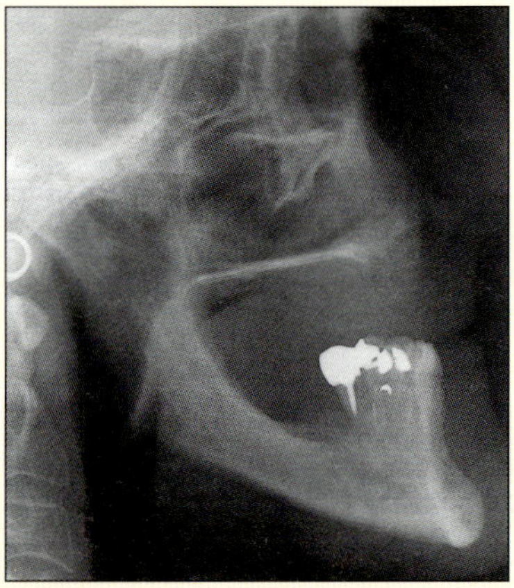

Fig 3-24 Preoperative profile.

Patient 4 (Routine Group) continued

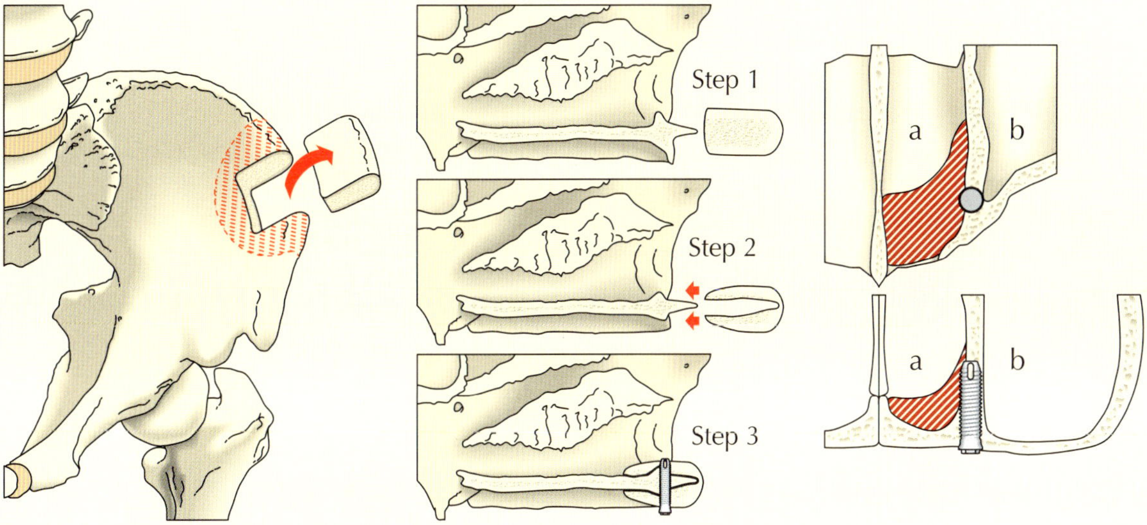

Fig 3-25 Grafting procedure (a—nasal cavity; b—maxillary sinus).

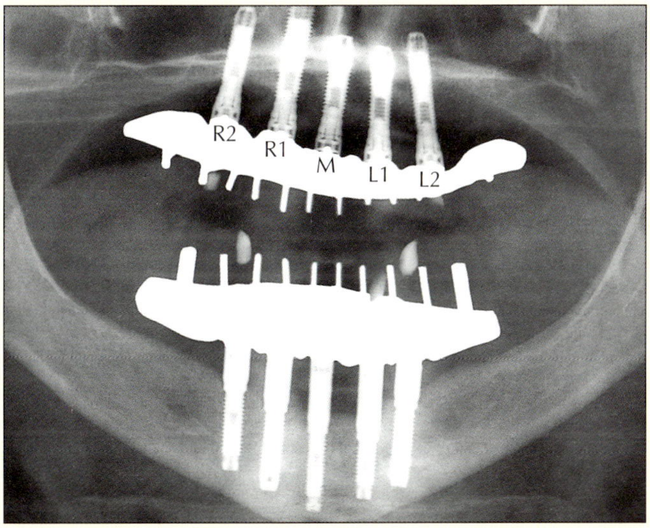

Fig 3-26 Connection of fixed prosthesis (1992).

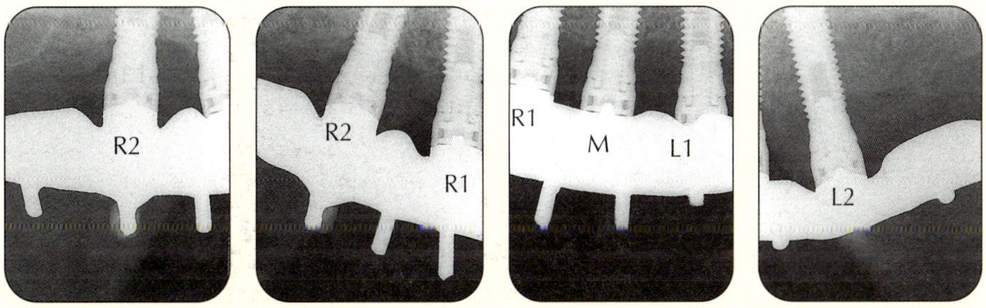

Fig 3-27 Connection of fixed prosthesis (1992).

Patient 4 (Routine Group) continued

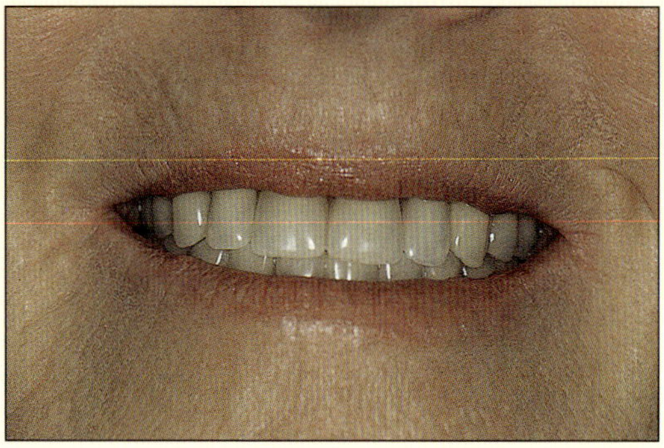

Fig 3-28 Clinical prosthetic appearance result (1992).

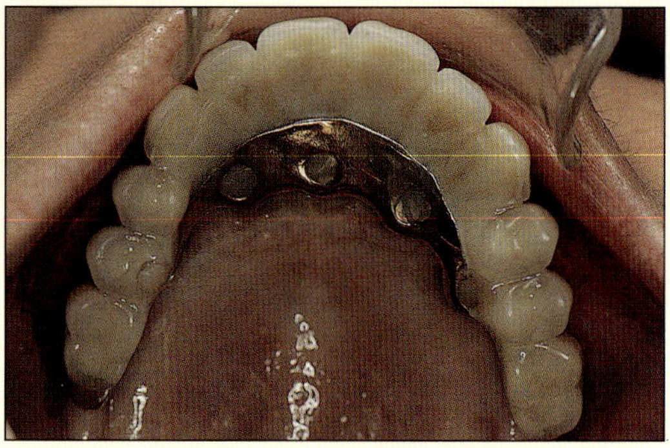

Fig 3-29 Intraoral clinical result (1992).

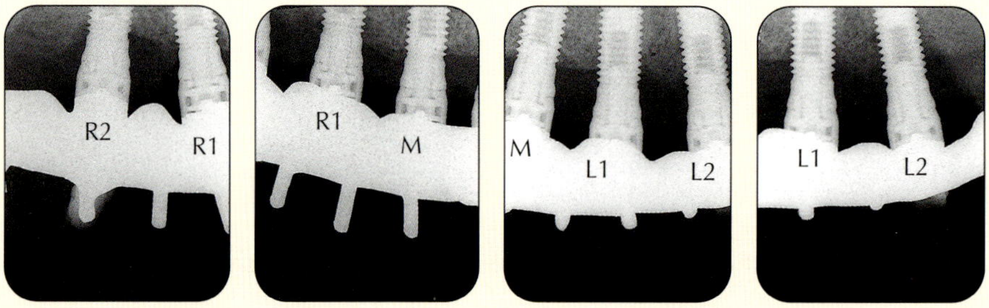

Fig 3-30 Fixed prosthesis at 7-year follow-up after conclusion of the study (1999).

Patient 5 (Routine Group)

Background

This female patient was born in 1939. She was edentulous in the mandible at the age of 23 (1962). The mandible was rehabilitated in 1980 with a fixed prosthesis with extensive cantilevers (Fig 3-31).

Preoperative comments

The bone height available for fixture anchorage was 6 mm. The patient exhibited a resorption pattern equivalent to type III and a sinus configuration equivalent to type C (see Figs 2-1 and 2-2).

Surgical procedure

Surgery was performed in May 1982, when the patient was 43 years old. The anatomy only allowed for placement of four 15-mm self-tapping conical fixtures to attach the graft taken from the left lateral ilium. The two distal fixtures had to be anchored in the canine region. Excellent primary stability was achieved for all four fixtures.

Postoperative comments

At the time of connection of the fixed prosthesis, the distance between the reference point and the marginal bone was 2.2 mm (Fig 3-35). A thin radiolucent zone was noted up to the first thread of some of the conical fixture heads.

Considering that the marginal portion of the grafted bone is the last to revascularize, it is hard to completely avoid bone loss in that region. In this case, the mean bone loss between connection of the fixed prosthesis and the 10-year follow-up visit was 1.4 mm (Fig 3-36). The marginal bone level remained above the first thread throughout the study period. This was probably the result of fixture support provided from both basal and grafted bone, which in turn resulted in adequate remodeling stimulus of the graft.

That the maxillary fixed prosthesis (anchored on four fixtures and with 10-mm extensions bilaterally) could survive in occlusion with the bone-anchored mandibular fixed prosthesis demonstrates that four maxillary fixtures can suffice in compromised situations[28] (see also patient 7 [routine group] and patient 4 [unusual group]). During the study period, there was a notable increase of bone density at the border between the basal and grafted bone (Fig 3-37).

Today a patient under similar circumstances would be treated with a less invasive grafting procedure, two zygoma fixtures, and four standard fixtures.

Patient 5 (Routine Group)

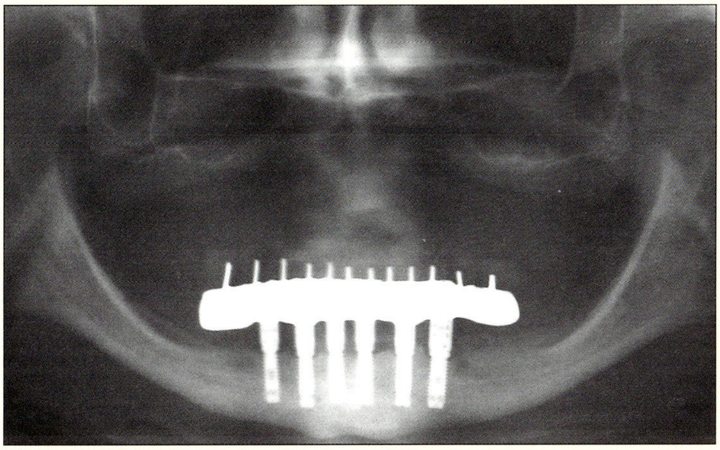

Fig 3-31 Preoperative panoramic view.

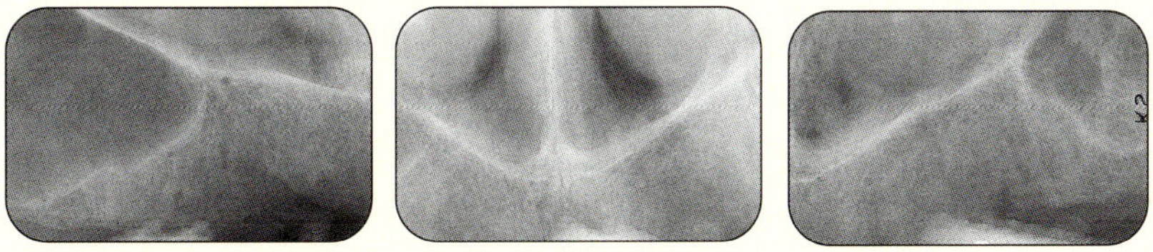

Fig 3-32 Preoperative intraoral radiographs.

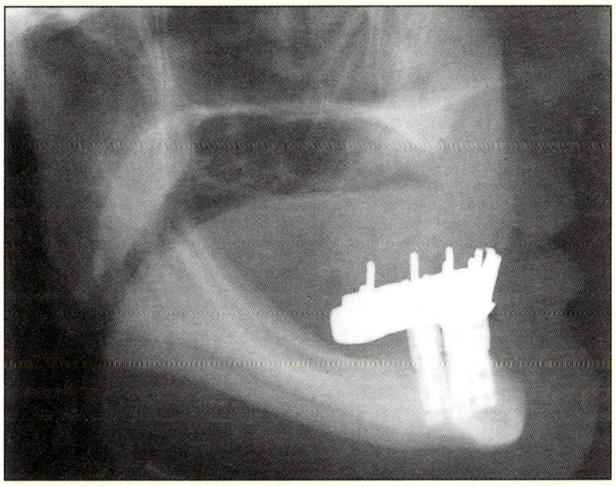

Fig 3-33 Preoperative profile.

Patient 5 (Routine Group) continued

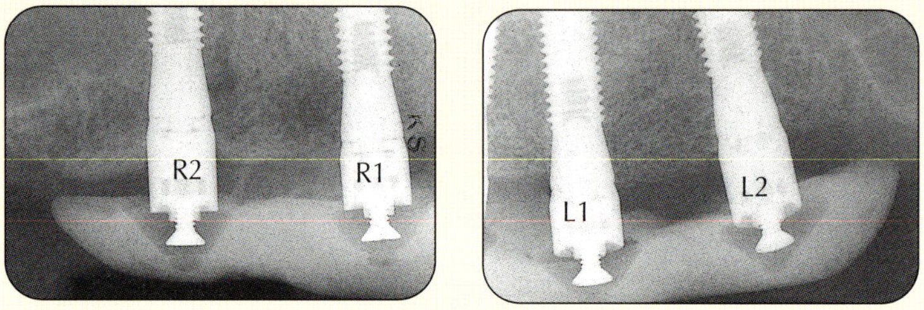

Fig 3-34 Abutment connection (1987).

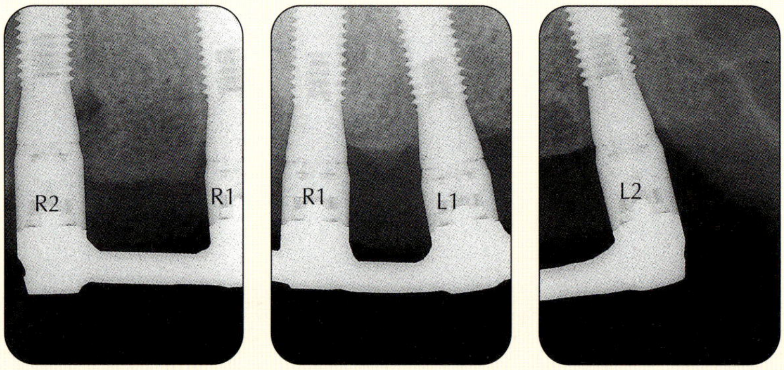

Fig 3-35 Connection of the provisional fixed prosthesis (1988).

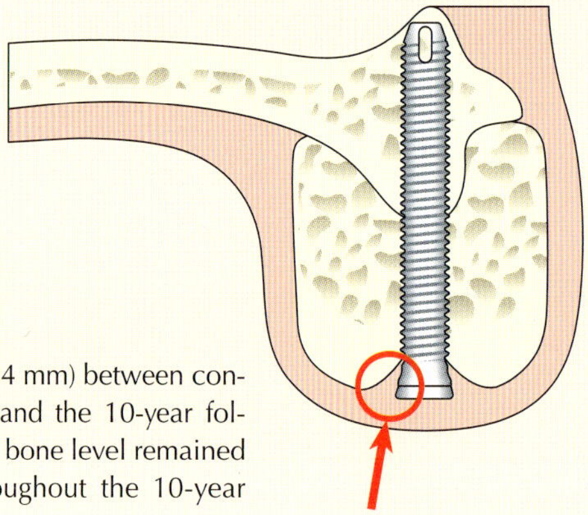

Fig 3-36 Mean bone loss (1.4 mm) between connection of fixed prosthesis and the 10-year follow-up (1997). The marginal bone level remained above the first thread throughout the 10-year period.

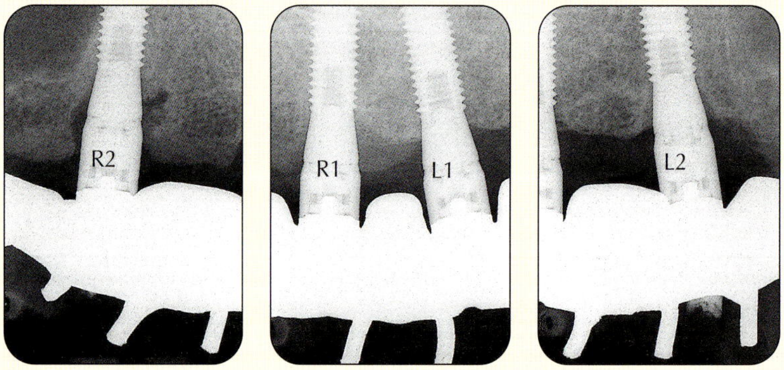

Fig 3-37 Fixed prosthesis at the 10-year follow-up (1997).

Patient 6 (Routine Group)

Background

This male patient was born in 1921 and had been edentulous in the maxilla since the age of 43 (1964). He received a bone-anchored prosthesis in the mandible in 1984. The patient was neither a bruxist nor a smoker.

Preoperative comments

The severe maxillary resorption (especially in the frontal region) was characteristic of a patient with a remaining partial dentition in the mandible. The anterior bone was about 2 to 3 mm wide and 2 mm in height. The patient exhibited a resorption pattern equivalent to type IV and a sinus configuration equivalent to type B (see Figs 2-1 and 2-2).

Surgical procedure

Surgery was conducted in June 1987, when the patient was 66 years old. The bone was of moderate strength and vascularity. The thin graft, taken from the left lateral ilium, was attached to the maxillary base with five self-tapping conical fixtures (10 and 13 mm). Good primary stability was achieved for all fixtures.

Postoperative comments

At the time of connection of the fixed prosthesis, the mean distance between the reference point and the marginal bone level was 1.1 mm. Between connection of the fixed prosthesis and the 5-year follow-up, the mean bone loss was 1.0 mm.

As seen in the radiographs from 1993 (Fig 3-44), the marginal bone level between the fixtures was highly distinct, indicating that the functional load placed upon the bone was sufficient to maintain its original density. The relatively short fixtures functioned well, in spite of the fact that they were placed in a very thin graft.

The patient died prior to the 1998 recall visit.

Patient 6 (Routine Group)

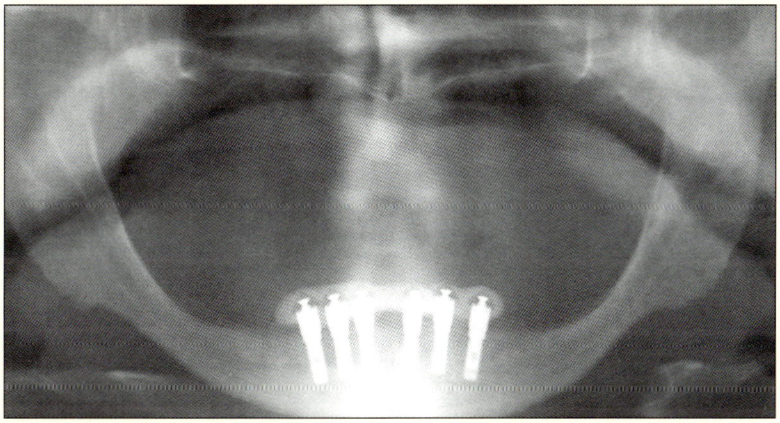

Fig 3-38 Preoperative panoramic view.

Patient 6 (Routine Group) continued

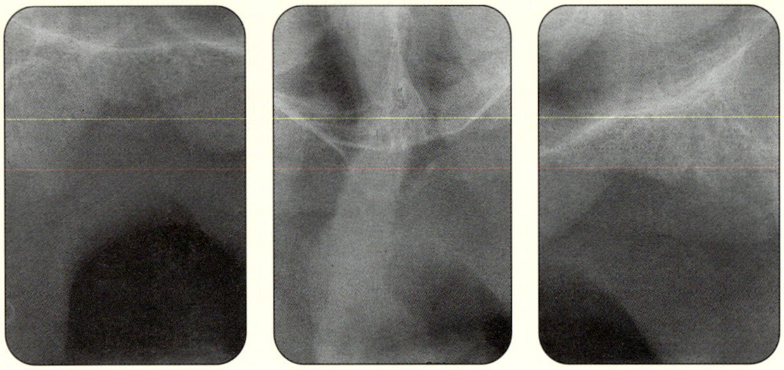

Fig 3-39 Preoperative intraoral radiographs.

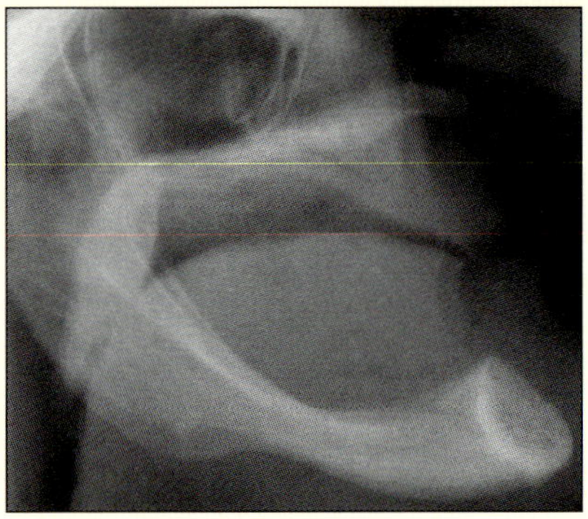

Fig 3-40 Preoperative profile.

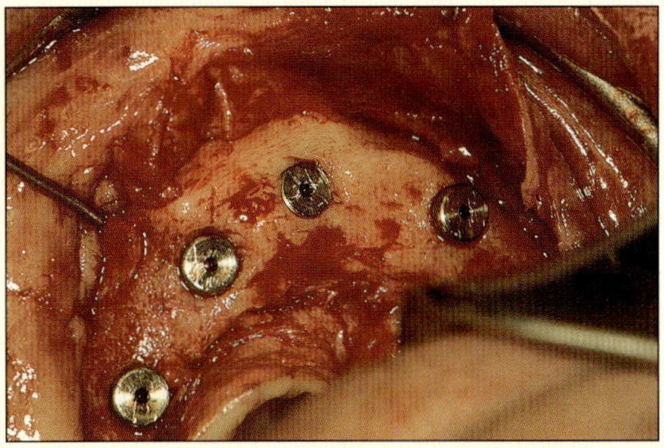

Fig 3-41 The very thin onlay graft attached with fixtures.

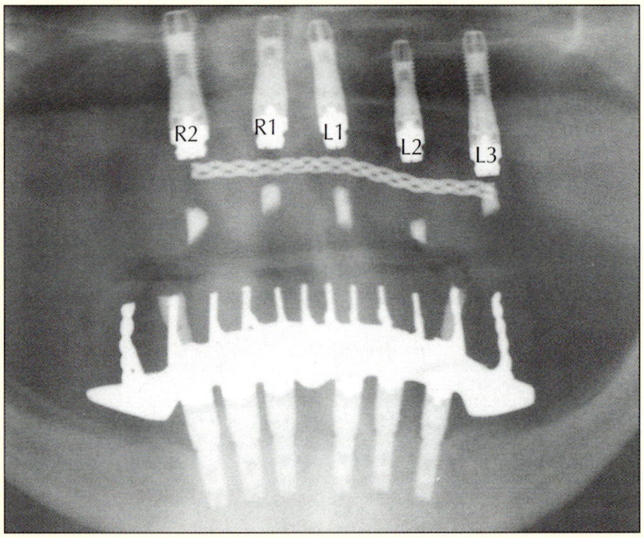

Fig 3-42 Connection of the provisional fixed prosthesis (1988).

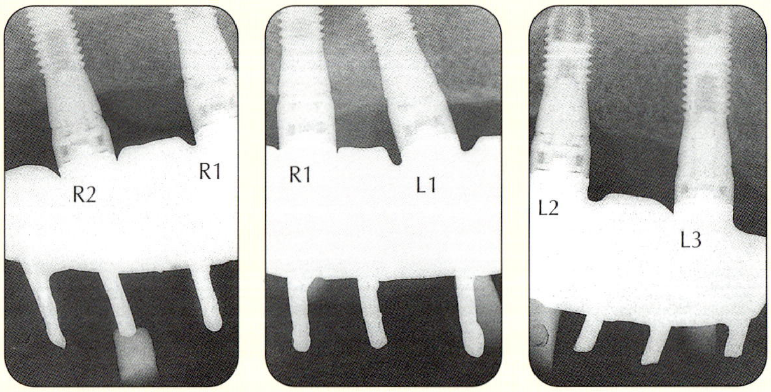

Fig 3-43 Connection of the fixed prosthesis (1988).

Patient 6 (Routine Group) continued

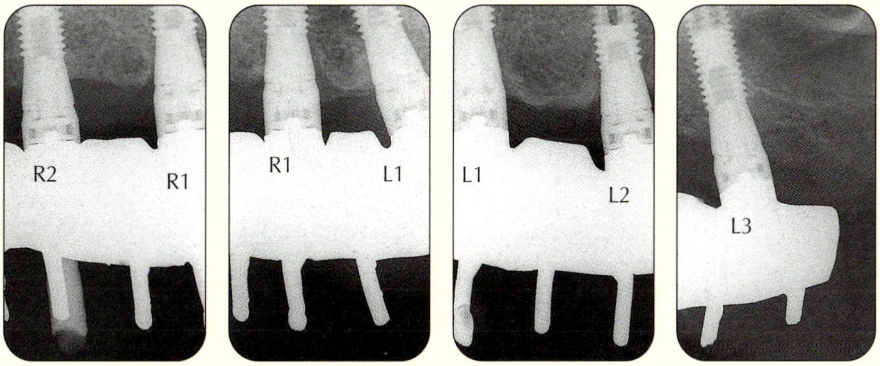

Fig 3-44 Fixed prosthesis at 5-year follow-up (1993).

Patient 7 (Routine Group)

Background

This female patient, born in 1925, had been edentulous in the maxilla since the age of 35 (1960). She had a dysfunctional, removable partial prosthesis in the mandible. The periodontal status of the remaining teeth was acceptable. Therefore a fixed prosthesis was carefully designed and mandibular fixture surgery was avoided.

Preoperative comments

The radiographic bone height was 5 to 6 mm, but the crest was thin and more pronounced resorption could be seen in the frontal region, which is common when a small anterior partial mandibular dentition remains. The patient had a wide incisive canal. The bony septum between the maxillary sinus and the nasal cavity was bilaterally judged capable of supporting the most distal fixture. The patient exhibited a resorption pattern equivalent to type III and a sinus configuration equivalent to type A (see Figs 2-1 and 2-2).

Surgical procedure

Surgery was performed in October 1981, when the patient was 56 years old. The onlay graft taken from the left lateral ilium was attached with four standard fixtures (10 and 12 mm).

Postoperative comments

The mean marginal bone loss was 0.3 mm during the 10-year follow-up period. It had primarily affected the two fixtures on the left (Fig 3-49). As noted in the radiographs, the bone margin was very distinct between and around the fixtures, which was indicative of proper functional loading. The case demonstrates that four fixtures can be used for long-term support of a bone-anchored prosthetic device as long as the overall occlusion and loading conditions are considered in the initial treatment planning.[29]

Today a patient under similar circumstances would be treated with a smaller graft, two zygoma fixtures, and four standard fixtures.

Patient 7 (Routine Group)

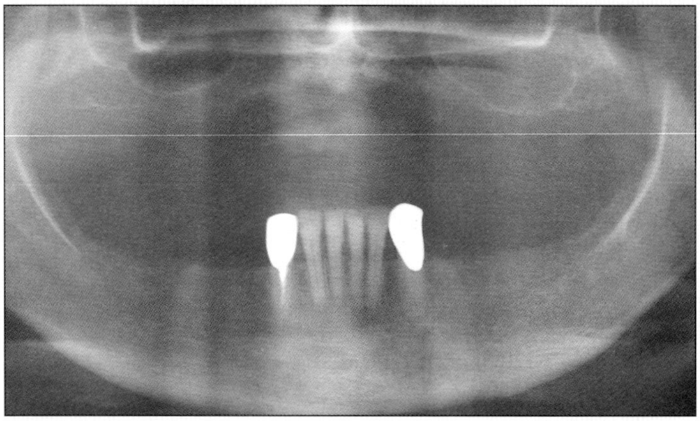

Fig 3-45 Preoperative panoramic view.

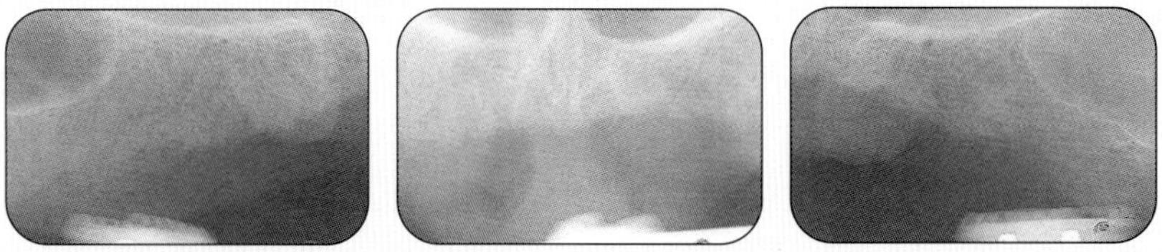

Fig 3-46 Preoperative intraoral radiographs.

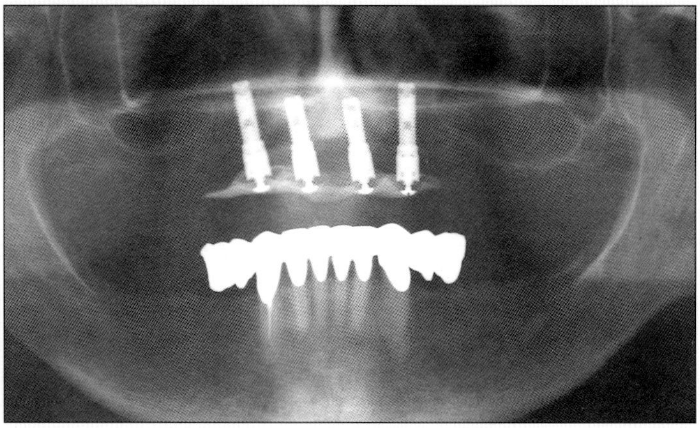

Fig 3-47 Abutment connection (1982).

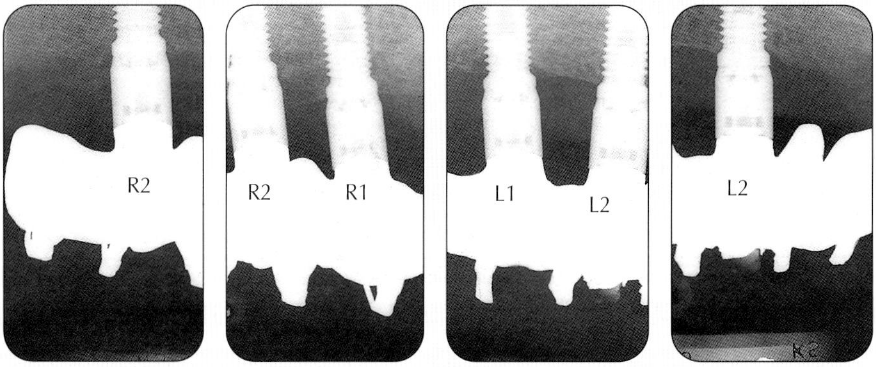

Fig 3-48 Connection of fixed prosthesis (1983).

Patient 7 (Routine Group) continued

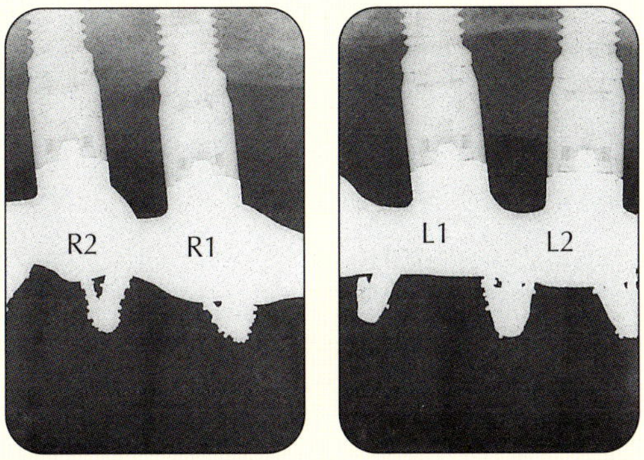

Fig 3-49 Fixed prosthesis at 10-year follow-up (1993).

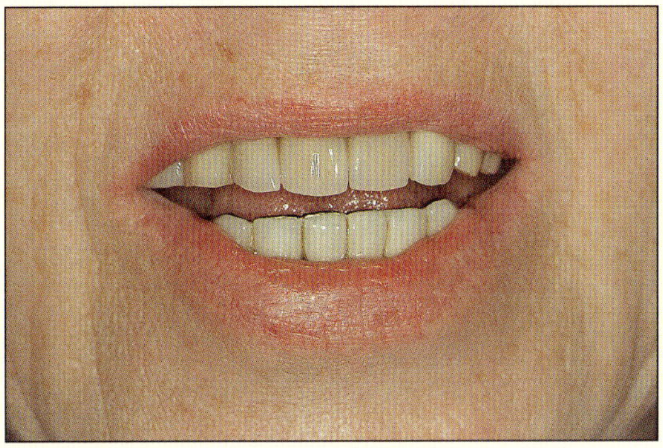

Fig 3-50 Clinical result (1993).

Patient 8 (Routine Group)

Background

This female patient, born in 1948, smoked 20 cigarettes per day prior to surgery. The partial mandibular dentition needed endodontic treatment (left second premolar) as well as fixture reinforcement (Fig 3-51).

Preoperative comments

The patient demonstrated moderate resorption and the alveolar crest varied in height between 10 and 15 mm. The left intraoral side was characterized by a number of rifts. The smoking most likely also had an adverse effect on the intraoral environment. The patient exhibited a resorption pattern equivalent to type III and a sinus configuration equivalent to type A (see Figs 2-1 and 2-2).

Surgical procedure

Surgery was performed in May 1989, when the patient was 41 years old. Onlay grafts and a nasal inlay graft were taken from the left medial ilium. No inlay was performed on the left side because of the rifts in that region and the consequent risk for accidental perforation of the nasal floor, which in turn could lead to fistula formation.

The maxillary grafts were attached with five self-tapping, swan-neck fixtures (10, 13, and 15 mm); the two distal fixtures penetrated the sinus. Two 10-mm standard fixtures were installed without nerve transposition in the distal right mandible.

Postoperative comments

At the 2-year follow-up, the mean marginal bone level was 2.7 mm below the reference point (Fig 3-54). The same figure after 6 years was 3.3 mm (Fig 3-55).

The L2 fixture was placed in limited basal bone. In 1996, the fixed prosthesis construction appeared to have been exposed to primary contact and L2 showed signs of lost osseointegration (Fig 3-55). In 1999 (after the conclusion of the study), the L2 fixture failed. R2 also showed increased bone loss. The altered occlusion and bending forces resulted in bone loss on the mandibular fixtures, where the marginal bone level was located at the sixth thread in 1999 (Fig 3-56).

The case demonstrates the essential need for proper occlusion and fit of the fixed prosthesis construction with careful consideration given to bending forces. If the problems persist, two zygoma fixtures will be installed. The existing fixed prosthesis would then act as a provisional prosthesis during healing. If zygoma fixtures had been installed from the beginning, the two distal fixtures would not have been required.

Patient 8 (Routine Group)

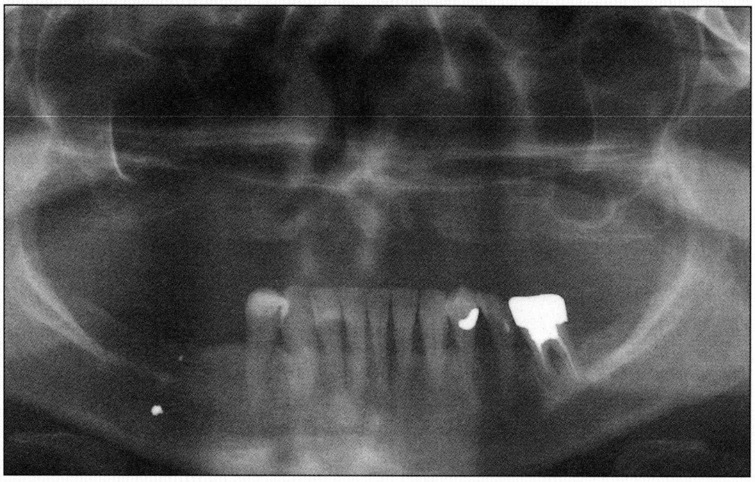

Fig 3-51 Preoperative panoramic view.

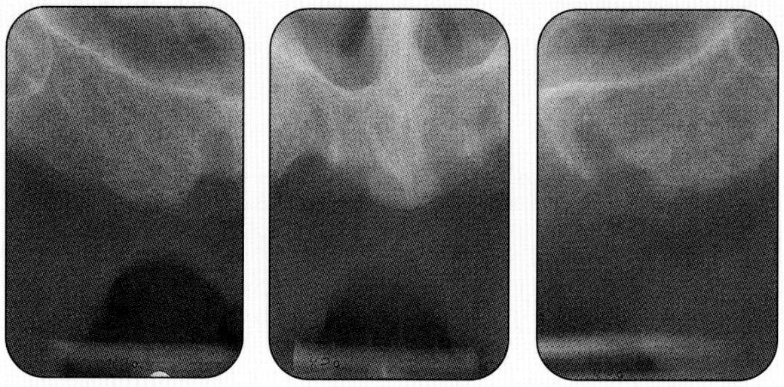

Fig 3-52 Preoperative intraoral radiographs.

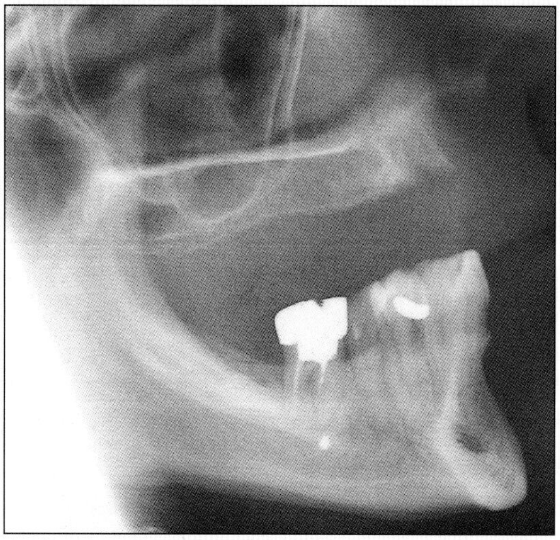

Fig 3-53 Preoperative profile.

Patient 8 (Routine Group) continued

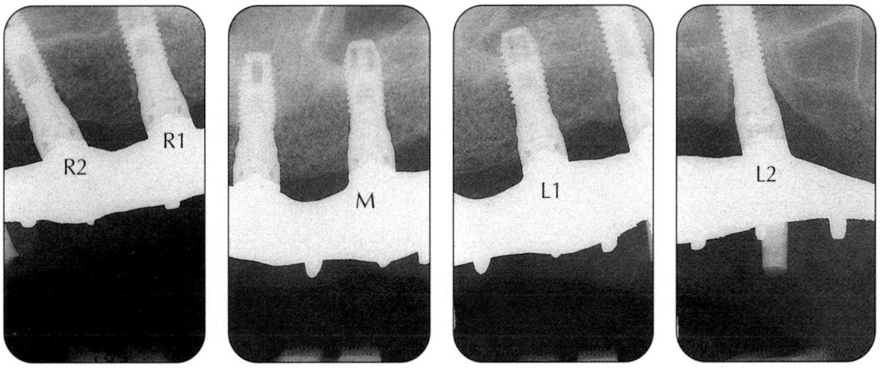

Fig 3-54 Two-year follow-up (1992).

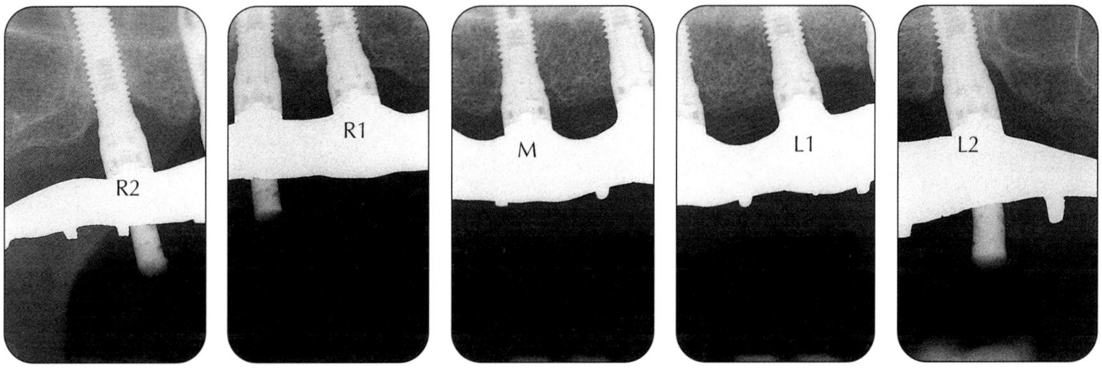

Fig 3-55 Six-year follow-up (1996).

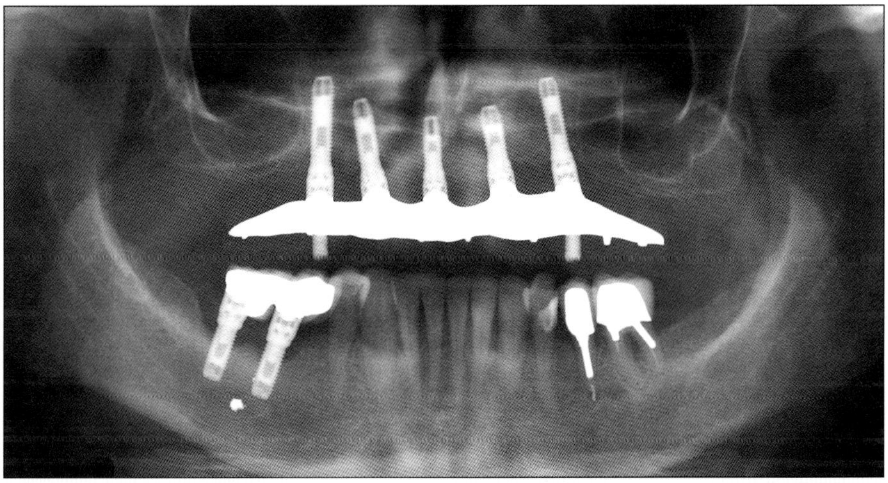

Fig 3-56 Eight-year follow-up after conclusion of the study (1999).

Patient 9 (Routine Group)

Background

This female patient was born in 1935 and had been edentulous in the maxilla since the age of 23 (1958). Her edentulism had caused her significant social and dietary problems. The dentition in the mandible required fixture reinforcement.

Preoperative comments

The alveolar crest varied in height from 2 to 7 mm. The available bone above the mandibular canal was 4 mm on the right and 8 mm on the left side, where the crest was also extremely thin (Fig 3-57). Therefore, a mandibular nerve transposition was indicated.[38] The patient exhibited a resorption pattern equivalent to type IV and a sinus configuration equivalent to type A (see Figs 2-1 and 2-2).

Surgical procedure

Surgery was performed in September 1989, when the patient was 54 years old. The onlay graft was taken from the left lateral ilium. The basal maxillary bone was of adequate strength and properly vascularized. Five self-tapping, swan-neck fixtures were installed in the maxilla (10, 13, and 15 mm). The 13-mm fixture was 4 mm in diameter and placed in the midline. Four self-tapping fixtures (13 and 15 mm) were installed in the mandible after bilateral nerve transposition.[38] The mandibular fixtures were designed with a smooth, unthreaded portion to minimize abrasive contact when placed adjacent to the nerve (Fig 3-59).

Postoperative comments

The distance between the marginal bone level and the reference point was 3.8 mm after 3 years. At the 9-year radiographic evaluation in 1999 (after the conclusion of the study), bone loss was primarily noted adjacent to the R1 and L1 fixtures, where the distance from the marginal bone to the reference point was 3.4 mm for R1 and 4.8 mm for L1. Minor bone loss was noted for the other fixtures. At the last examination, the distance from the marginal bone to the reference point was 3.4 mm for R2, 2.8 mm for M, and 3.4 mm for L2 (Fig 3-64).

Patient 9 (Routine Group)

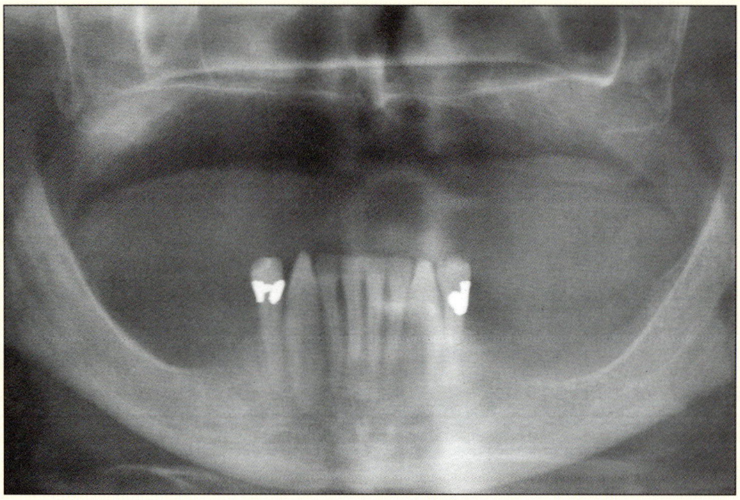

Fig 3-57 Preoperative panoramic view.

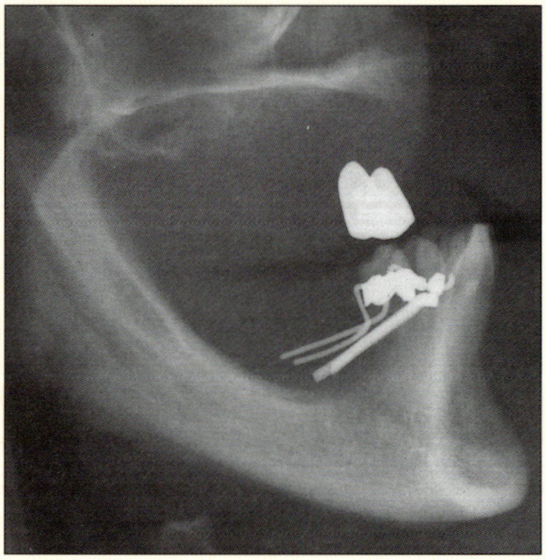

Fig 3-58 Preoperative profile.

Patient 9 (Routine Group) continued

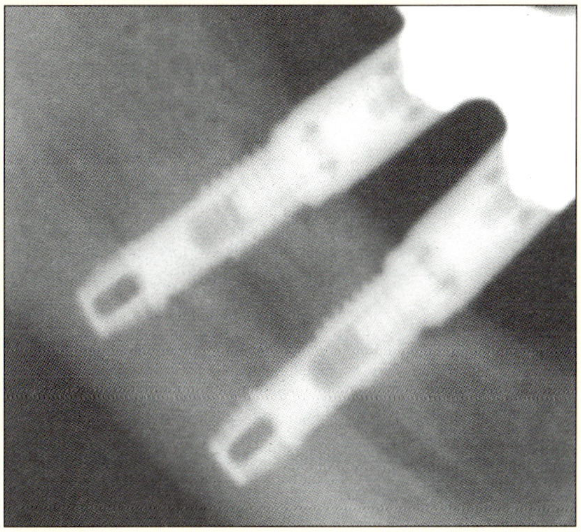

Fig 3-59 Special mandibular fixtures developed for use in nerve transposition procedures.

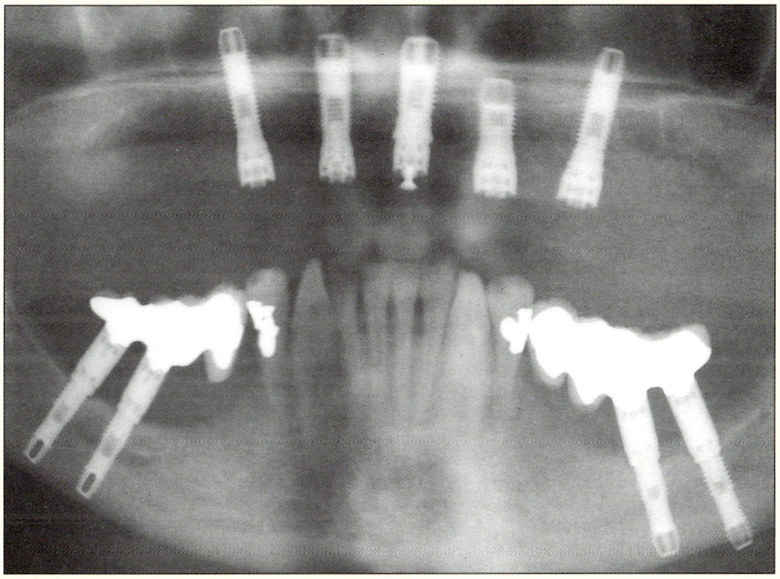

Fig 3-60 Abutment connection (1989).

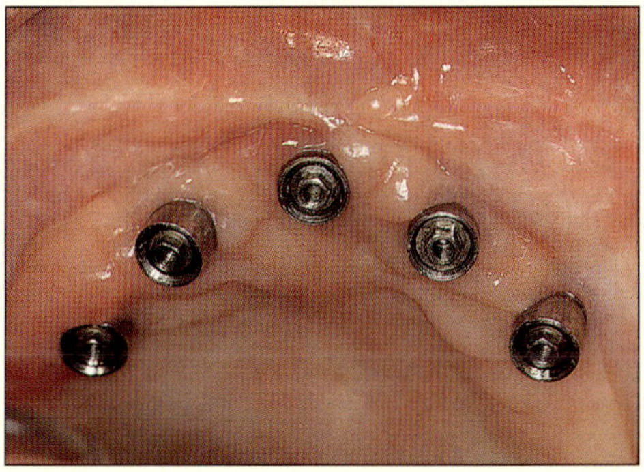

Fig 3-61 Abutment connection (1989).

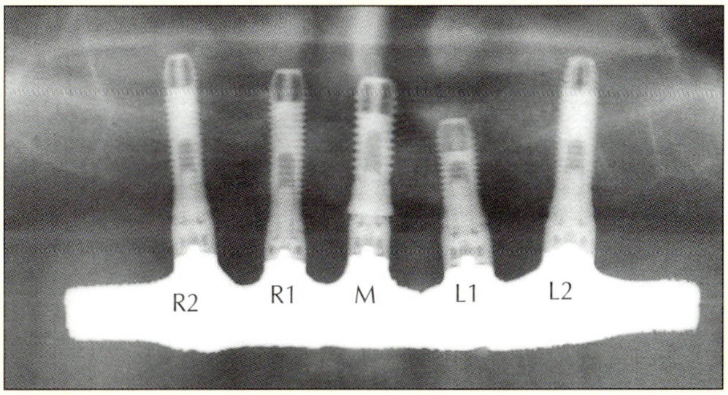

Fig 3-62 Connection of the fixed prosthesis (1990).

Patient 9 (Routine Group) continued

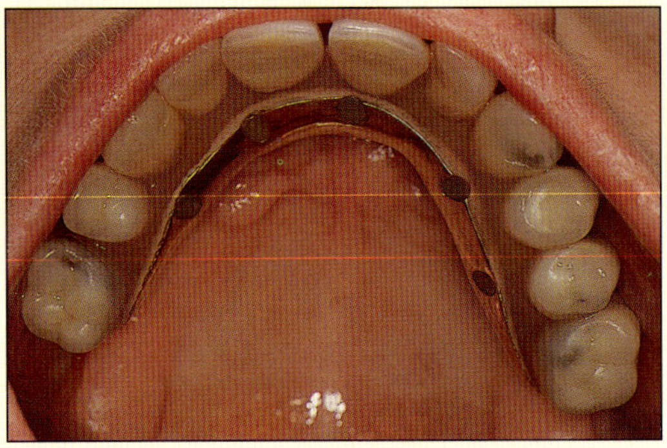

Fig 3-63 Connection of the fixed prosthesis (1990).

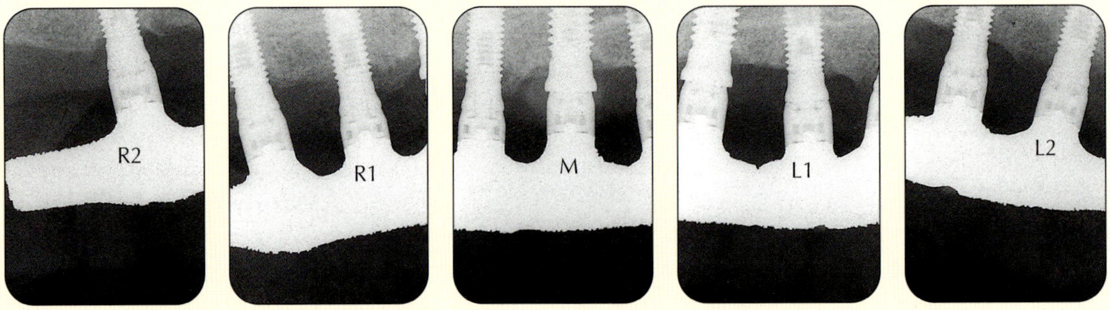

Fig 3-64 Fixed prosthesis at the 9-year follow-up after conclusion of the study (1999).

Patient 10 (Routine Group)

Background

This female patient was born in 1921 and had been edentulous in the maxilla since the age of 60 (1981). She received a mandibular fixed prosthesis in 1981 (Fig 3-66).

Preoperative comments

The alveolar height varied from 6 to 8 mm. A wide incisive canal was noted. The mandibular fixture-supported fixed prosthesis had extensive cantilevers. The patient exhibited a resorption pattern equivalent to type III and a sinus configuration equivalent to type B (see Figs 2-1 and 2-2).

Surgical procedure

Surgery was performed in January 1986, when the patient was 65 years old. The onlay graft was taken from the left lateral ilium. Five self-tapping, conical 13-mm fixtures were installed. One fixture was placed in the midline after the incisive canal had been cleaned out and filled with particulated bone and marrow. Good primary stability was achieved for the fixtures and the graft.

Postoperative comments

At connection of the fixed prosthesis, the mean marginal bone level was located 0.3 mm below the reference point. The patient had headaches after connection of the fixed prosthesis. These were reversed after a malocclusion was resolved.

At the 10-year follow-up in 1996, the mean marginal bone loss was 3.2 mm. A thin radiolucency was noted around the conical portion of some fixtures (eg, R1). This finding is in contrast to other cases where the marginal bone level remained unaltered adjacent to the conical portion of the fixture head. The grafted bone retained its degree of mineralization and highly distinct marginal bone could be seen between the fixtures at the 10-year follow-up visit (Fig 3-69).

Patient 10 (Routine Group)

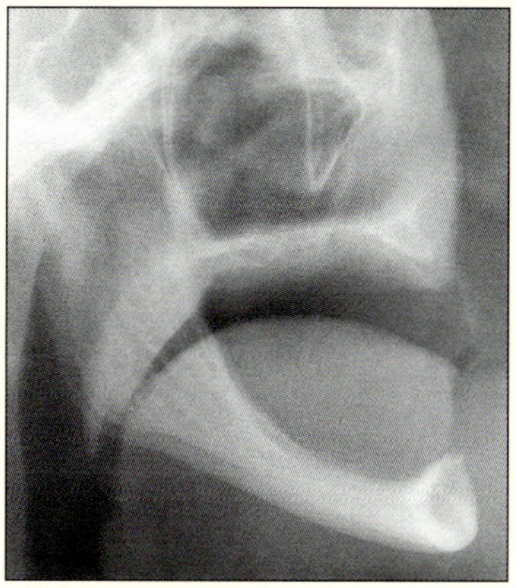

Fig 3-65 Profile prior to mandibular rehabilitation (1981).

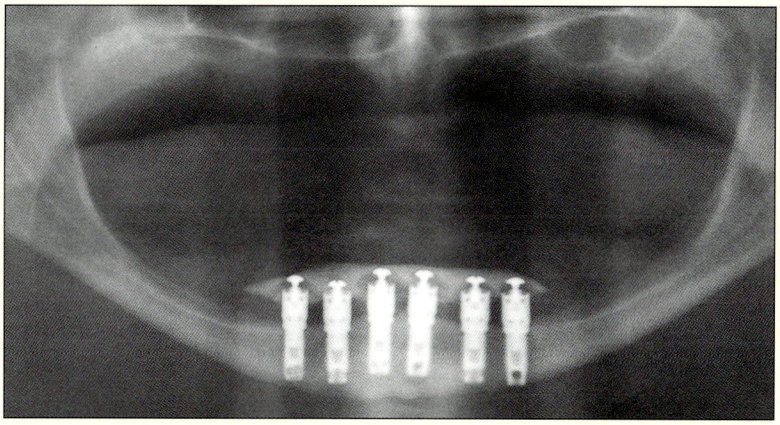

Fig 3-66 Panoramic view after mandibular abutment connection.

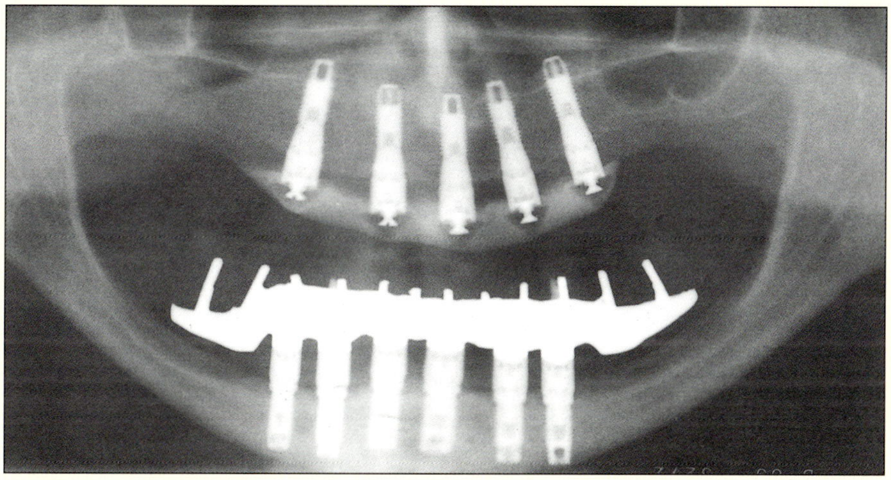

Fig 3-67 Abutment connection (1986).

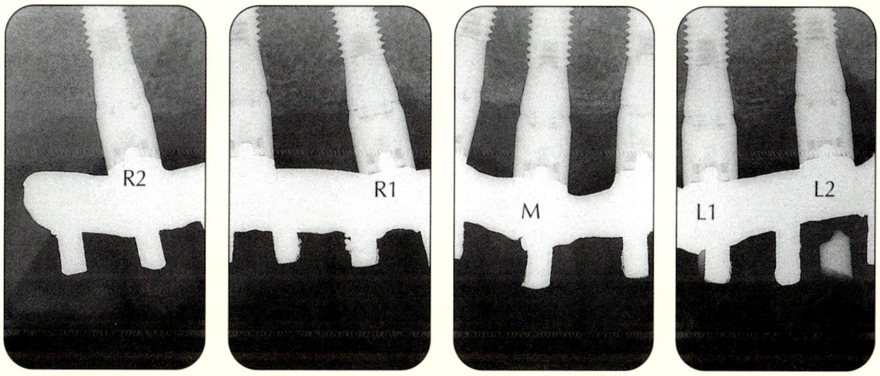

Fig 3-68 Connection of the fixed prosthesis (1986).

Patient 10 (Routine Group) continued

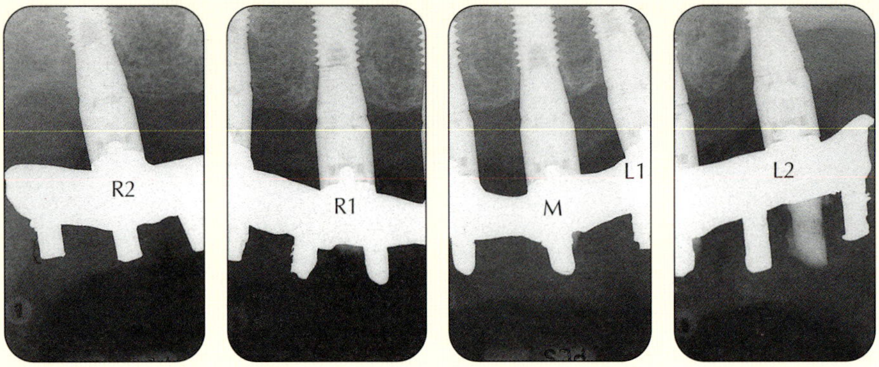

Fig 3-69 Fixed prosthesis at the 10-year follow-up (1996).

Patient 11 (Routine Group)

Background

This female patient was born in 1925. The maxilla had been severely resorbed for many years, whereas the mandible had been rehabilitated with a bone-anchored prosthesis in 1978. The mandibular fixed prosthesis had an extensive cantilever on the right side.

Preoperative comments

The height of the alveolar crest varied from 10 to 12 mm, but it was so thin that only 5 mm was available for fixture anchorage (Figs 3-70 and 3-71). The patient exhibited a resorption pattern equivalent to type V and a sinus configuration equivalent to type C (see Figs 2-1 and 2-2).

Surgical procedure

Surgery was performed in August 1983, when the patient was 58 years old. The onlay graft was taken from the left lateral ilium and attached with six self-tapping fixtures (13 and 15 mm). The L3 fixture perforated the sinus. Good stability was obtained.

Postoperative comments

At abutment connection in March 1984, instability of R3 and L3 was noted, although by percussion they appeared adequate. The residual maxillary bone in this region was only 5 mm in height. To avoid bending forces, it was decided to install a provisional fixed prosthesis until complete bone remodeling had occurred.

Note that if a so-called torque test[38] had been applied to these fixtures, it would have caused them to fail, whereas they now remained stable in the axial direction. After 6 months, all fixtures in question were well osseointegrated and a permanent fixed prosthesis construction was delivered.

The mean distance between the marginal bone level and the reference point was 1.1 mm at the time of connection of the fixed prosthesis, compared to 1.2 mm after 10 years. During the 15-year follow-up, the grafted bone demonstrated a distinct increase in density, particularly in the R3 and R1 regions (Fig 3-76). The increased mineralization was likely the response to adequate functional loading. After 15 years in function, the bone remained in close apposition to the smooth collars of the fixture heads (eg, in the R3 position).

Patient 11 (Routine Group)

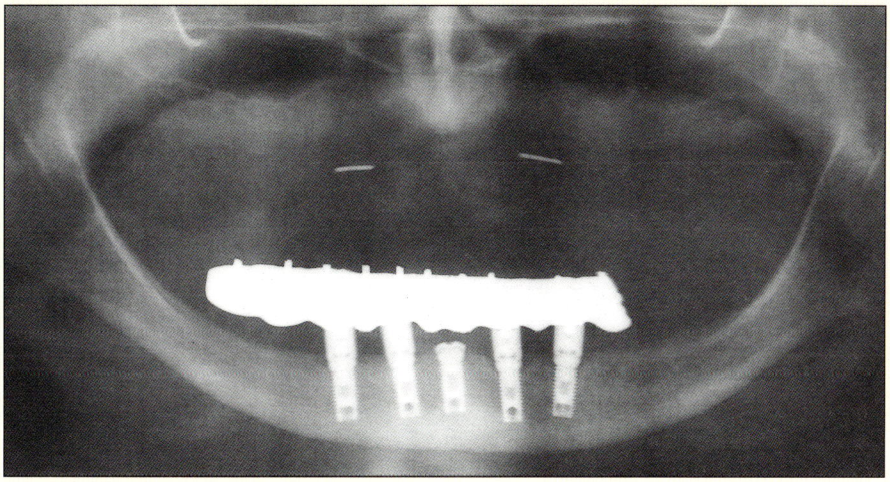

Fig 3-70 Preoperative panoramic view.

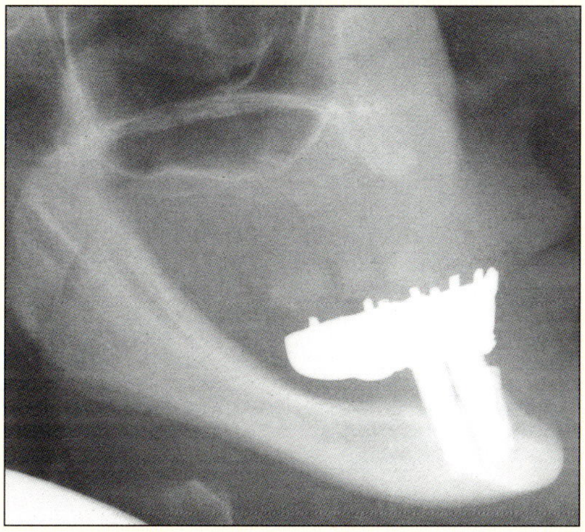

Fig 3-71 Preoperative profile.

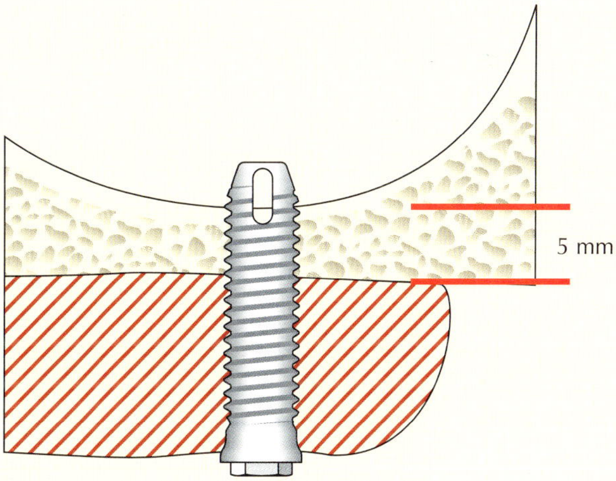

Fig 3-72 Fixture supported by grafted bone and only 5 mm basal bone.

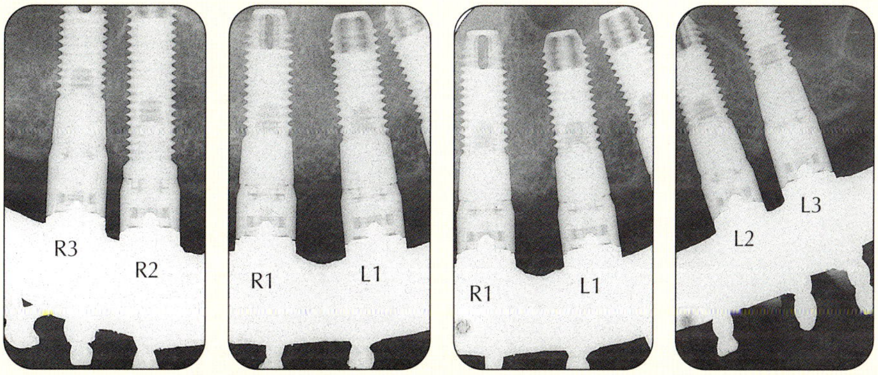

Fig 3-73 Connection of the fixed prosthesis (1984).

Patient 11 (Routine Group) continued

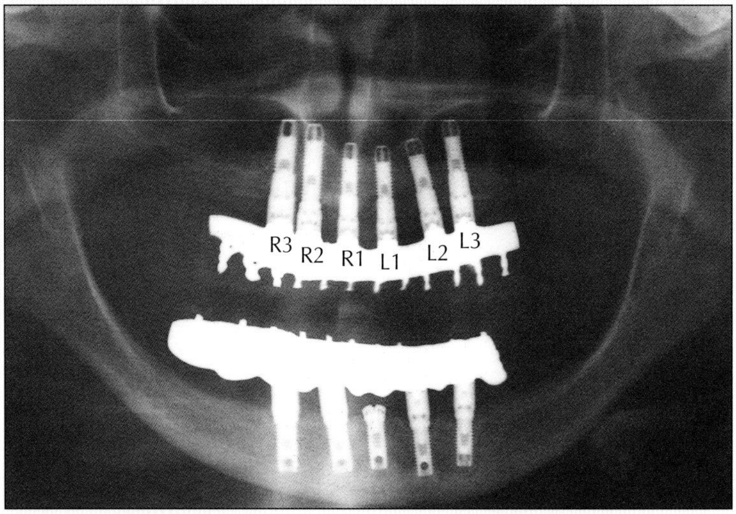

Fig 3-74 Connection of the fixed prosthesis in the maxilla (1984).

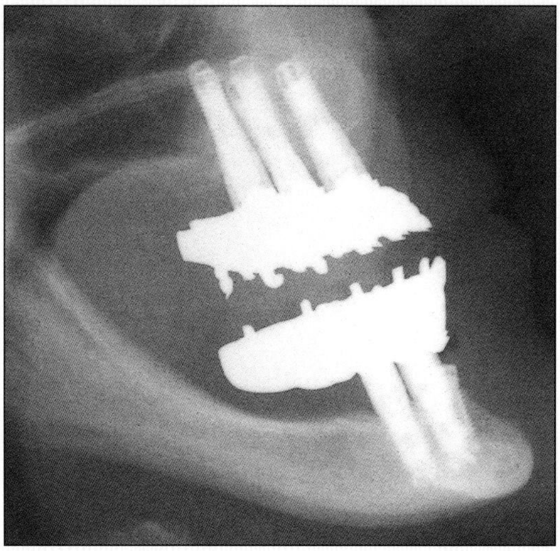

Fig 3-75 Profile at connection of the fixed prosthesis (1984).

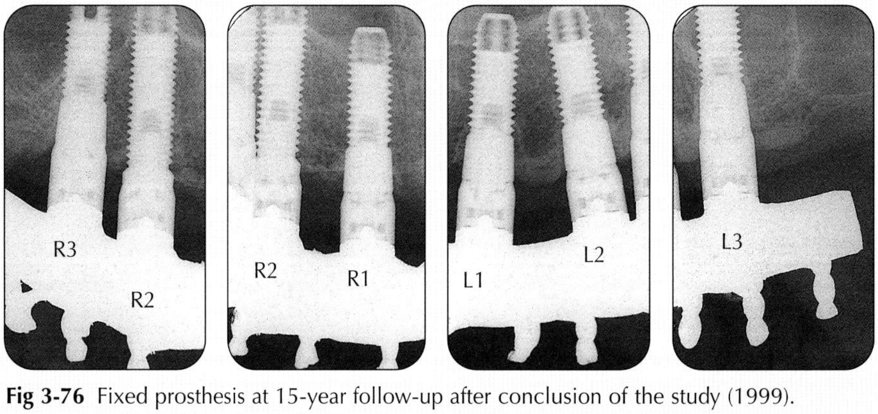

Fig 3-76 Fixed prosthesis at 15-year follow-up after conclusion of the study (1999).

Patient 12 (Routine Group)

Background

This female patient was born in 1931. She had been edentulous in the maxilla since the age of 51 (1982). The dentition in the mandible remained functional, although adequate support was missing in the left posterior mandible.

Preoperative comments

The alveolar bone height was 13 mm, but the crest was extremely thin because of advanced buccolabial resorption. Only 5 mm of bone was available for fixture anchorage. Limited expansion of the sinus was seen bilaterally. A defect caused by previous removal of a radicular cyst was present in the left canine area. The patient exhibited a resorption pattern equivalent to type V and a sinus configuration equivalent to type A (see Figs 2-1 and 2-2).

Surgical procedure

Surgery was performed in January 1986, when the patient was 55 years old. The bone was of good strength and adequately vascularized. The onlay graft was taken from the left lateral ilium and stabilized with six self-tapping conical fixtures (13 and 15 mm). Good primary stability was achieved for all fixtures.

Postoperative comments

The R1 fixture was lost during the initial healing period. It was not replaced because adequate stability of the fixed prosthesis could be obtained on the five remaining fixtures. The mean bone loss was 2 mm during the 10-year follow-up. Four of the five fixtures demonstrated marginal bone levels at the first thread. Distinct crestal margins were noted at the last follow-up visit. An increased density was also seen, particularly in the R3 and L2 regions (Figs 3-82 and 3-83). The marginal bone level adjacent to the L3 fixture was equivalent to baseline; that is, it was located at the conical portion of the fixture head (Figs 3-84 and 3-85).

Today a patient under similar circumstances would also receive two fixtures in the left posterior mandible to optimize occlusion and minimize bending moments.

Patient 12 (Routine Group)

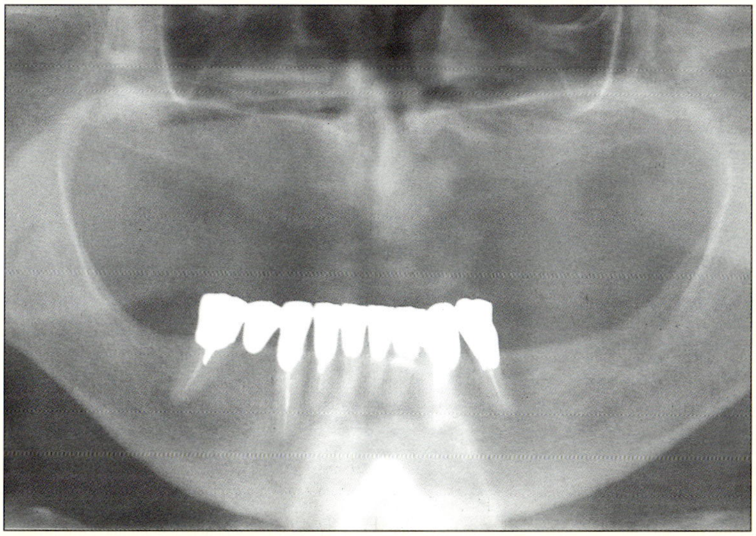

Fig 3-77 Preoperative panoramic view.

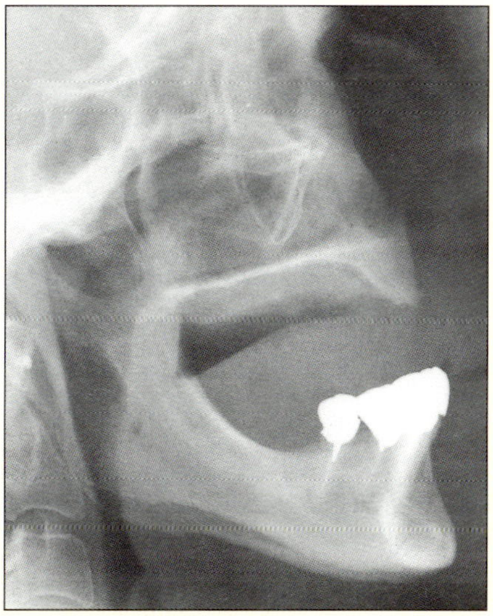

Fig 3-78 Preoperative profile.

Patient 12 (Routine Group) continued

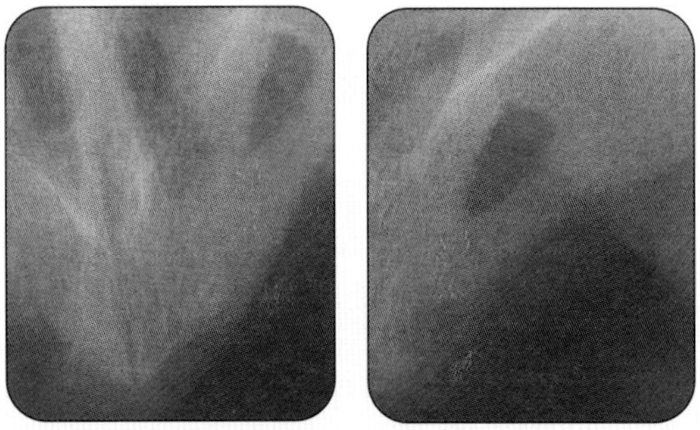

Fig 3-79 Preoperative intraoral radiographs.

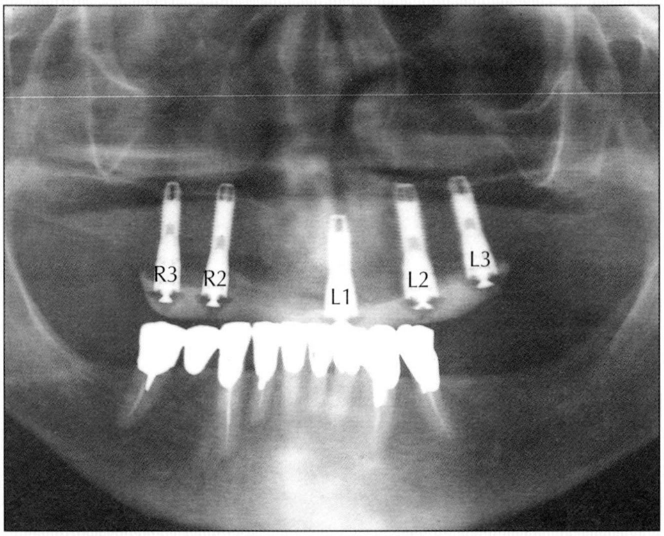

Fig 3-80 Abutment connection (1986). The R1 fixture had failed.

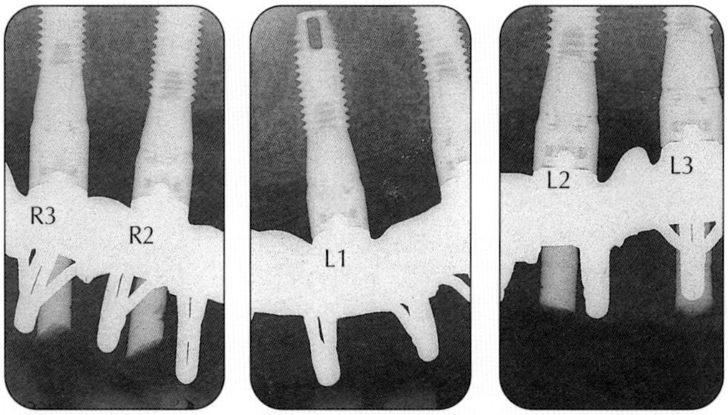

Fig 3-81 Connection of the fixed prosthesis (1986).

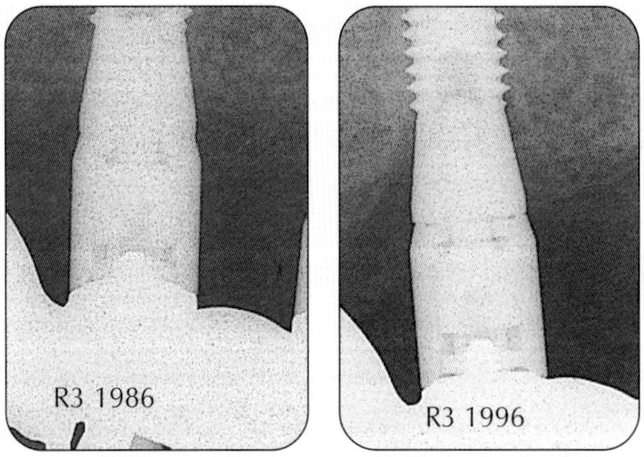

Fig 3-82 R3 1986 vs 1996.

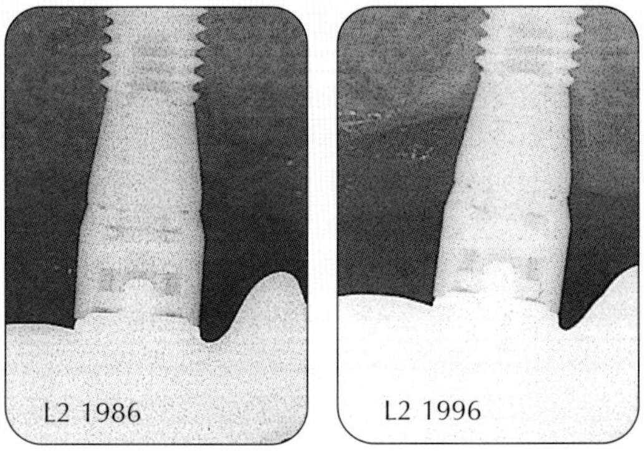

Fig 3-83 L2 1986 vs 1996.

Patient 12 (Routine Group) continued

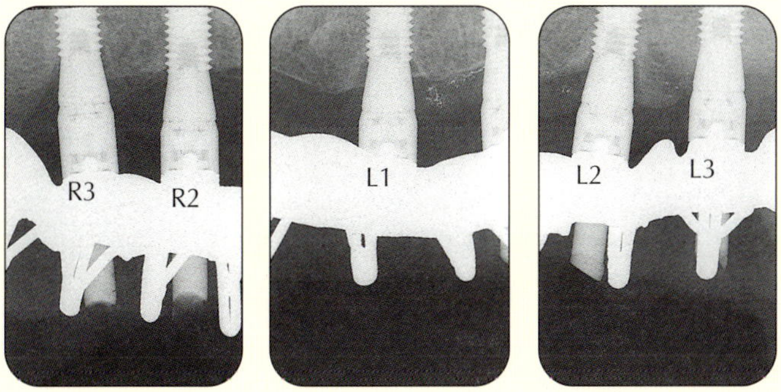

Fig 3-84 Ten-year follow-up (1996).

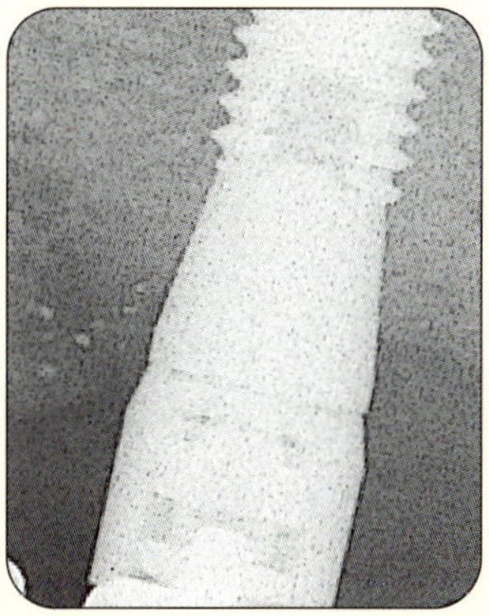

Fig 3-85 Enlargement of L3 from Fig 3-84.

Patient 13 (Routine Group)

Background

This female patient was born in 1942. In 1979, at the age of 37, she was rehabilitated with a mandibular bone-anchored prosthesis with extensive cantilevers. She requested a fixed solution in the maxilla.

Preoperative comments

The alveolar bone height was 16 mm, but the crest was paper thin. Only 6 mm was available for fixture anchorage when measured at the midline. Limited expansion of the sinus was seen bilaterally. The patient exhibited a resorption pattern equivalent to type V and a sinus configuration equivalent to type A (see Figs 2-1 and 2-2).

Surgical procedure

Surgery was performed in May 1985, when the patient was 43 years old. The crest was almost transparent and the basal bone was compact with acceptable vascularity. The thin marginal bone was used to stabilize the onlay graft taken from the left lateral ilium (see Fig 2-3).

The graft was secured with six self-tapping standard fixtures (13 and 15 mm). The R3 and L3 fixtures penetrated the sinus. R3 was stable. The L3 fixture was primarily supported by the bony septum, which made the fixture less stable than the other fixtures.

Postoperative comments

At connection of the fixed prosthesis, the mean marginal bone level was 0.1 mm from the reference point (Fig 3-89). After 9 years, the corresponding value was 2.9 mm. The bone loss (mean 2.4 mm) primarily occurred during the first year after connection of the fixed prosthesis. The most pronounced bone loss was seen adjacent to R2, where the marginal bone level was apical to the abutment screw. The resorption most likely originated from insufficient dynamic loading or overload of the grafted bone in this region.

The thick cortical zone around R3 and R2 diminished over time. The L3 fixture that penetrated the sinus remained stable throughout the study period (Fig 3-91).The bone loss around the mandibular fixtures–particularly those in the midline–may have resulted from bending forces initiated by the extensive fixed prosthesis cantilevers.

Patient 13 (Routine Group)

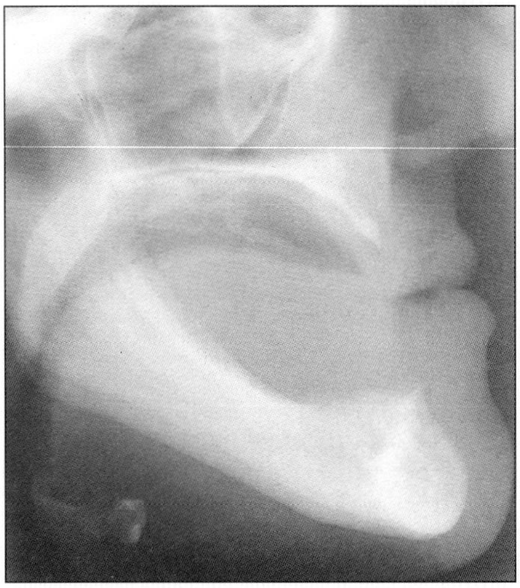

Fig 3-86 Profile before mandibular fixture treatment.

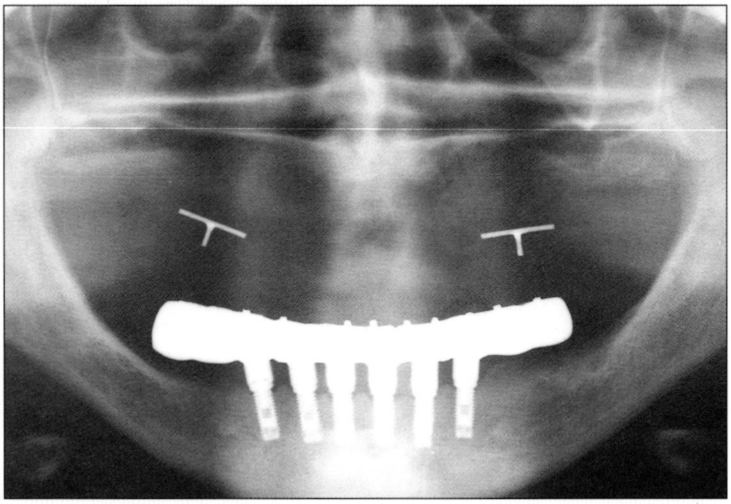

Fig 3-87 Preoperative panoramic view (1985). The mandibular rehabilitation took place in 1979.

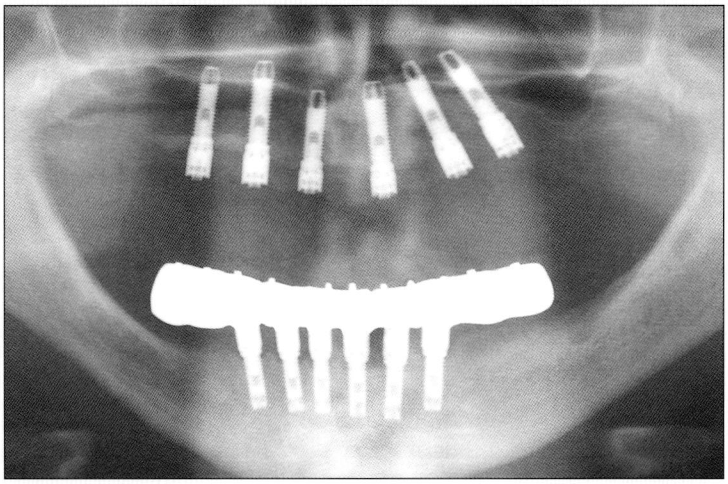

Fig 3-88 Abutment connection (1986).

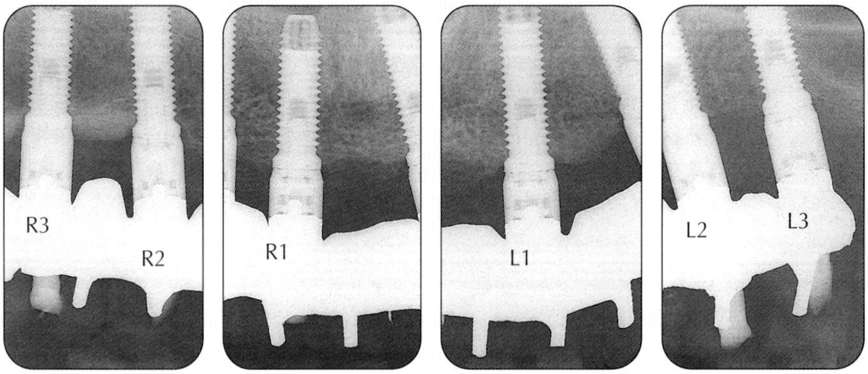

Fig 3-89 Connection of the fixed prosthesis (1986).

Patient 13 (Routine Group) continued

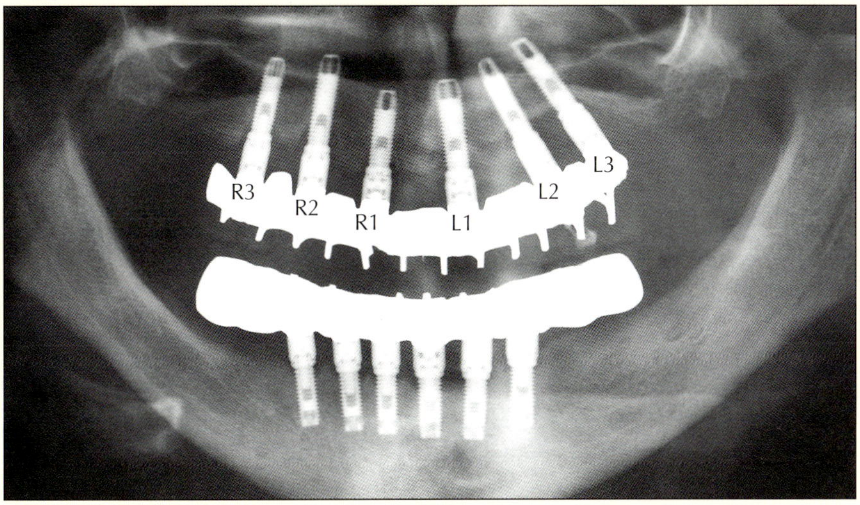

Fig 3-90 Fixed prosthesis at the 5-year follow-up (1991).

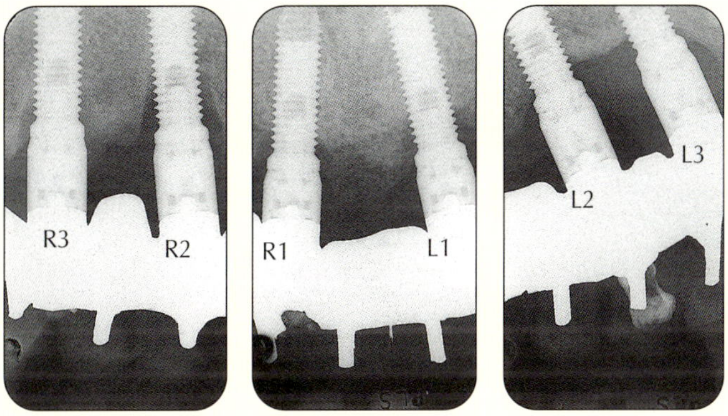

Fig 3-91 Nine-year follow-up (1995).

CHAPTER 4

Compromised Case Presentations

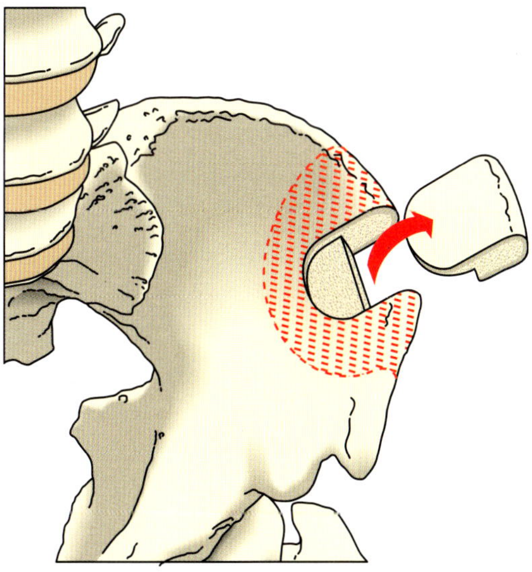

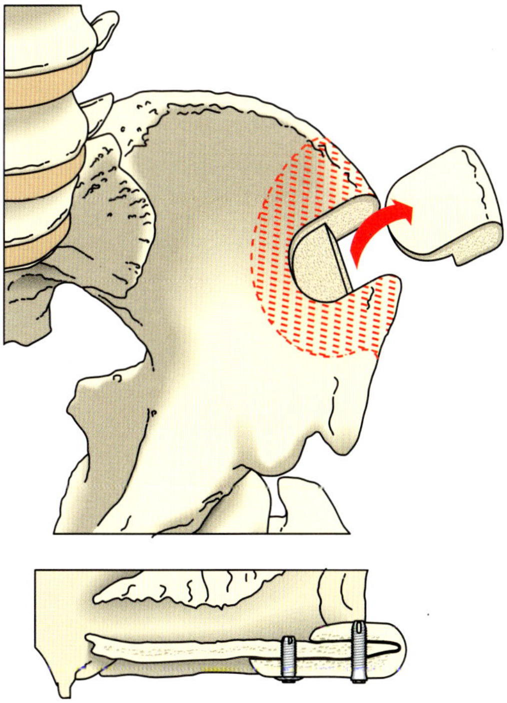

These patient presentations describe some of the more difficult challenges that were faced during the onlay grafting study. The severe complications originated from causes such as existing communication between the nasal and oral cavity, unfavorable occlusion, or poor graft quality.

Patient 1 (Compromised Group)

Background

This male patient, born in 1939, was a smoker. He had lost all his maxillary teeth because of periodontal disease in 1959, at the age of 20. He had suffered extensively from his oral handicap.

Preoperative comments

Prior to the current grafting procedure, the patient had a bone-anchored fixed prosthesis for 13 years in the maxilla and a removable partial denture in the mandible. When the fixed prosthesis failed in 1985, the patient wore a conventional denture until a grafting procedure could be carried out in 1989. The patient exhibited a resorption pattern equivalent to type IV and a sinus configuration equivalent to type A (see Figs 2-1 and 2-2).

Surgical procedure

In October 1989, an onlay graft was taken from the left medial ilium and attached to the maxillary bone with six self-tapping fixtures, 13, 15, 18, and 20 mm in length. Good primary stability was obtained for all fixtures.

Complications

The patient had contacted his hometown dentist when a dehiscence occurred. The dentist failed to resuture, and 2 months after the grafting procedure, the patient returned to us with fistulae.

During a surgical intervention in December 1989, a mobile fixture (L2) and large amounts of granulation tissue and bone sequestrae were removed. Two weeks later, all the remaining fixtures had to be removed for the same reason.

Additional surgery

In January 1991, onlay and inlay blocks were taken from the right lateral ilium and anchored to the maxilla with five self-tapping and two 50-mm zygoma fixtures. Postoperative infection occurred again, manifested by suppuration from fistulae emerging from the treated region. Several unsuccessful attempts were made to isolate specific bacteria. The microbiological tests showed growth of bacteria sensitive to clindamycin. The wound was reopened and cleaned out with saline solution and 3% hydroperoxide. The patient was then placed on an intensive antibiotic regimen. After 6 weeks, the infection had subsided and the oral mucosa was healed and intact. The complications clarify the essential need for careful observation and maintained closure of the wound at the grafted donor site.

In January 1991, the bone graft was exposed bilaterally in the canine regions and the anterior part of the graft was found to be nonvital and mobile. The affected portion of the graft sequestrae and some granulation tissue were removed.

Nonintegrated fixtures in regions L1 and R1 were replaced by two new fixtures (10 and 13 mm). The remaining fixtures were clinically well integrated without adjacent marginal bone resorption. During surgery, an existent communication between the oral and nasal cavities was noted as the likely cause of the infection. The defect was closed with soft tissue release and thorough suturing.

At abutment connection in May 1991, all seven fixtures demonstrated excellent stability and were clinically well osseointegrated. The remaining graft was vital. The bone-anchored prosthesis was delivered to the patient in June 1991.

In November 1991, the R2 fixture was mobile and therefore replaced with a wide diameter fixture.

Follow-up

At the 8-year follow-up visit in 1999, the radiographic examination revealed a minor marginal bone reduction, but with a distinct bone level. The patient exhibited mucosal swelling of the left sinus, which was also present in sinus scanograms taken in 1991. Similar symptoms seen in the right sinus in 1991 had disappeared at the last follow-up visit.

At the last clinical evaluation, the functionality of the fixed prosthesis was excellent and the patient was pleased with the appearance of his fixed prosthesis. He spontaneously commented on the enhanced quality of life he had experienced over the past 8 years.

Patient 1 (Compromised Group)

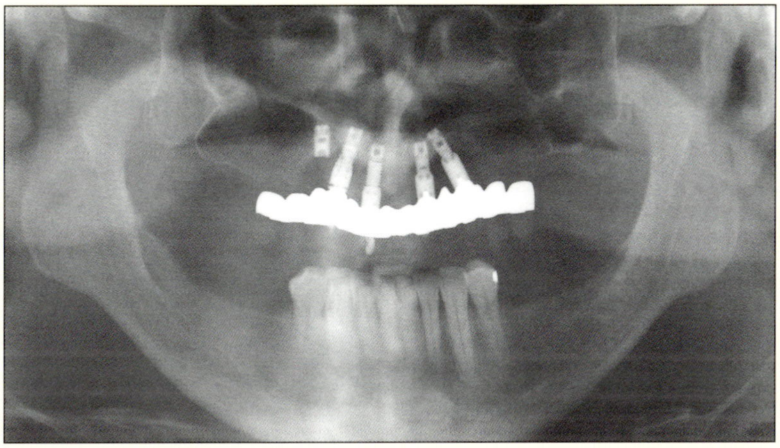

Fig 4-1 Panoramic view (December 1985). Attempted repairs had failed or were failing.

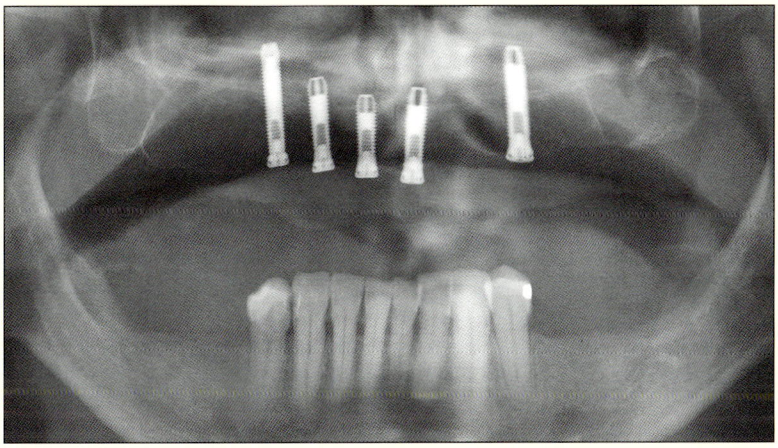

Fig 4-2 Panoramic view (December 1989). Fistulae appeared and the fixtures were lost.

Patient 1 (Compromised Group) continued

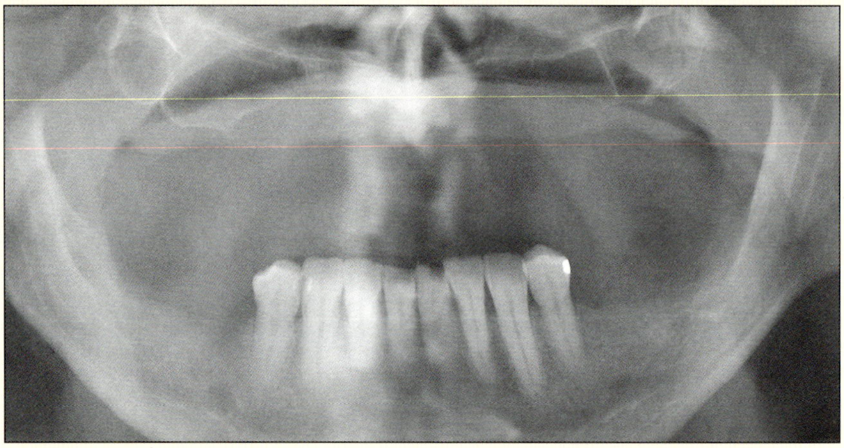

Fig 4-3 Panoramic view from the preoperative examination (1990).

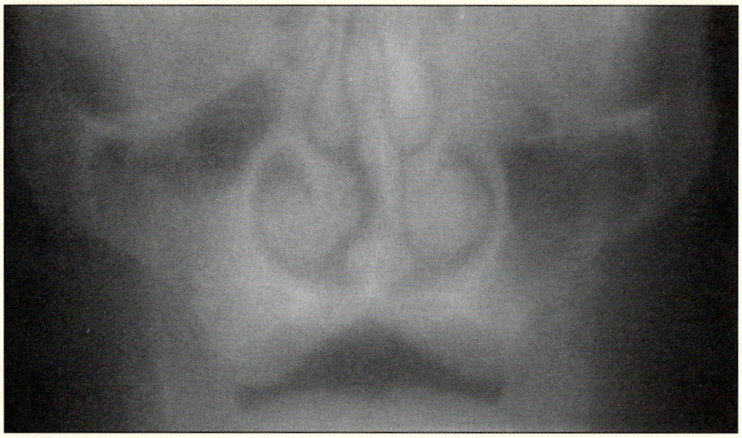

Fig 4-4 Conventional tomogram from the preoperative examination (1990).

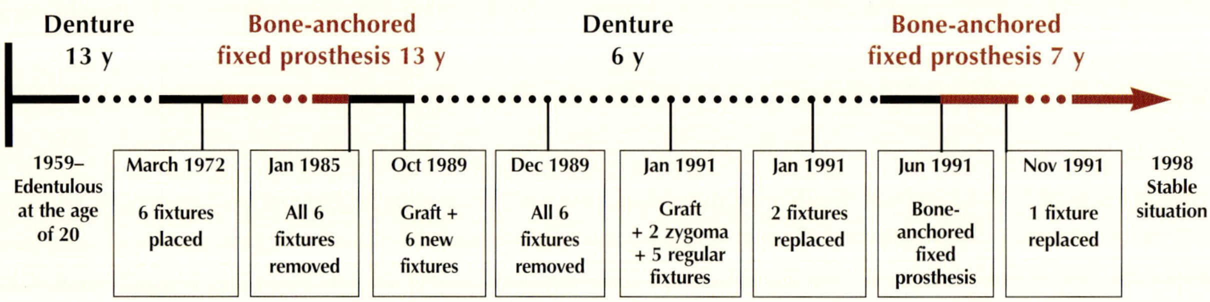

Fig 4-5 Schematic overview of the chain of treatments and follow-up.

Patient 1 (Compromised Group) continued

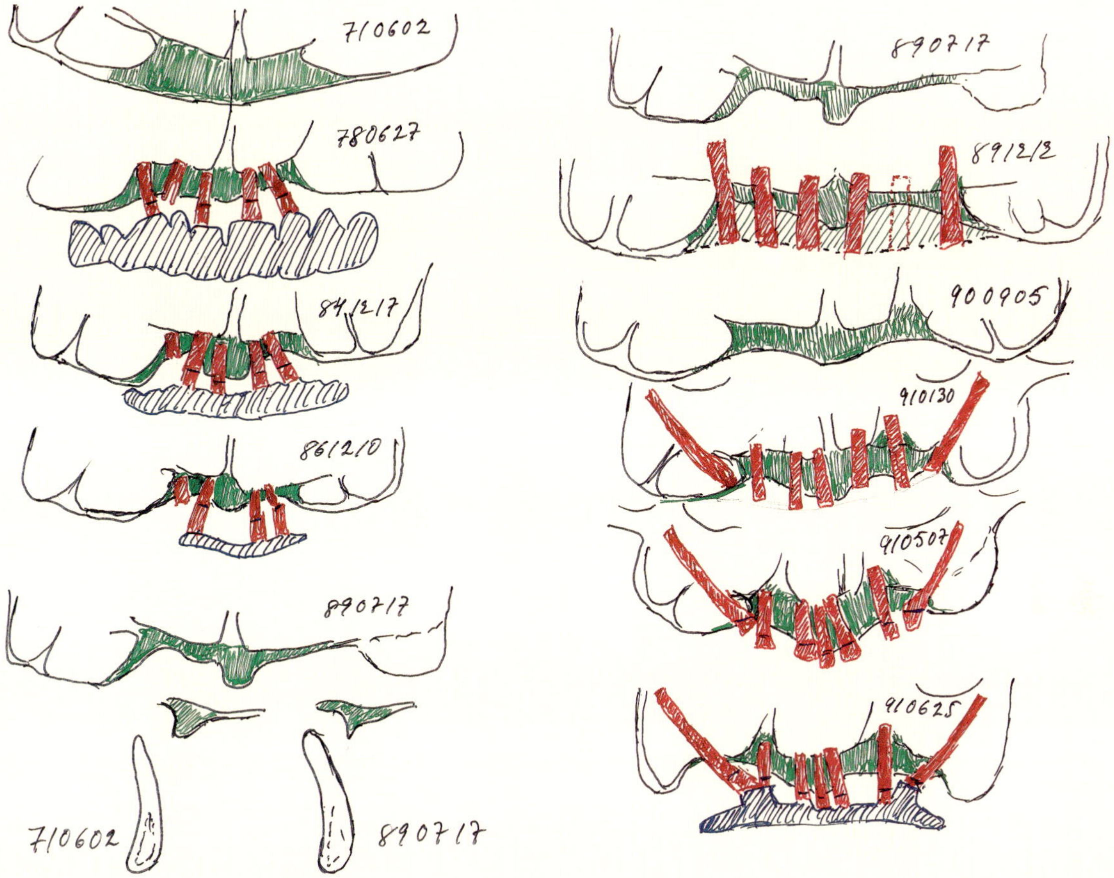

Fig 4-6 Chronological patient status as drawn by P-I Brånemark.

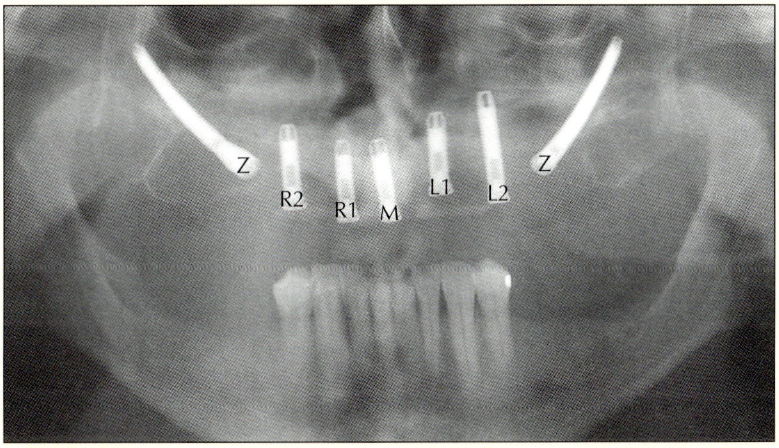

Fig 4-7 Fixture installation (January 1991).

Patient 1 (Compromised Group) continued

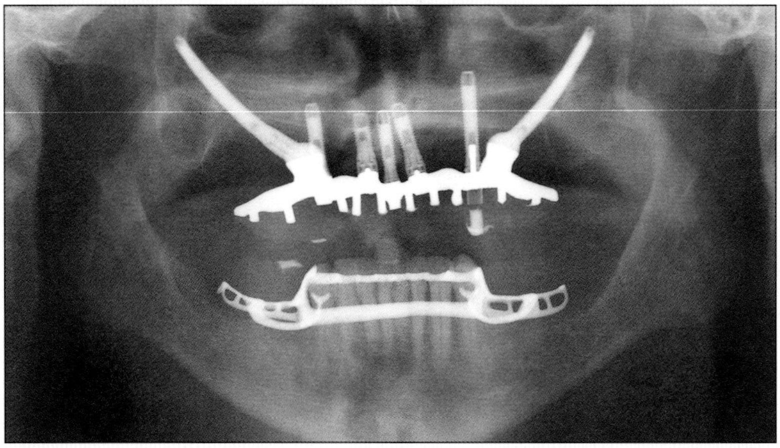

Fig 4-8 Connection of fixed prosthesis, June 1991 (after replacement of the R1 and L1 fixtures).

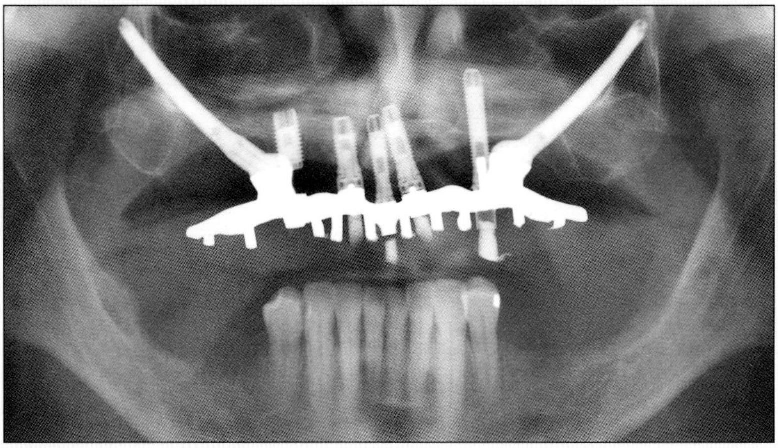

Fig 4-9 Four-year follow-up (1995).

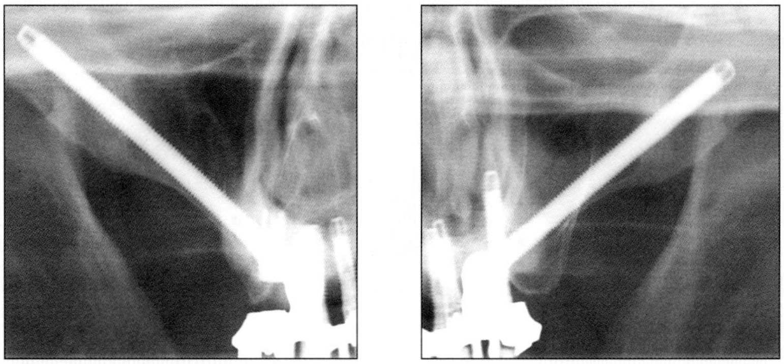

Fig 4-10 Right and left sinus views (1999).

Patient 1 (Compromised Group) continued

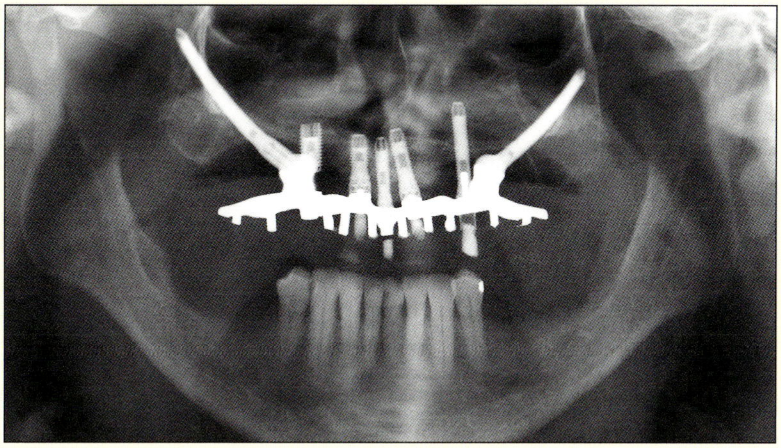

Fig 4-11 Eight-year follow-up after conclusion of the study (1999).

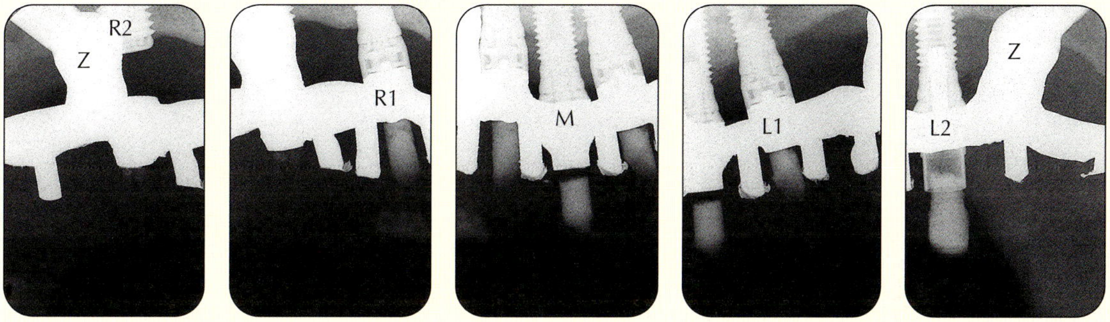

Fig 4-12 Eight-year follow-up after conclusion of the study (1999).

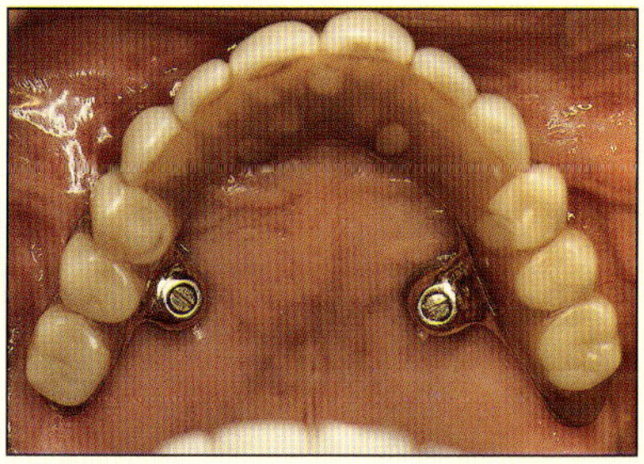

Fig 4-13 Intraoral view showing the exit points of the zygoma fixtures. These do not generate discomfort or dysfunction for the patient.

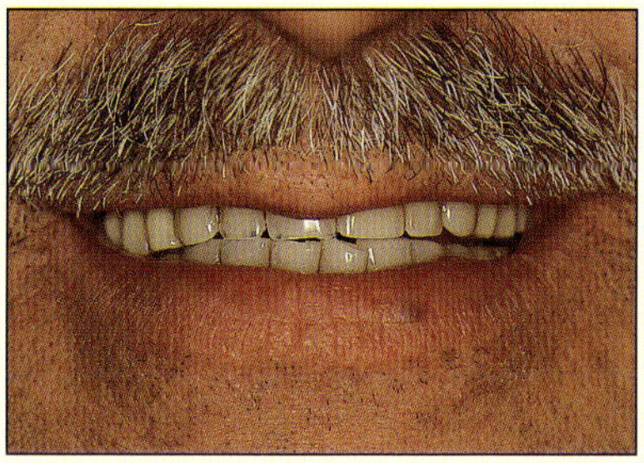

Fig 4-14 Clinical result.

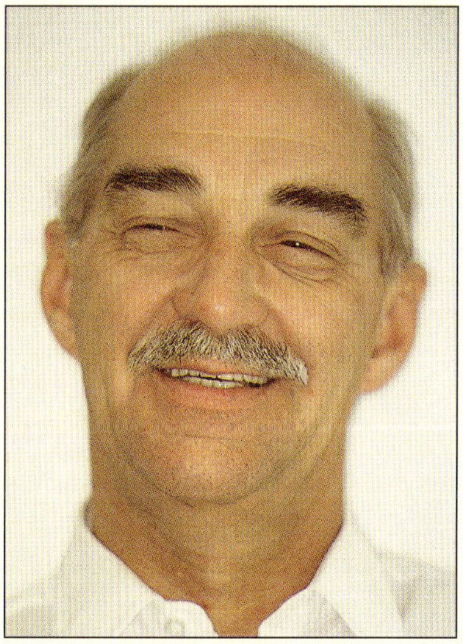

Fig 4-15 Clinical result. After years of pain and discomfort, the patient experienced a renewed quality of life.

Patient 2 (Compromised Group)

Background

This female patient was born in 1933. She suffered from long-term periodontitis, which resulted in complete maxillary edentulism when she was 54 years old (1987). She wore a prosthesis in the mandible, where some of the teeth were mobile. She exhibited clear signs of bruxism.

Preoperative comments

The patient had a wide incisive canal. The total bone height varied, but only 2 mm was available for fixture support on the right side of the midline. The patient exhibited a resorption pattern equivalent to type III and a sinus configuration equivalent to type B (see Figs 2-1 and 2-2).

Surgical procedure

The initial surgery took place in March 1992 when onlay and nasal inlay grafts were taken from the left medial and lateral ilium. The bone was of good strength and vascularity. Six swan-neck fixtures in lengths of 13 and 15 mm were installed in association with the grafting procedure. Adequate primary stability was achieved.

Complications

At abutment connection, the first fixture on the right side (R1) was mobile, and loss of osseointegration was verified radiographically. It was also noted that 3 to 4 mm of the grafted bone had resorbed. The R1 fixture was removed, and a fixed prosthesis was constructed on the remaining five fixtures in September 1992.

After 1 year of adequate functioning, the fixed prosthesis and all fixtures became mobile in September 1993. The radiographic examination verified lost osseointegration of all five fixtures.

The partial dentition in the mandible was scheduled for rehabilitation in the patient's hometown prior to maxillary reconstruction. This procedure was never carried out. Unfavorable loading of the grafted maxilla resulted from the bruxism and malocclusion. The unfavorable occlusion with the limited and somewhat mobile dentition in the mandible was considered the primary cause of the failure.

Additional surgery

In October 1993, two 10-mm flange fixtures were installed in the midline and one 40-mm zygoma fixture was placed on each side. The zygoma fixture on the right could only be anchored in 5 to 6 mm of bone because of the extension of the sinus.

The fixture on the right was placed close to a defect caused by one of the failed fixtures. This site was carefully cleaned out and filled with bone chips harvested from the alveolar crest prior to fixture placement. The abutments were connected after a 7-month healing period.

Restoration and follow-up

The patient received a fixed prosthesis in 1994. The radiographic examination after connection of the fixed prosthesis verified the difference in bone support for the zygoma fixtures between the right and the left side (5 to 6 vs 15 mm). At this time, the right maxillary sinus demonstrated normal conditions whereas a mucosal swelling was seen along the lateral wall of the left sinus.

At the last examination in October 1999 (5 years after revision surgery), the maxillary right sinus still showed normal condition. An increased density of the inferior part of the left sinus was noted.

Patient 2 (Compromised Group)

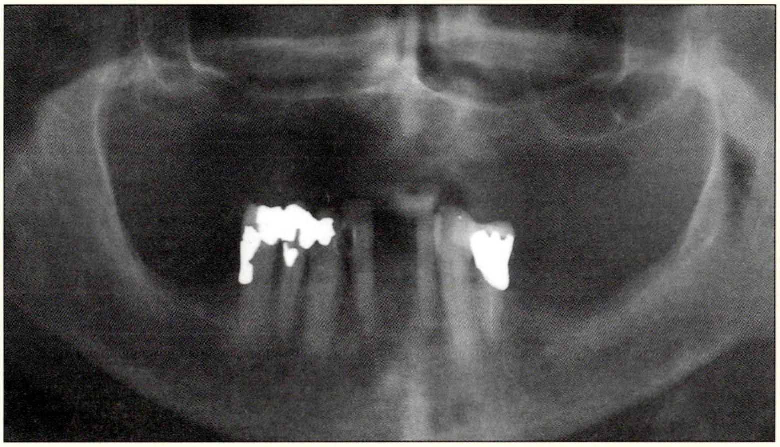

Fig 4-16 Preoperative panoramic view.

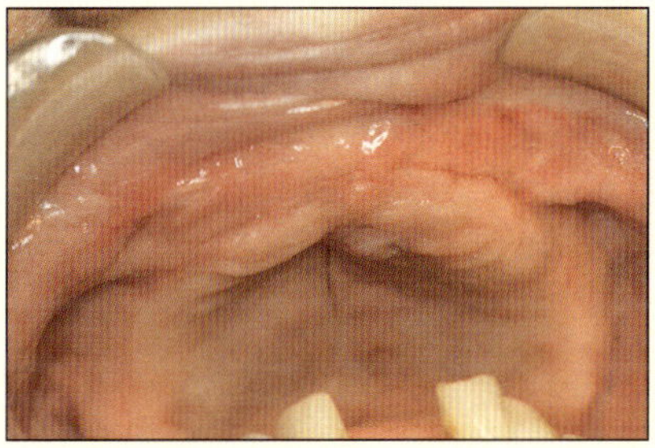

Fig 4-17 Preoperative view of the edentulous maxilla.

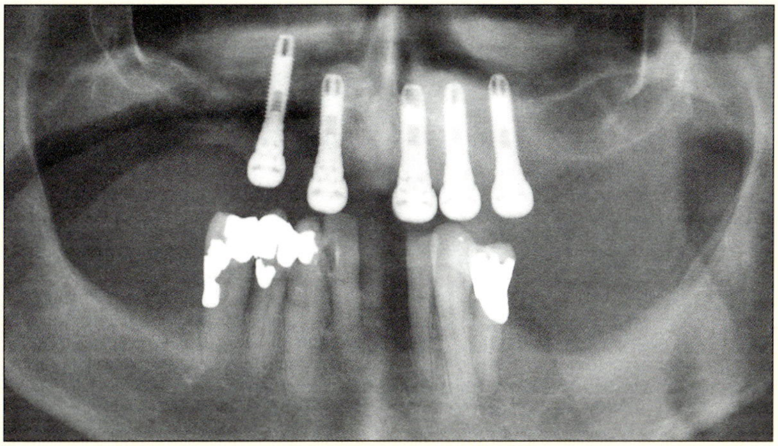

Fig 4-18 Abutment connection (1992). R1 had been removed.

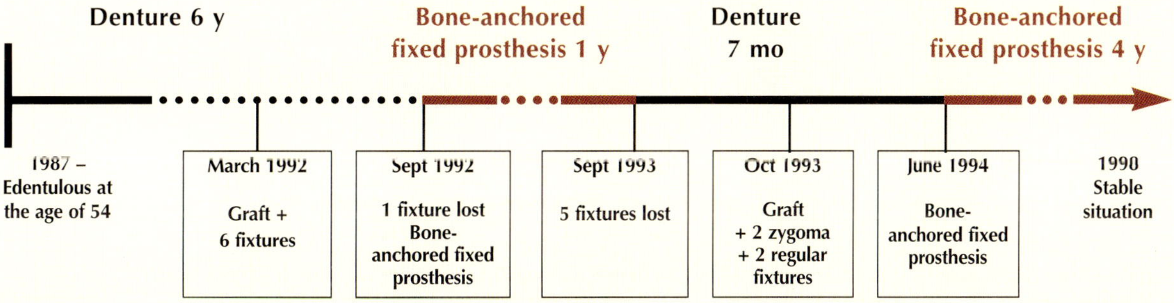

Fig 4-19 Schematic overview of the chain of treatments and follow-up.

Patient 2 (Compromised Group) continued

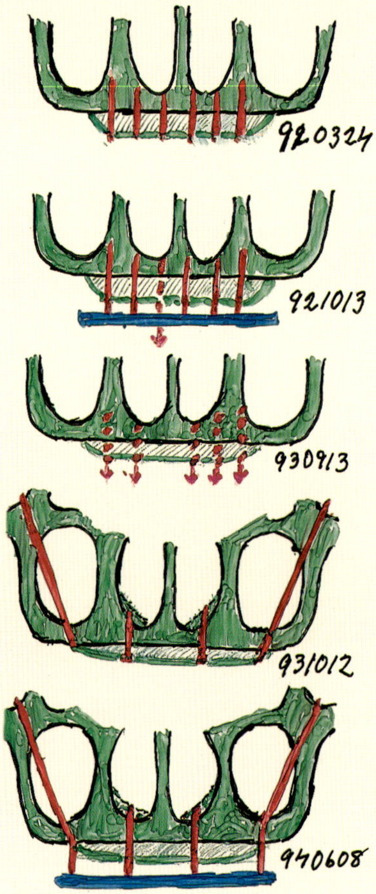

Fig 4-20 Chronological patient status as drawn by P-I Brånemark.

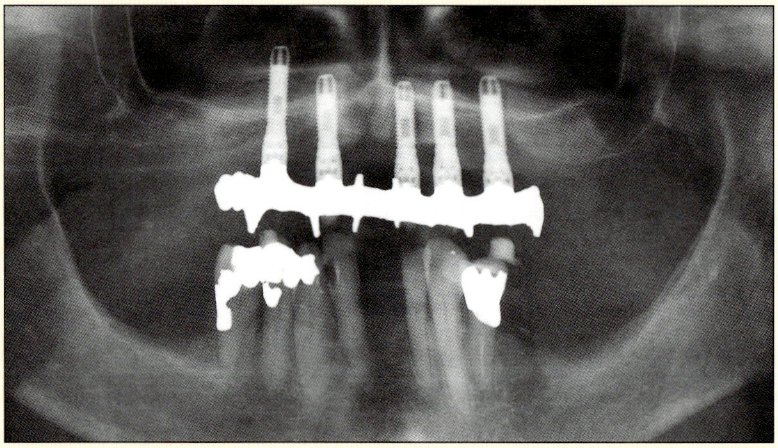

Fig 4-21 Panoramic view showing the presence of complications (September 1993).

Patient 2 (Compromised Group) continued

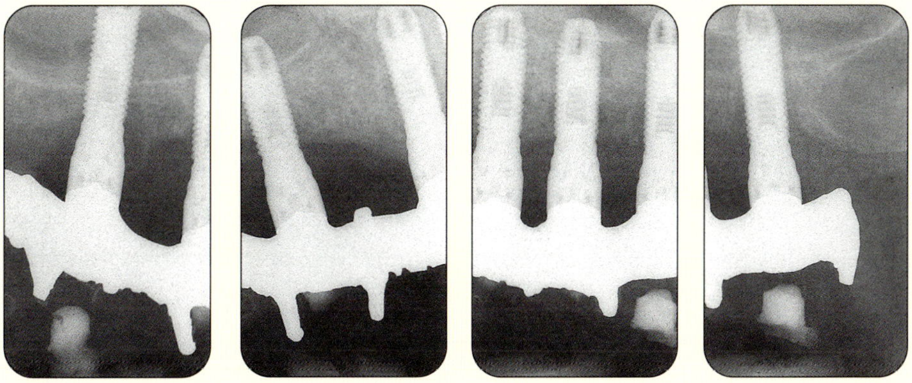

Fig 4-22 Intraoral radiographs (September 1993).

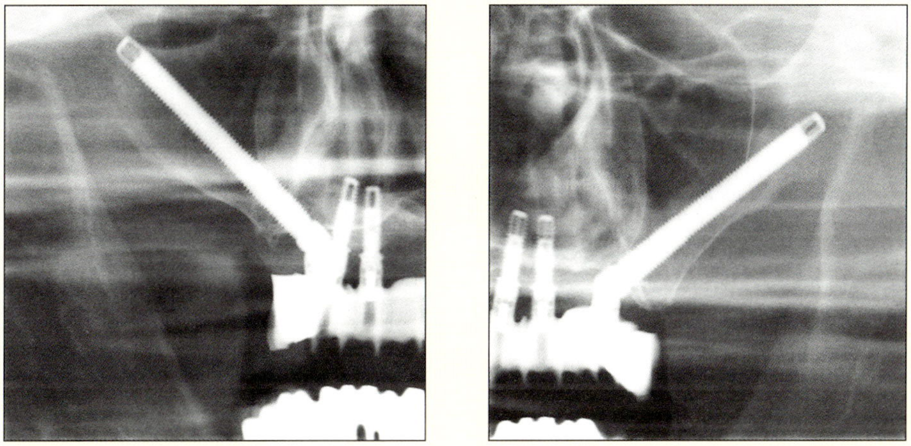

Fig 4-23 Sinus views taken at connection of fixed prosthesis (1994).

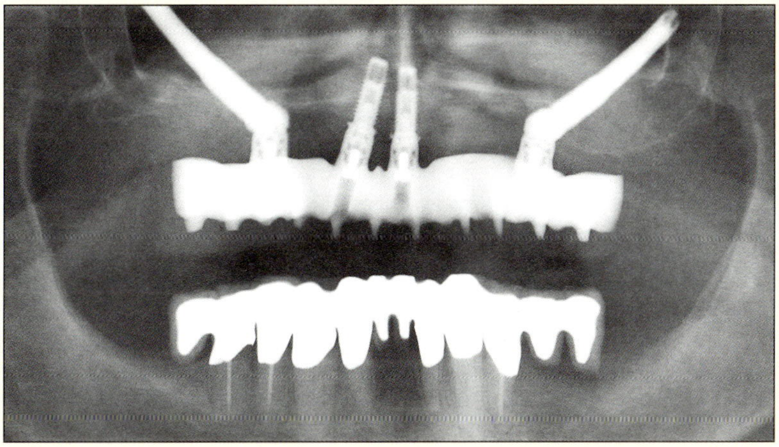

Fig 4-24 Connection of fixed prosthesis after revision surgery (1994).

Patient 2 (Compromised Group) continued

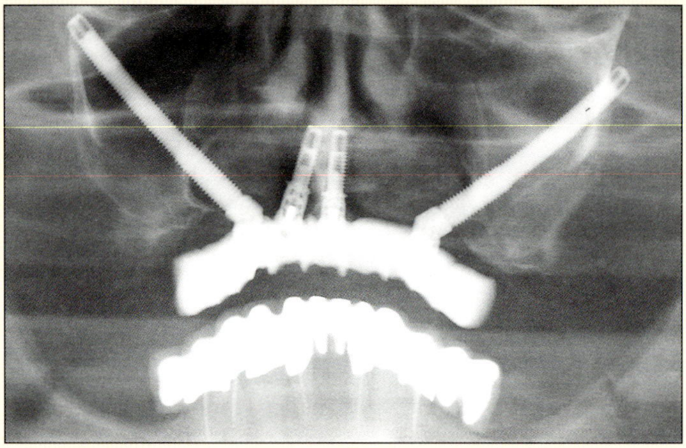

Fig 4-25 Mid-face (frontal) panoramic view after conclusion of the study (1999).

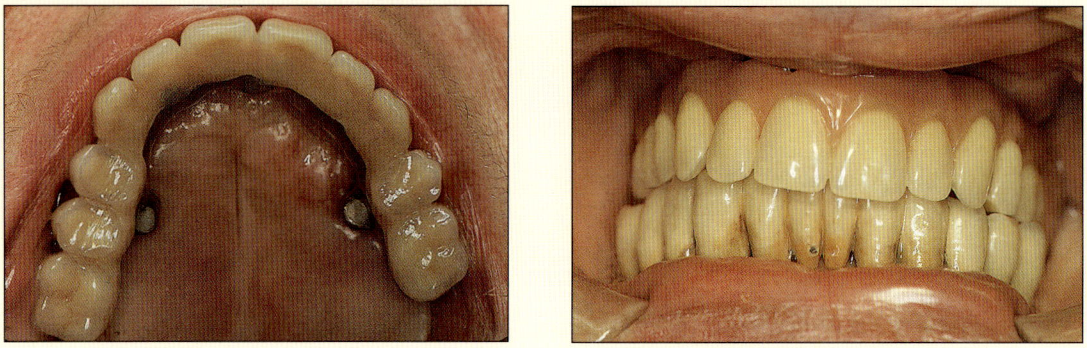

Figs 4-26a and 4-26b Postoperative clinical status (1997).

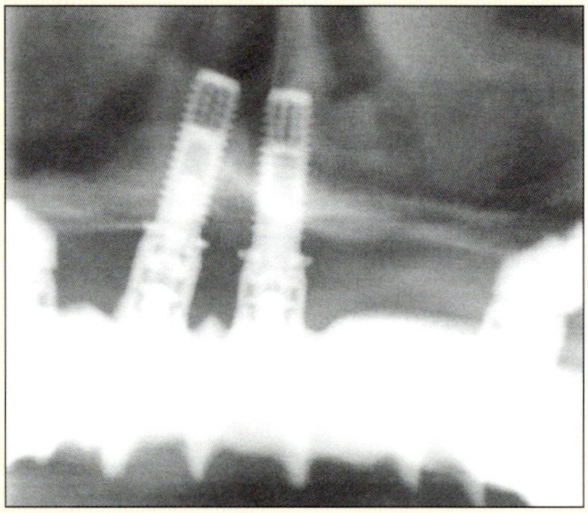

Fig 4-27 Dental scanogram at the 5-year follow-up after conclusion of the study (1999).

Patient 2 (Compromised Group) continued

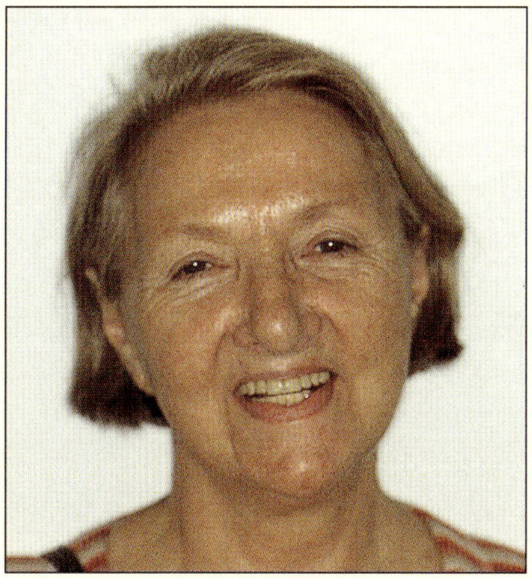

Fig 4-28 The patient at the 5-year follow-up visit.

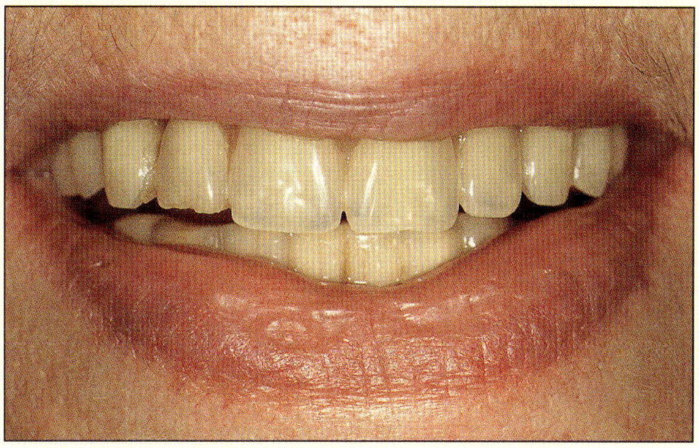

Fig 4-29 Clinical result. The patient remains satisfied with the esthetic appearance of her fixed prosthesis.

Patient 3 (Compromised Group)

Background

This female patient was born in 1942 and had been edentulous in the maxilla all of her adult life. The patient smoked occasionally. She had a complete denture in the maxilla and a partial denture in the mandible.

Preoperative comments

The alveolar crest was extremely resorbed with a total bone height of 3 to 8 mm. The mandible was characterized by protruding incisors. The patient exhibited a resorption pattern equivalent to type IV and a sinus configuration equivalent to type A (see Figs 2-1 and 2-2).

Surgical procedure

The initial surgery was performed in April 1992 when the patient was 50 years old. The maxillary bone was extremely resorbed but of good quality and vascularity. Patches of fibrous tissue were noted. This was partially caused by previous osteotomies and three cerclage wires that were removed from the frontal area. A small defect was seen on the left posterior sinus wall and an even larger defect was present on the right side. Sinus inlay and onlay grafts were taken from the left lateral and medial ilium. These were secured with seven swan-neck fixtures according to a "sandwich" approach (see Fig 3-25). A sinus inlay was attached with the most distal fixture on the right. Good primary stability was obtained.

Complications and additional surgery

The patient returned after 1 month (May 1992) with a fistula. The incision was made and the area was cleaned of granulation tissue. The grafted bone remained vital in all engaged areas and the fixtures were stable. The sinus graft was also in good condition. The incision was resutured to adequate closure.

A radiographic evaluation in June 1992 indicated some disturbances on the right side with resorption of the inferior part of the graft. Increased density of the maxillary sinus was also noted. In addition, the cover screw on the L1 fixture was incorrectly seated. Later that month, the R2, R1, and L1 fixtures were removed because of mobility. R1 and L1 were replaced with new fixtures.

The distal fixture on the right (R4) was lost in August 1992. It was replaced with a shorter fixture in November 1992 in association with abutment connection of the R1 and L1 fixtures.

Restoration and follow-up

The patient received a provisional fixed prosthesis in November 1992. When she was examined a few days later, the tissue was in excellent shape and no complications were noted. The recently installed distal fixture on the right side remained unloaded until April 1993. It was then incorporated into a permanent fixed prosthesis construction in May 1993.

The initial complications had led to advanced bone resorption, as noted at the radiographic examination performed in association with delivery of the fixed prosthesis. Most bone loss was noted adjacent to the R2, R1, and L2 fixtures, and the bone graft had resorbed on the right side (Fig 4-40).

During the following years, the patient had some sinus discomfort. A sinus radiograph taken in 1998 showed a completely dense right sinus. The condition was treated with conventional antibiotics. No further bone loss was seen during the 5-year follow-up period.

The protruding mandibular teeth were extracted in October 1998. At that time, the patient received a fixed prosthesis on three fixtures according to the Brånemark Novum same-day teeth procedure.

Patient 3 (Compromised Group)

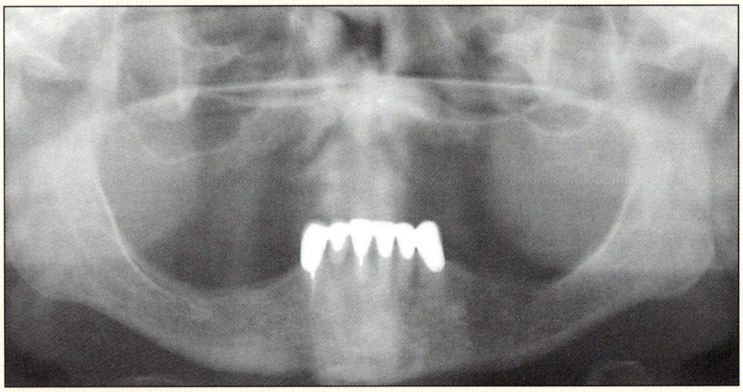

Fig 4-30 Preoperative panoramic view.

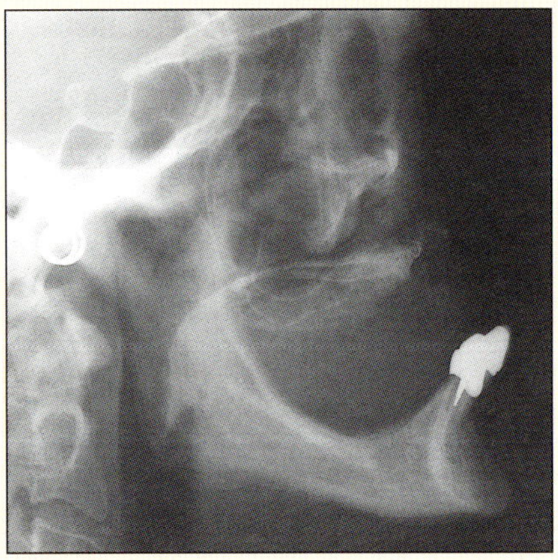

Fig 4-31 Preoperative profile.

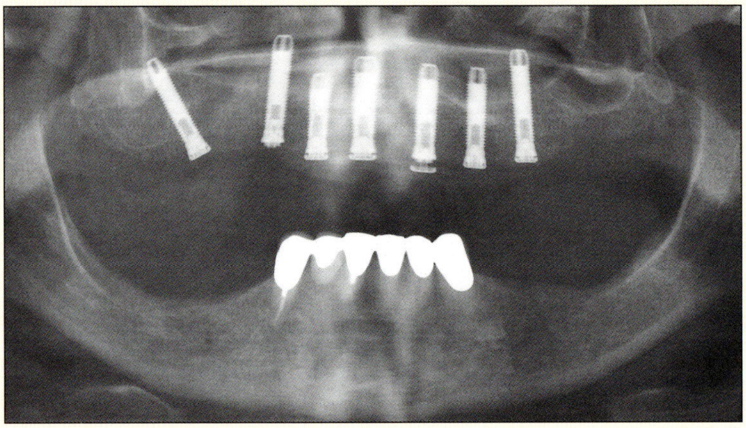

Fig 4-32 Panoramic view (June 1992). A fistula had appeared and resorption of the inferior part of the sinus inlay graft was noted. The R4 fixture was later replaced.

Patient 3 (Compromised Group) continued

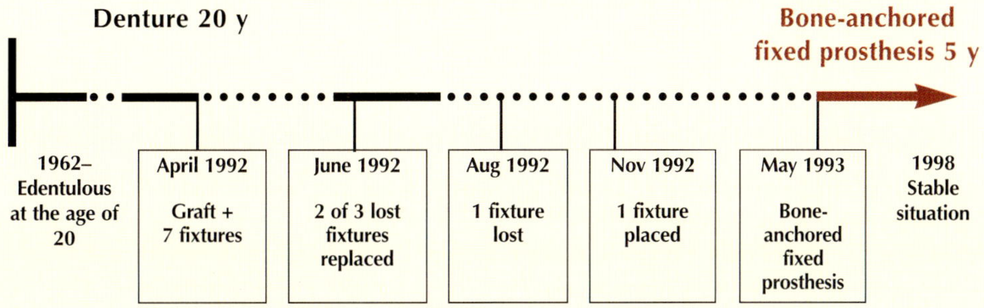

Fig 4-33 Schematic overview of the chain of treatments and follow-up.

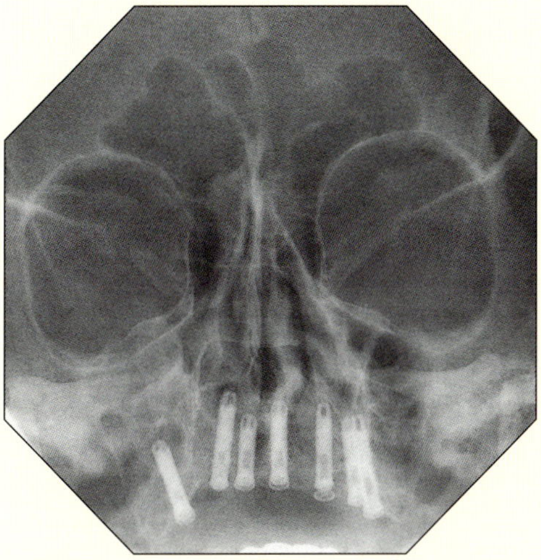

Fig 4-34 Posteroanterior (Caldwell) view showing increased density of the right sinus (June 1992).

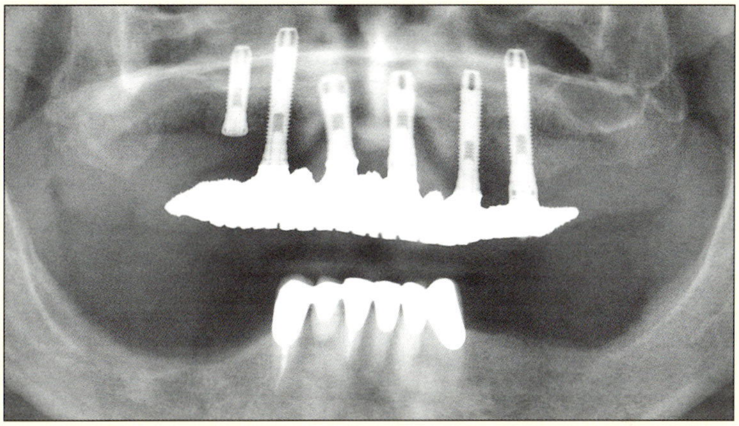

Fig 4-35 Connection of fixed prosthesis (November 1992). The recently installed fixture remained unloaded until April 1993.

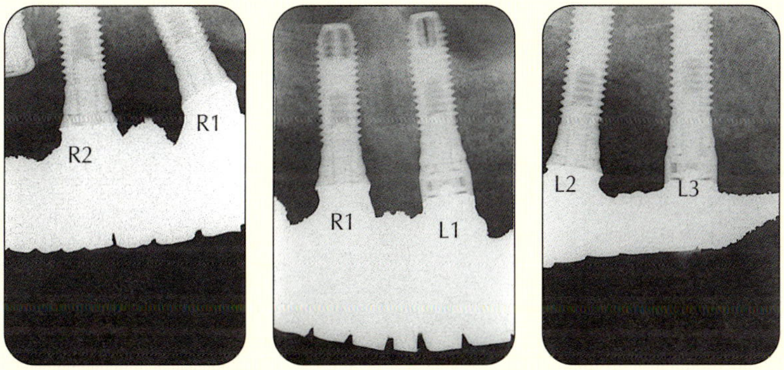

Fig 4-36 Connection of fixed prosthesis (November 1992).

Patient 3 (Compromised Group) continued

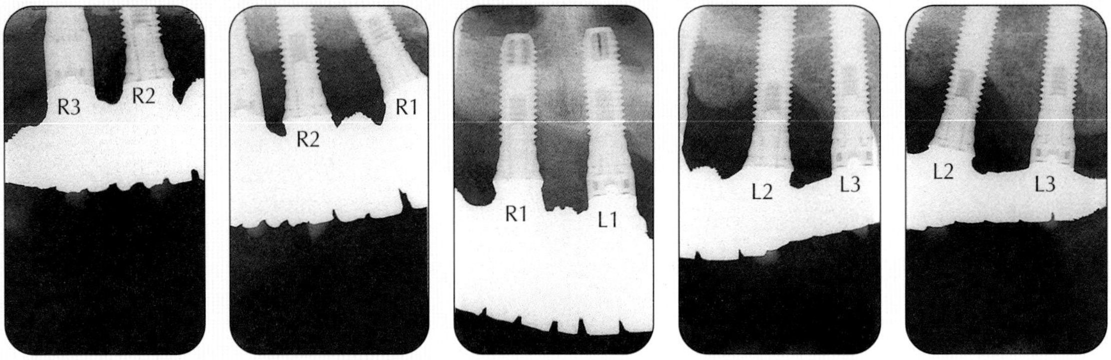

Fig 4-37 Fixed prosthesis at 4-year follow-up (1997).

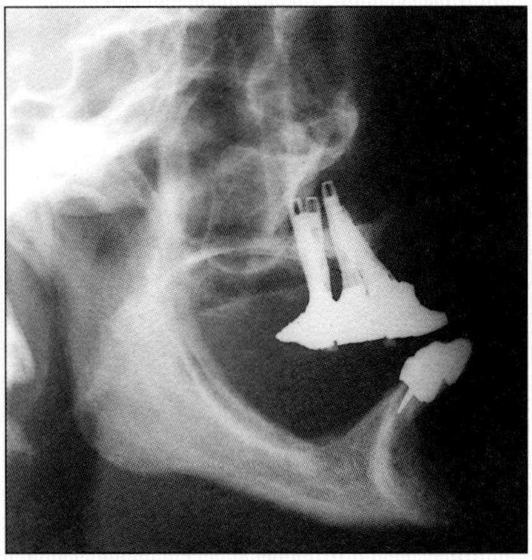

Fig 4-38 Profile at 4-year follow-up (1997).

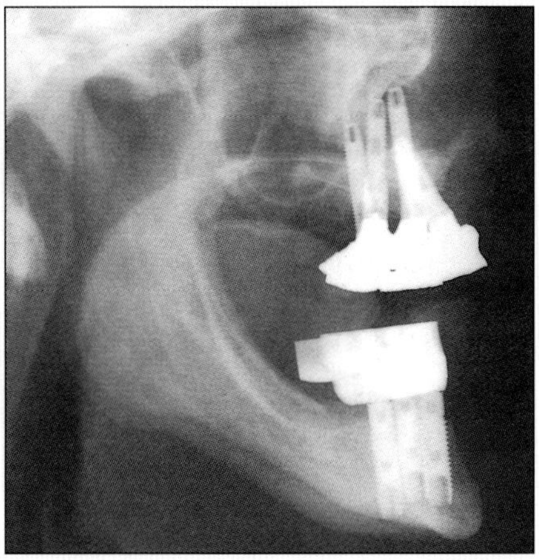

Fig 4-39 Profile in October 1998. The patient had just received a mandibular Brånemark Novum bridge to improve jaw relations.

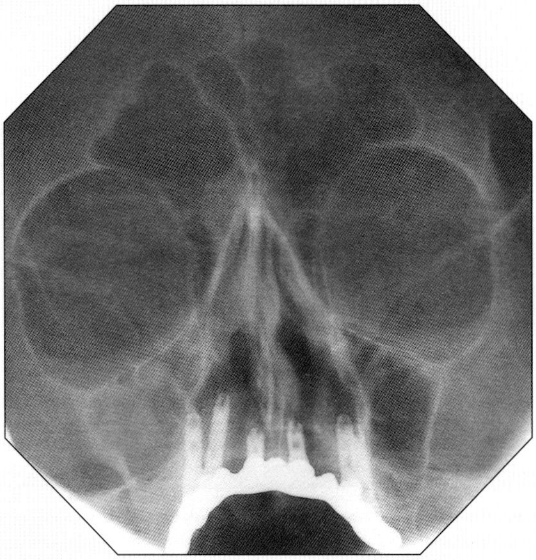

Fig 4-40 Occipitomental (Waters) view taken at the last follow-up visit (1998).

Patient 3 (Compromised Group) continued

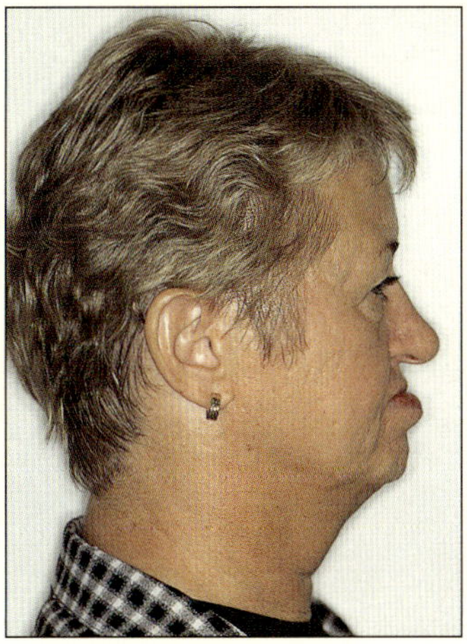

Fig 4-41a Preoperative profile.

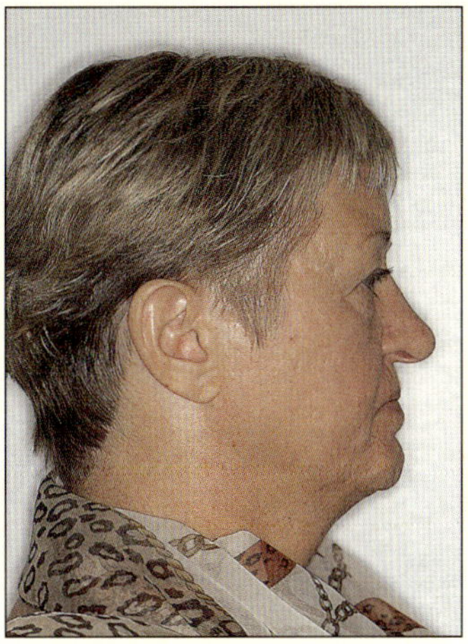

Fig 4-41b Profile at the 5-year follow-up (1998).

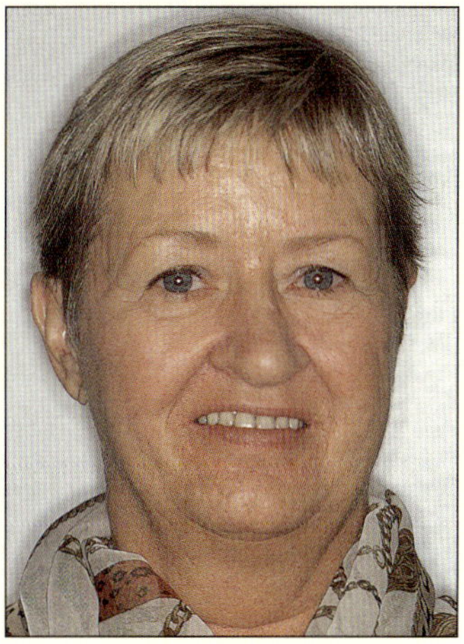

Fig 4-42 Facial view at the 5-year follow-up (1998).

Patient 4 (Compromised Group)

Background

This female patient was born in 1928. She smoked approximately 30 cigarettes per day. When first examined in January 1994, she exhibited advanced periodontitis in the maxilla. All her maxillary teeth were therefore extracted in February 1994.

Preoperative comments

The total bone height was 10 mm. The patient exhibited a resorption pattern equivalent to type III and a sinus configuration equivalent to type A (see Figs 2-1 and 2-2).

Surgical procedure

The initial surgery was performed in May 1994 when the patient was 66 years old. She received six swan-neck fixtures in combination with an onlay bone graft from the medial ilium. The marginal portion of the alveolar crest had been ground into bone chips and packed in the fixture sites to enhance stability. The incisive canal was thoroughly debrided of all soft tissue. The distal fixture on each side was then placed slightly in the distal direction to obtain anchorage in the bony septum between the sinus and the nasal cavity. Abutments were connected in October 1994.

Complications and additional surgery

In November 1994, the patient received a porcelain-fused-to-metal fixed prosthesis. The prosthesis exhibited less than optimal biomechanical properties because it did not fit passively. Signs of lost osseointegration were seen at the first annual radiographic examination in December 1995, particularly adjacent to the R3 and L3 fixtures. Clinical signs of mobility of the fixed prosthesis were also noted.

When the patient underwent surgery again in March 1997, it became clear that the system failure was attributable to bilateral communication between the oral cavity and the maxillary sinus. Careful curettage of the fixture sites was performed. A small rift on the left side was sutured after part of the thick hypertrophic sinus mucosa had been removed on the lateral side.

The extreme resorption in the anterior region motivated a nasal inlay/onlay grafting procedure of the "sandwich" type (see Fig 3-25). The inlay and onlay grafts taken from the left iliac crest were of good density and vascularity.

Two zygoma fixtures (50 and 45 mm) and three standard fixtures that engaged both the inlay and onlay grafts were installed. Excellent stability was obtained for both fixtures and grafts. Abutment connection was performed in September 1997. The abutments were rigidly connected with a bar (Fig 4-54).

Restoration and follow-up

The patient received her new fixed prosthesis in November 1997. An occlusal night guard was also provided. The first annual control was performed in October 1998, at which time the prosthetic construction was functioning well.

Patient 4 (Compromised Group)

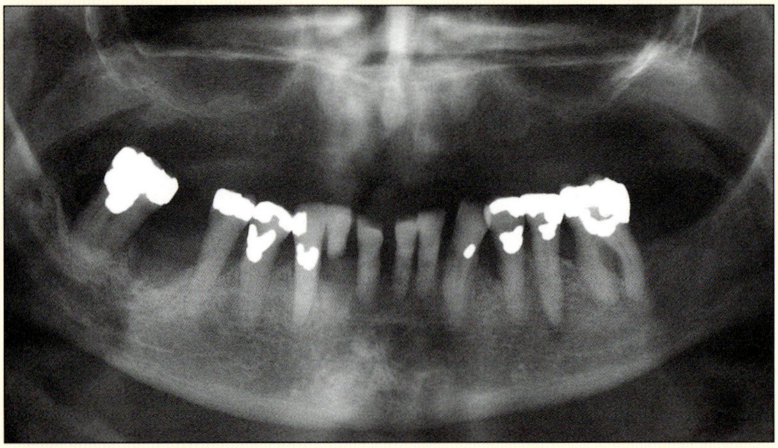

Fig 4-43 Preoperative panoramic view.

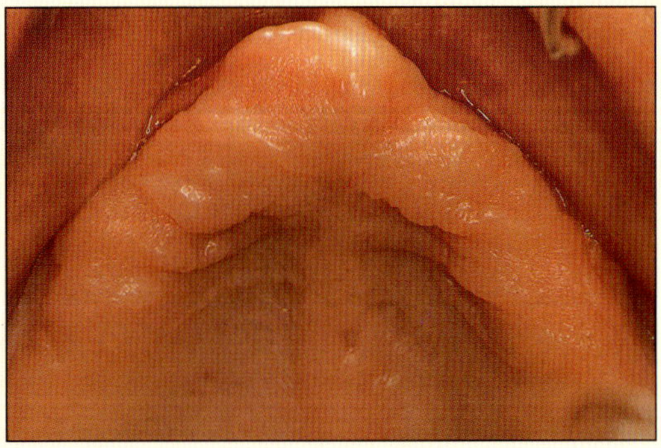

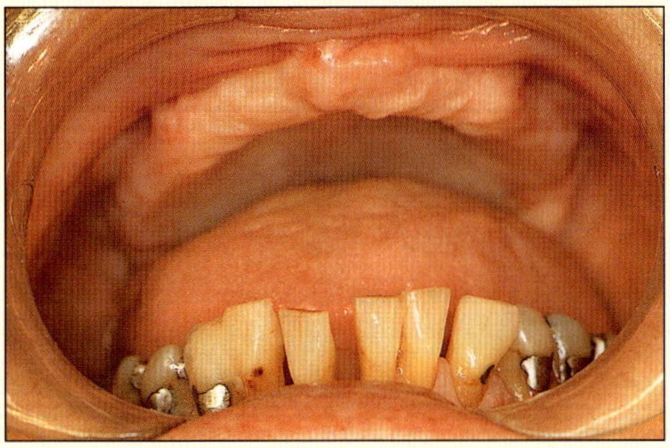

Figs 4-44a and 4-44b Preoperative clinical view.

Patient 4 (Compromised Group) continued

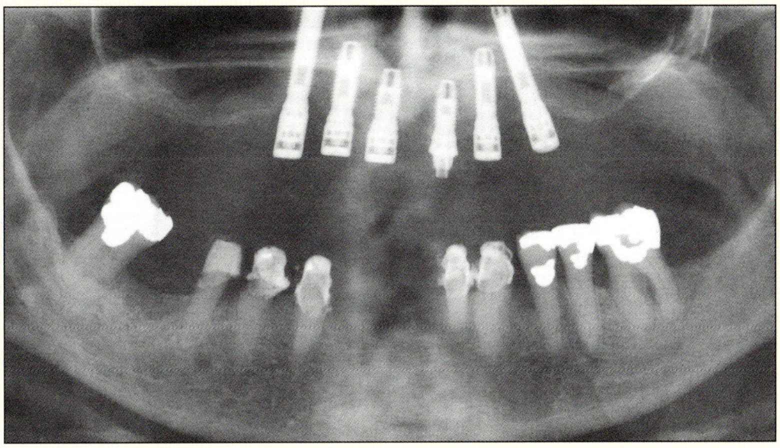

Fig 4-45 Abutment connection (1994).

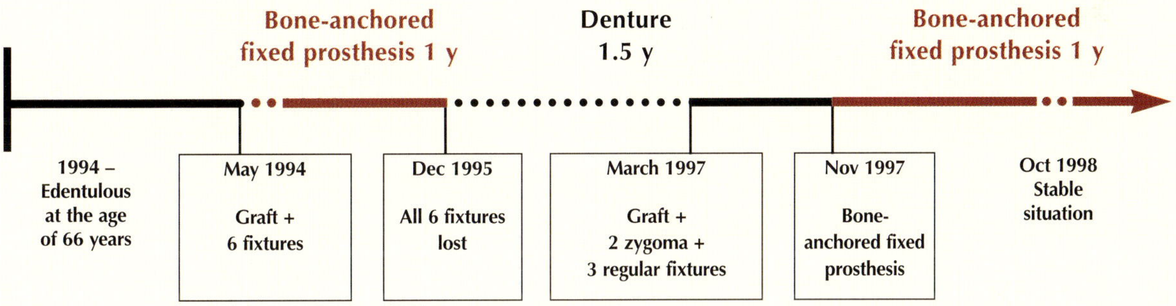

Fig 4-46 Schematic overview of the chain of treatments and follow-up.

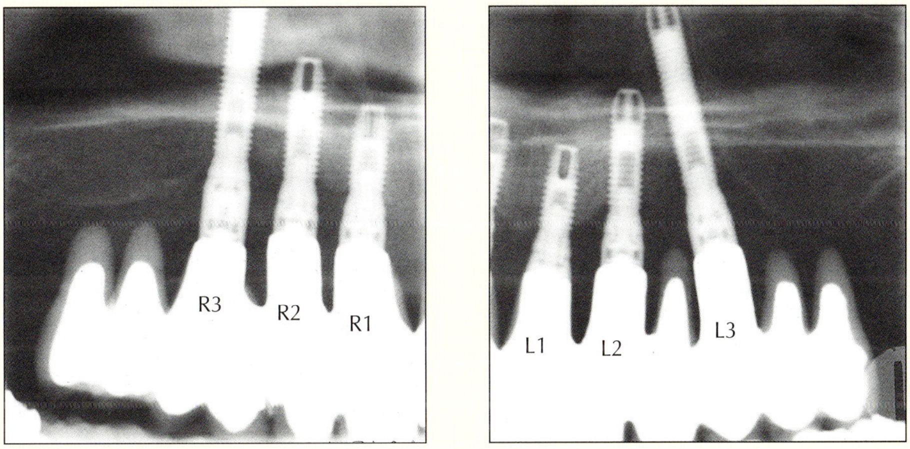

Fig 4-47 Dental scanograms at the 1-year follow-up revealing signs of lost osseointegration of R3 and L3 (1995).

Patient 4 (Compromised Group) continued

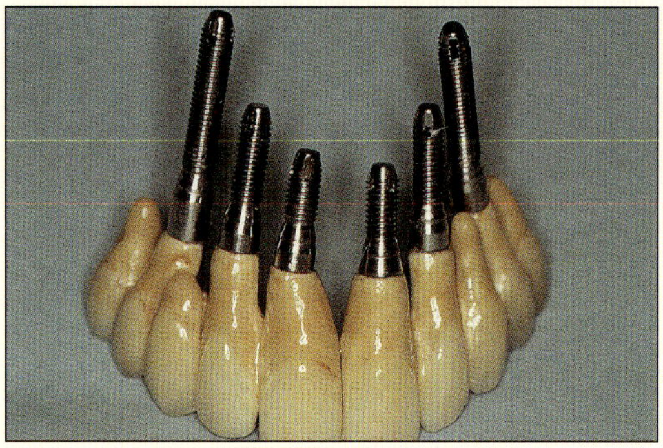

Fig 4-48 Removed prosthetic construction with fixtures (December 1995).

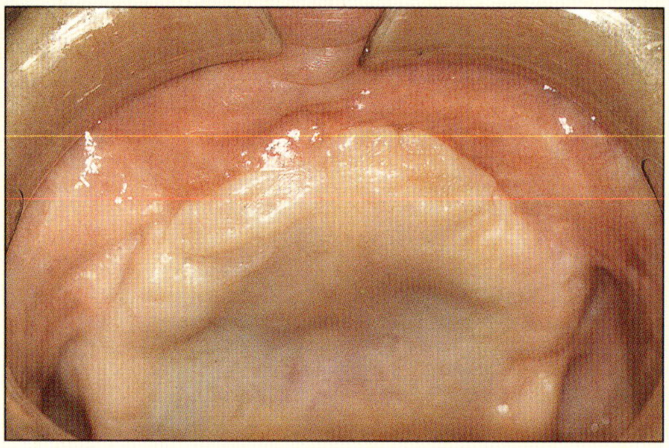

Fig 4-49 Edentulous maxilla after removal of fixtures (December 1995).

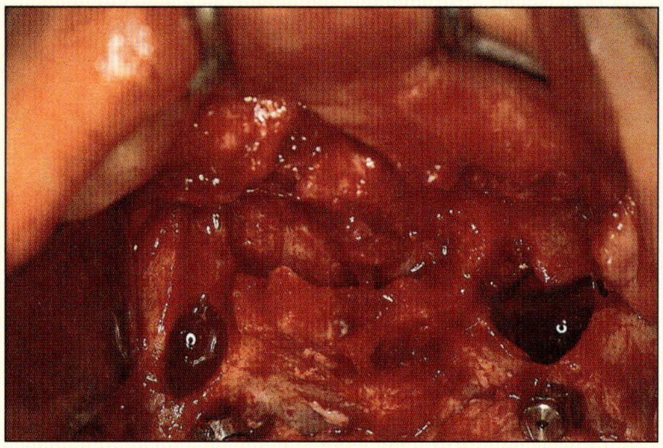

Fig 4-50 Recipient site during surgical procedure (March 1997).

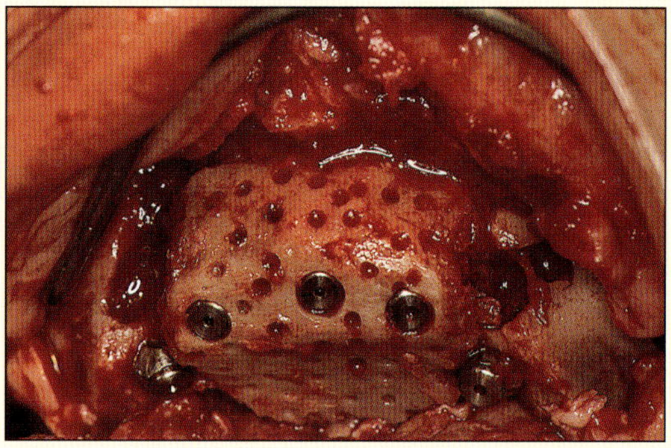

Fig 4-51 The graft in place, secured with fixtures.

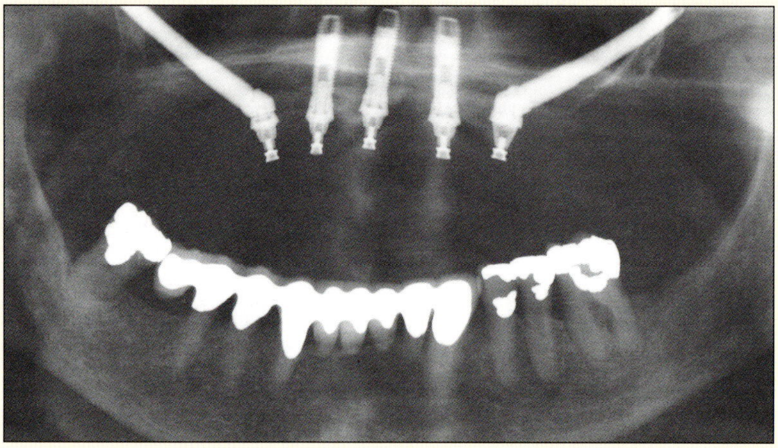

Fig 4-52 Panoramic view of abutment connection (September 1997).

Patient 4 (Compromised Group) continued

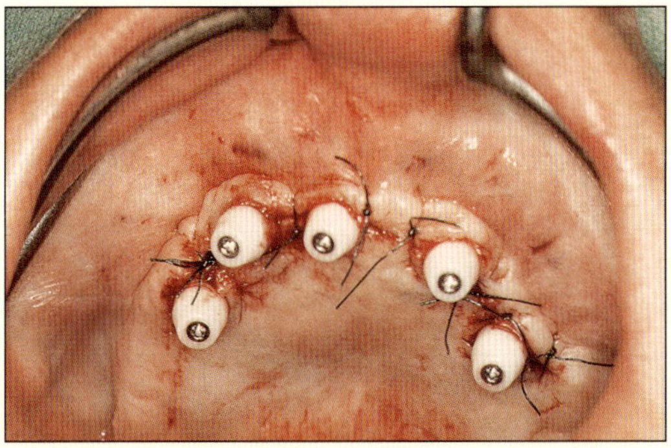

Fig 4-53 Abutment connection.

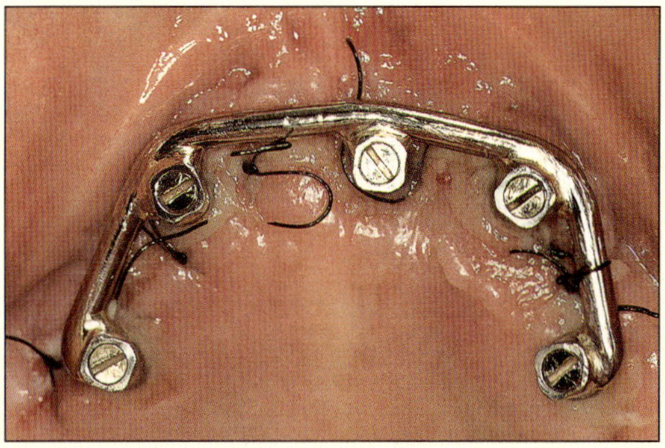

Fig 4-54 Rigid bar in place to stabilize the fixtures and prevent torque and bending forces.

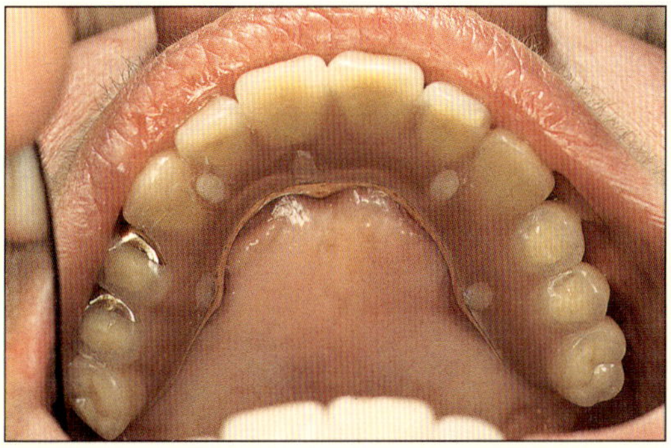

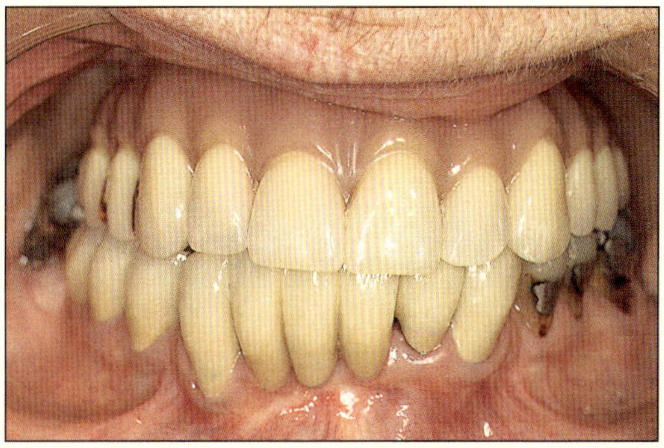

Figs 4-55a and 4-55b Connection of fixed prosthesis (November 1997).

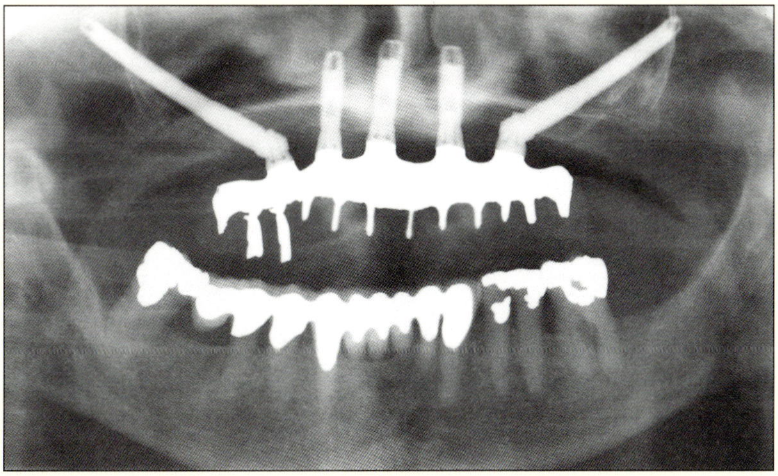

Fig 4-56 Panoramic view of connection of fixed prosthesis (November 1997).

Patient 4 (Compromised Group) continued

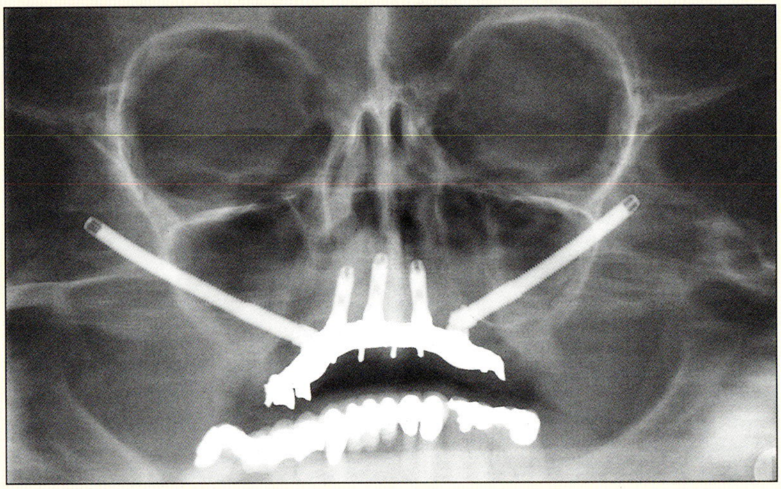

Fig 4-57 Mid-face panorama (frontal view) revealing a stable situation (1998).

Patient 5 (Compromised Group)

Background

This female patient was born in 1933. She had all her maxillary teeth extracted and received a removable denture in 1965. She had a fixed prosthesis in the mandible supported by only four teeth. The patient was a smoker.

Preoperative comments

The maxilla was extremely resorbed and characterized by bilateral sinus expansion. There was only 1 mm of available bone for fixture support. The patient exhibited a resorption pattern equivalent to type IV and a sinus configuration equivalent to type B (see Figs 2-1 and 2-2).

Surgical procedure

During the initial surgery in October 1990, an onlay graft was taken from the left medial ilium. It was secured to the premaxilla with five 18-mm swan-neck fixtures and two zygoma fixtures (30 and 40 mm). A partially fractured distal segment of the graft was attached with a locking screw.

Complications and additional surgery

At abutment connection in May 1991, three anterior fixtures (R1, L1, and L2) were mobile and removed. The bone graft and parts of the thin residual bone had resorbed. The nasal mucosa was exposed in the incisor regions.

The bone surrounding the R2 fixture had resorbed to only 4 to 5 mm. The fixture was mobile and disappeared into the sinus cavity with only a light touch. It was removed in association with a Caldwell-Luc procedure during which the zygoma fixtures were inspected as well. To replace the R2 fixture, a new site was prepared in the triangular bone of the anterior sinus wall. A 15-mm swan-neck fixture could then be installed with good primary stability. In September 1991 the original L3 fixture was removed because of mobility.

An abutment was connected to the new R2 fixture in November 1991. At that time, the bone thickness to the left of the midline and distally toward the anterior sinus wall was only 1 to 2 mm. Yet it was possible to place a 7-mm flange fixture in the septum between the nasal cavity and the sinus. A standard 7-mm fixture was also placed anterior of the flange fixture. Acceptable primary stability was achieved. Some hyperplastic mucosa was extirpated around the zygoma fixtures. Shortly thereafter, an alveolar bar construction was fitted on the three exposed abutments to enable the patient to wear a removable denture during the prolonged healing period.

In April 1992, the two 7-mm fixtures were uncovered and both were well integrated. The additional L1 fixture in the frontal region that had helped support the provisional bar construction was mobile and therefore removed. The bone density was still acceptable. After careful curettage of the site, a wide-diameter fixture (5 x 10 mm) could be installed with good stability.

Abutment connection of the wide-diameter fixture occurred in June 1992, but at this time the left anterior 7-mm fixture was mobile and had to be removed. The remaining four fixtures were stable. The patient received a new provisional overdenture with Ceka attachments, which required frequent adjustments during the following 10 months.

In May 1993, the two fixtures remaining between the zygoma fixtures were removed because of lack of integration. No signs of infection were noted. The cause of failures was believed to be overload of the fixtures.

A new attempt to solve this difficult case involved a grafting procedure 10 days later. During the surgery, it was noted that the lateral basal bone was only 1 mm in height, but the bone tissue demonstrated better mechanical capacity during this grafting procedure compared to the previous operation. The enhanced bone density may have resulted from altered smoking habits.

Nasal inlay and maxillary onlay grafts were harvested from the right medial ilium. A 7-mm flange fixture and four swan-neck fixtures (20 and 13 mm) were installed between the two remaining zygoma fixtures. The swan-neck fixtures were placed through the graft and reached up in the anterior-lateral nasal walls. Excellent primary stability was obtained. Two standard fixtures (15 and 18 mm) were also installed bilaterally in the mandible.

At abutment connection in November 1993, the bone grafts were vital and well incorporated and all fixtures were osseointegrated.

Restoration and follow-up

In December 1993, the patient could finally receive the fixed prosthesis for the maxilla and the mandible. The maxillary prosthesis was screw-retained while the mandibular reconstruction was cast in one piece and cemented onto the four telescopic crowns on the remaining natural teeth.

In May 1995, the patient underwent bilateral rhinoscopy and sinoscopy. The nasal mucosa was healthy and without signs of inflammation or irritation. A visual examination of the zygoma fixtures could be carried out internally from the sinuses. Healthy sinus mucosa was seen bilaterally. Dental scanograms taken in 1993 and 1997 revealed a stable situation without changes of the marginal bone level.

No complications occurred during the following 5 years. At the last clinical examination, the oral and masticatory systems were functioning well.

Patient 5 (Compromised Group)

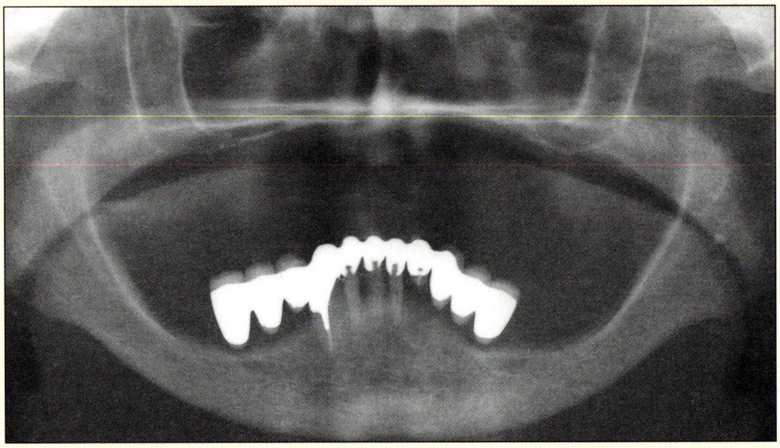

Fig 4-58 Preoperative panoramic view.

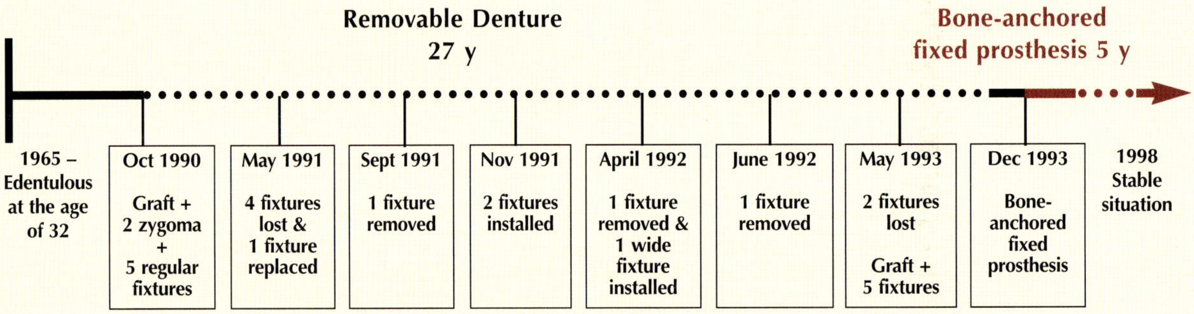

Fig 4-59 Schematic overview of the chain of treatments and follow-up events.

Patient 5 (Compromised Group) continued

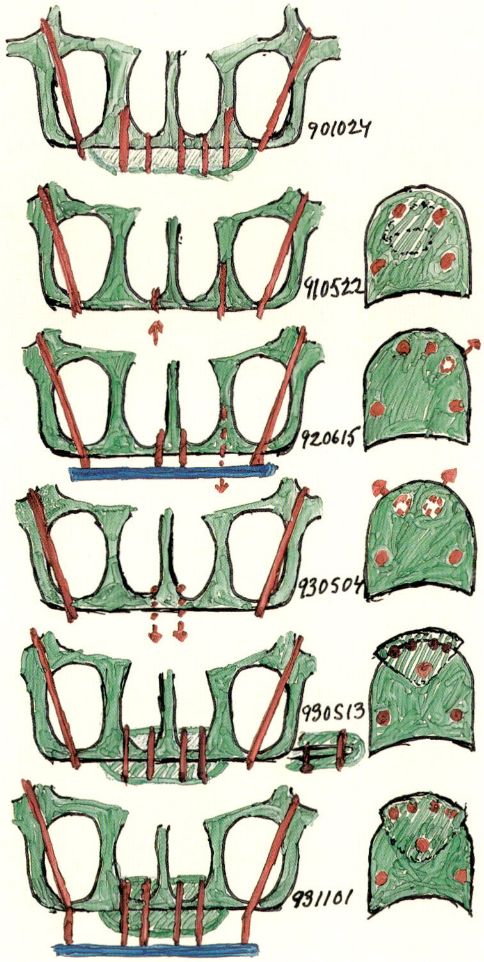

Fig 4-60 Chronological patient status as drawn by P-I Brånemark.

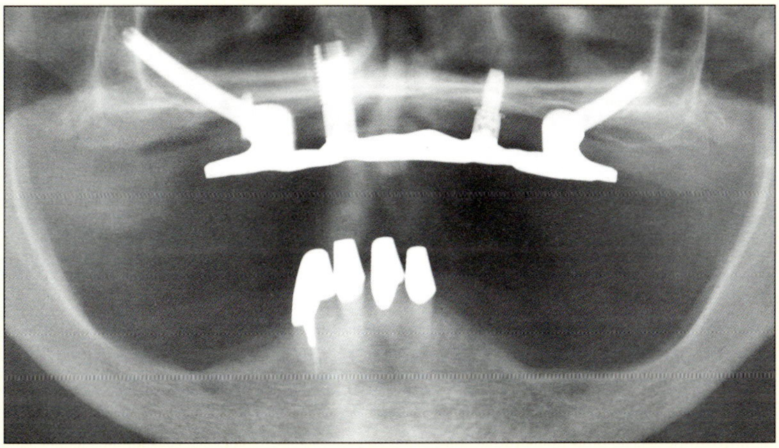

Fig 4-61 Temporary bar after fixture loss (June 1992). The two anterior fixtures are also failing.

Patient 5 (Compromised Group) continued

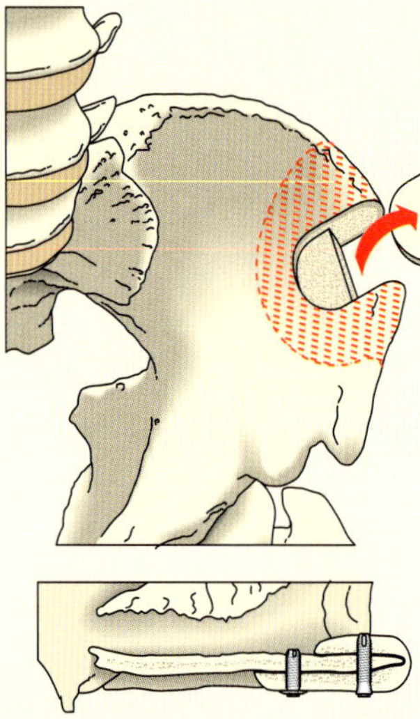

Fig 4-62 Nasal inlay and maxillary onlay with flange fixtures stabilizing the graft against the palate of the extremely resorbed maxilla.

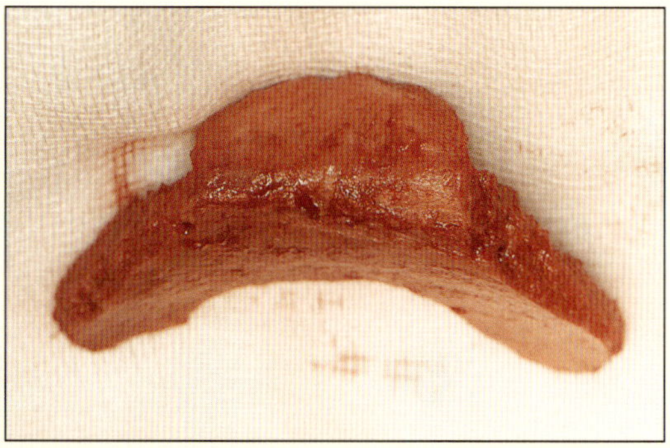

Fig 4-63 The detached graft.

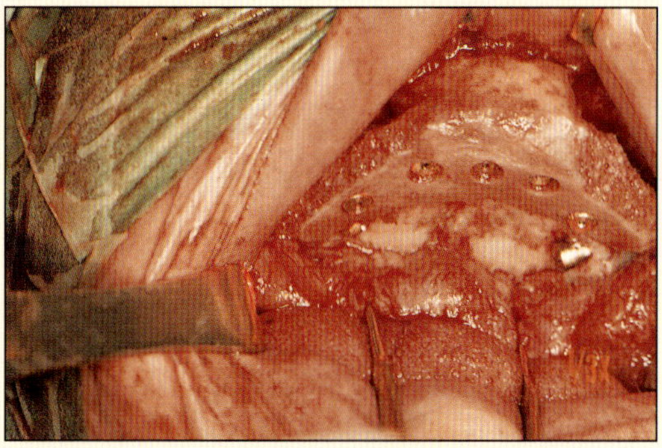

Fig 4-64 The graft in situ, stabilized with fixtures (October 1990).

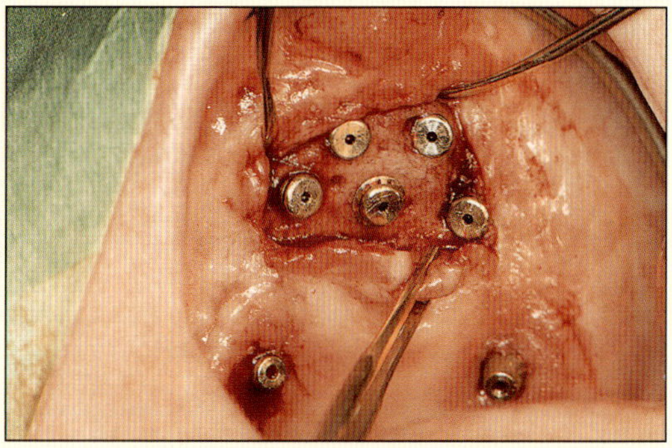

Fig 4-65 Additional fixtures installed. Note the flange fixture in the midline (May 1993).

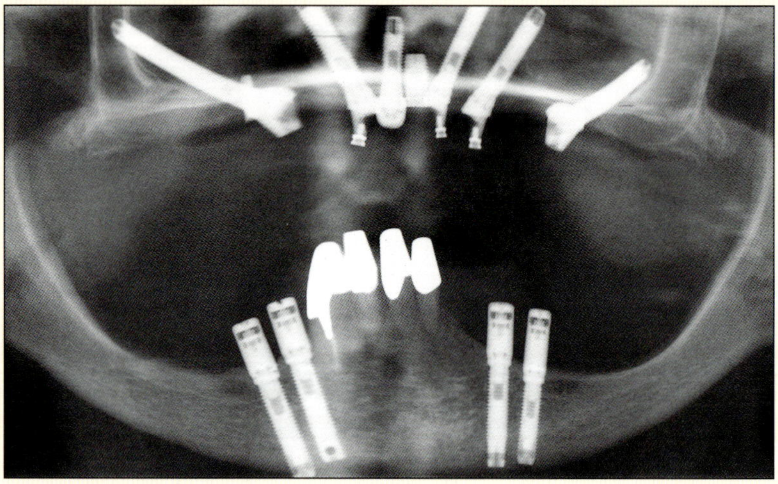

Fig 4-66 Abutment connection (1993).

Patient 5 (Compromised Group) continued

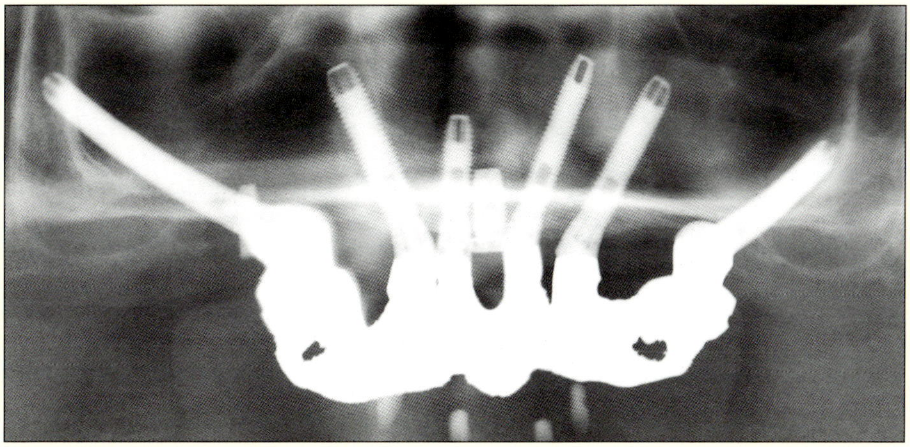

Fig 4-67 Two-year follow-up (1995).

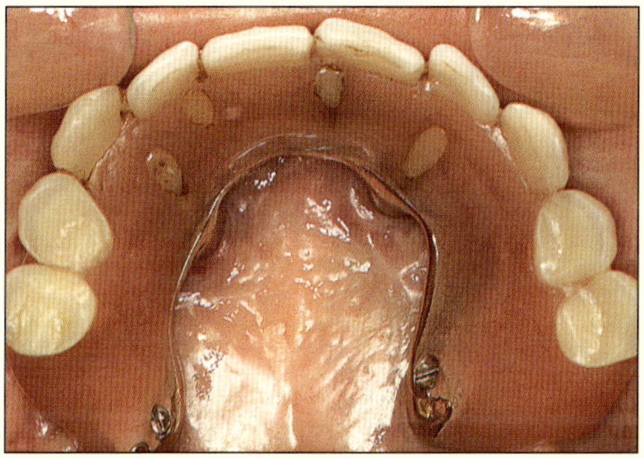

Fig 4-68 Intraoral view. The patient did not experience any discomfort from the two zygoma fixtures in the palate.

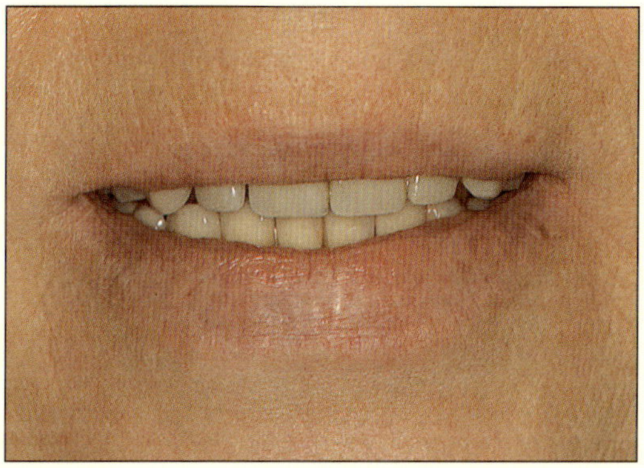

Fig 4-69 Clinical result at the 4-year follow-up.

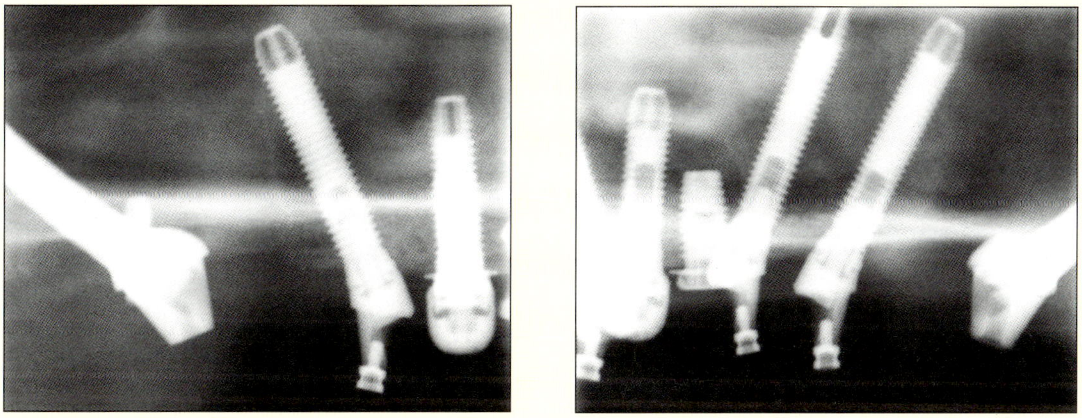

Fig 4-70 Dental scanograms (1993).

Patient 5 (Compromised Group) continued

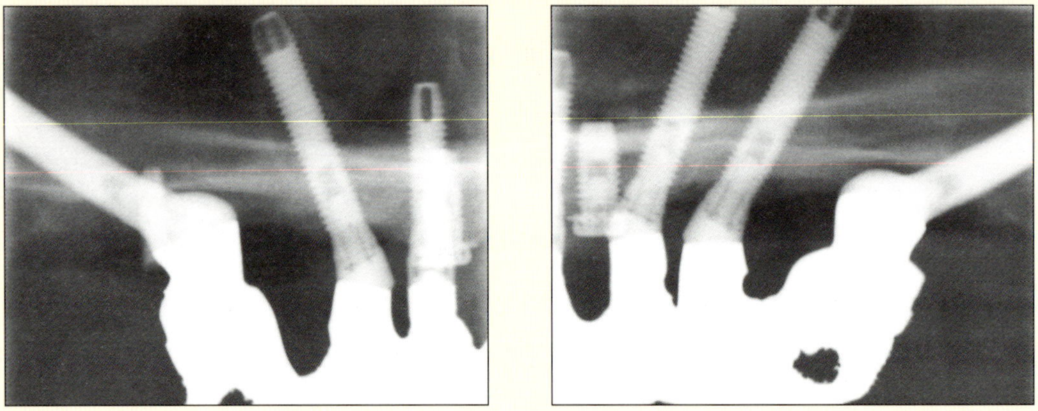

Fig 4-71 Dental scanograms (1997).

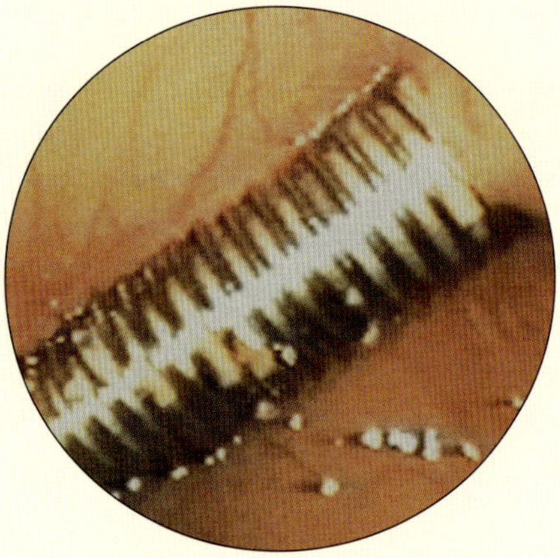

Fig 4-72 Photo obtained by B. Petruson during sinoscopy revealing a healthy mucosal status (1997).

CHAPTER 5

Unusual Case Presentations

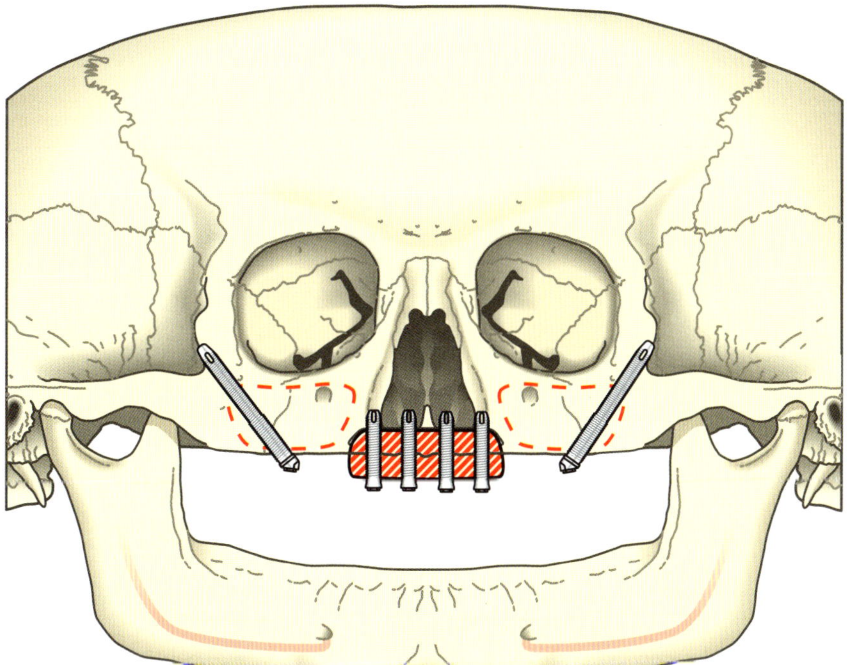

The following six patient presentations reveal some of the more unusual scenarios that were encountered during the study. They represent defect anatomies and reconstruction attempts that deviate considerably from what we have seen over a period of two decades of treating edentulous patients. The clinical outcome emphasizes that even nonconventional therapeutic procedures might work.

Patient 1 (Unusual Group)

Background

This female patient, born in 1939, became edentulous in the maxilla at the age of 25. In November 1984, she was rehabilitated elsewhere with a fixture-supported fixed prosthesis construction in the maxilla. Eventually only the fixtures in regions 14 and 24 remained. Because of the lack of bone support, she was forced to revert to a conventional denture. The patient exhibited a resorption pattern equivalent to type IV and a sinus configuration equivalent to type D (see Figs 2-1 and 2-2).

Surgical procedure

In January 1987, an onlay graft was taken from the left iliac crest. The graft was of moderate density and vascularity. It was attached to the maxillary base with three conical fixtures (10 and 13 mm). To incorporate the existing two fixtures in the new fixed prosthesis construction, an extension similar to a long abutment cylinder was attached to each fixture.

At the second stage in September 1987, all fixtures were well integrated. The patient was then referred back to her regular dentist for fixed prosthesis construction.

Follow-up

At the 3-year clinical follow-up visit, the patient was very satisfied and had not experienced any discomfort or complication. The clinical examination at the 12-year follow-up in 1999 (after conclusion of the study) revealed a stable fixed prosthesis and healthy soft tissue. The patient was pleased with all aspects of the prosthesis.

Patient 1 (Unusual Group)

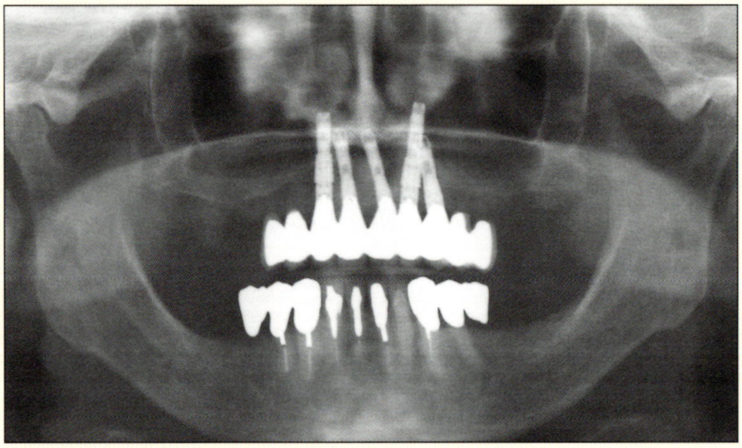

Fig 5-1 Connection of the fixed prosthesis (1987).

Patient 1 (Unusual Group) continued

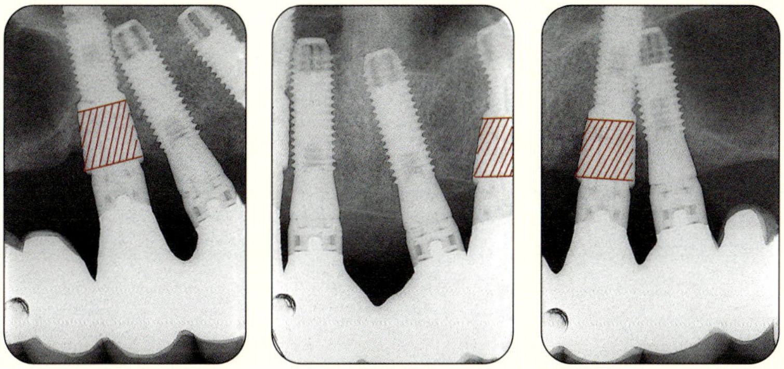

Fig 5-2 Three-year follow-up (1990). The special fixture extensions used to incorporate the two previously integrated fixtures into the new bridge are highlighted.

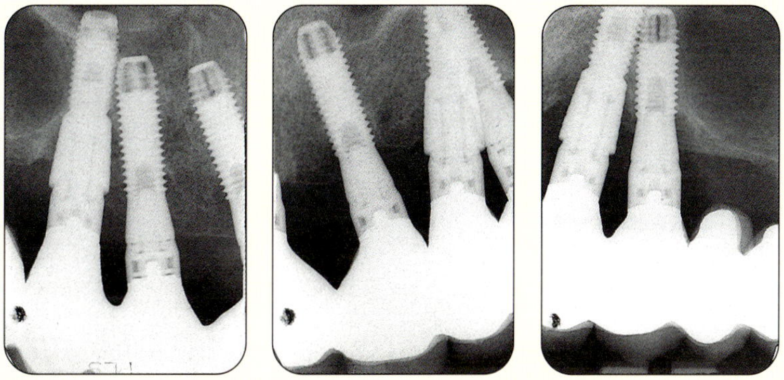

Fig 5-3 Twelve-year follow-up after conclusion of the study (1999).

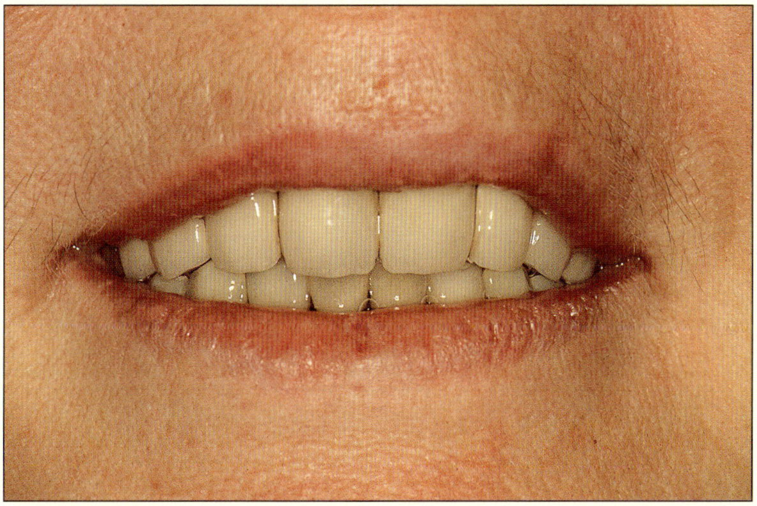

Fig 5-4 Clinical result.

Patient 2 (Unusual Group)

Background

This female patient was born in 1929. In 1987 she was treated by her local surgeon with a mandibular bone-anchored prosthesis with good function. In May of the same year she was also treated in her maxilla with four 7-mm fixtures without bone grafting. These fixtures and most of the alveolar bone were lost. In March 1991 she was subjected to additional treatment with four fixtures and a small inlay graft from her right ilium. When the patient first came to our clinic in 1993, only the two distal fixtures remained.

Preoperative comments

The patient had an extremely resorbed and thin maxilla with a resorption pattern equivalent to type IV and a sinus configuration equivalent to type B (see Figs 2-1 and 2-2).

Surgical procedure

In May 1993, the two existing maxillary fixtures were removed. A graft was then taken from the left medial ilium. The grafted bone was thin and of low density.

The graft was divided into two pieces: an onlay graft and an L-shaped nasal inlay. On the right side, two swan-neck fixtures were placed through the onlay graft, the premaxilla, and the nasal inlay (Fig 5-7). The stability was further enhanced with a zygoma fixture.

Because the left side was more compromised, it could only accommodate two regular fixtures and one zygoma fixture. The distal fixture was placed in the septum between the nasal cavity and the sinus with the apex penetrating into the sinus.

Complications

At abutment connection in January 1994, the second fixture on the left side had failed. A month later, the L1 fixture was also lost. The fixtures were not replaced because the patient did not wish to undergo additional surgery. The fixed prosthesis was instead constructed on the remaining four fixtures.

Follow-up

A dental scanogram taken at the 5-year follow-up visit showed minor bone loss adjacent to the R2 and R1 fixtures. A mid-face panorama demonstrated normal sinus conditions. Oral function was adequate.

Patient 2 (Unusual Group)

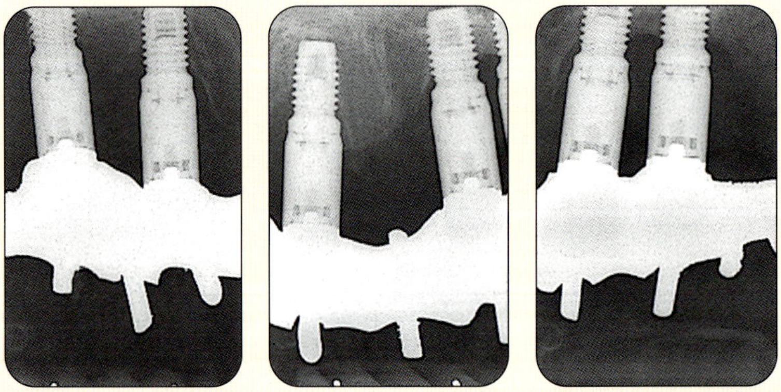

Fig 5-5 Four fixtures placed by the patient's hometown dentist in 1987.

Patient 2 (Unusual Group) continued

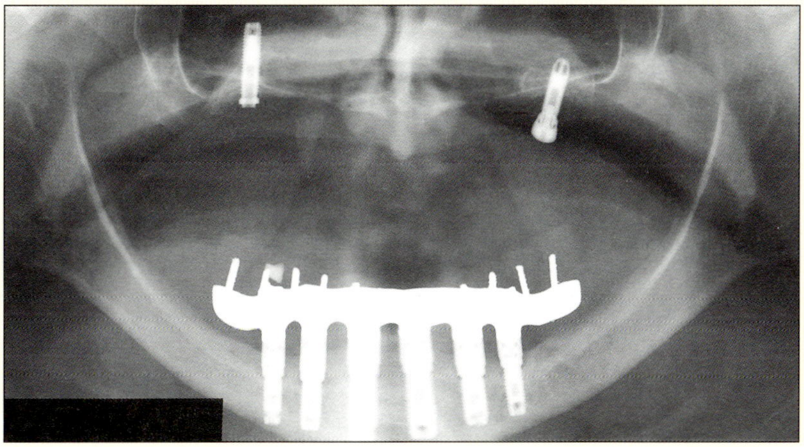

Fig 5-6 Status at initial visit (1993).

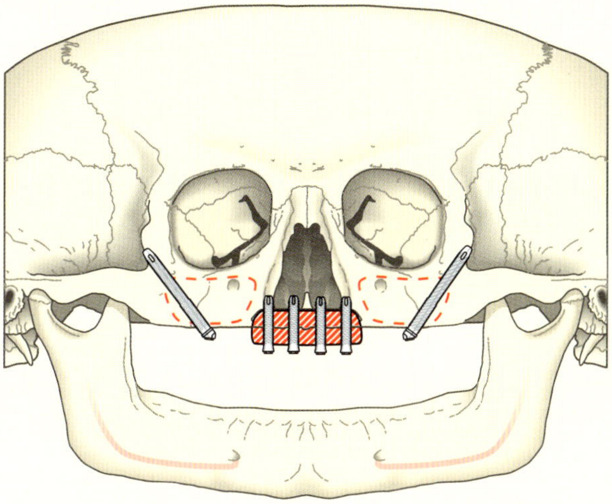

Fig 5-7 The "sandwich" approach. The anterior fixtures penetrate the onlay graft, the maxillary base, and the inlay graft.

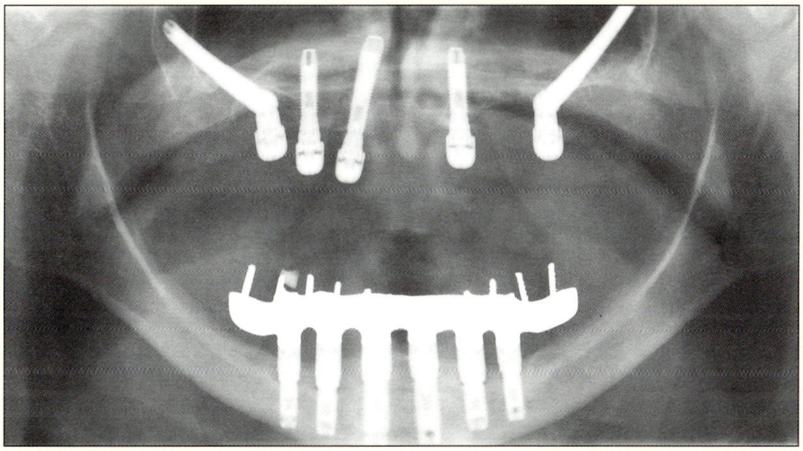

Fig 5-8 Abutment connection (January 1994).

Patient 2 (Unusual Group) continued

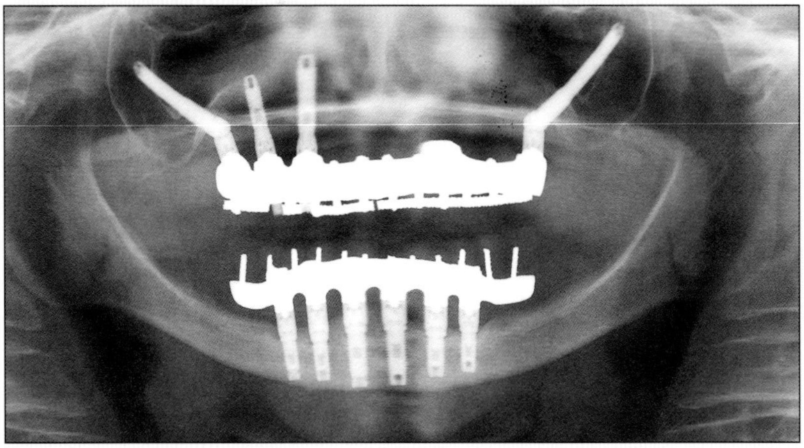

Fig 5-9 Five-year follow-up after conclusion of the study (1999).

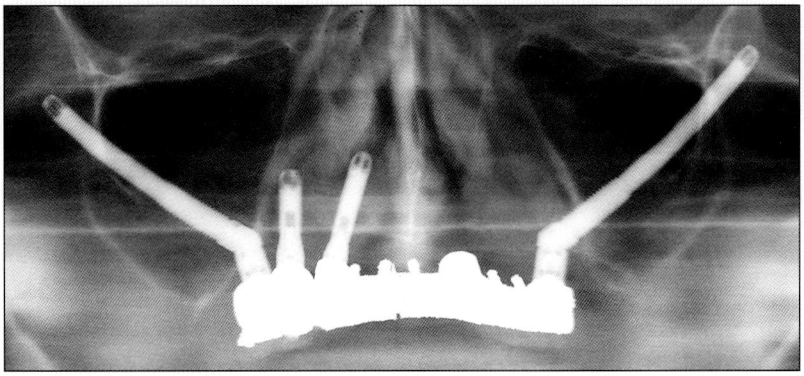

Fig 5-10 Mid-face (frontal) panorama demonstrating normal sinus conditions after conclusion of the study (1999).

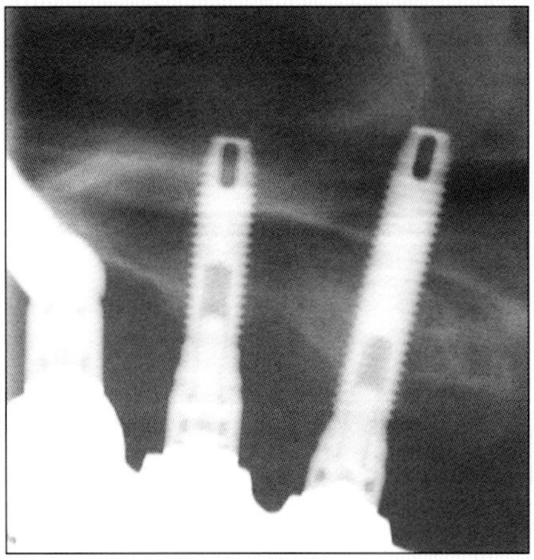

Fig 5-11 Dental scanogram after conclusion of the study (1999).

Patient 3 (Unusual Group)

Background

This female patient was born in 1934. She had been edentulous since 1962 when she was only 28 years old. She was a smoker. Her fixture-supported fixed prosthesis in the mandible was characterized by extensive cantilevers.

Preoperative comments

The sinus extended slightly in the anterior direction on both sides. The patient exhibited a resorption pattern equivalent to type III and a sinus configuration equivalent to type B (see Figs 2-1 and 2-2).

Surgical procedure

In February 1991, a thin onlay graft with a cortical layer was taken from the left ilium. It was stabilized with six swan-neck fixtures (13 and 20 mm). The two distal fixtures were placed in the bony septum between the sinus and nasal cavities. Good stability of graft and fixtures was achieved.

Follow-up

The patient was seen by her hometown dentist during the following 8 years. When she returned to us in May 1999, the R2 and L3 fixtures had been removed and replaced with two wide-diameter (5-mm) fixtures. The marginal bone level was located adjacent to the second thread of the R3 fixture, the third thread of the R2 fixture, and the first thread of the R1 and L3 fixtures. Oral function was adequate.

Patient 3 (Unusual Group)

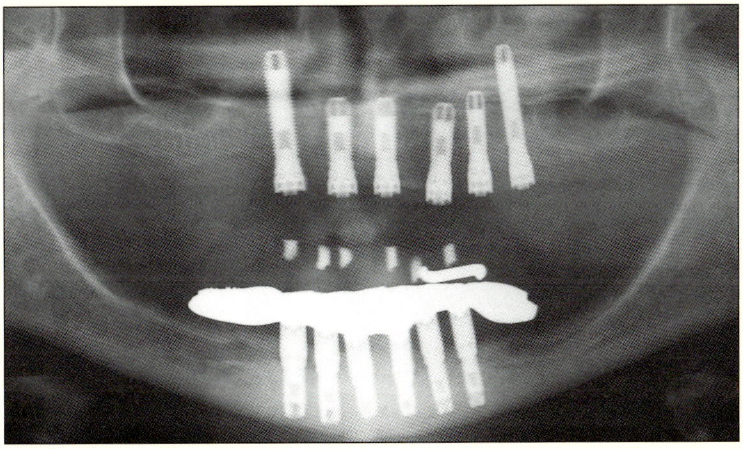

Fig 5-12 Abutment connection (1991).

Patient 3 (Unusual Group) continued

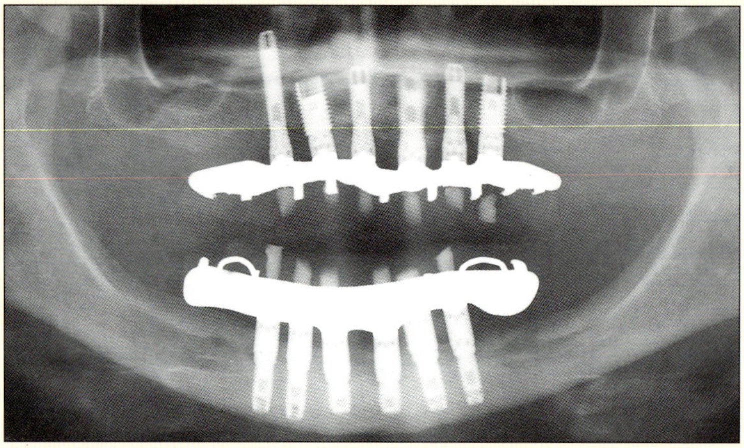

Fig 5-13 Panoramic image obtained at the 8-year examination after conclusion of the study (1999).

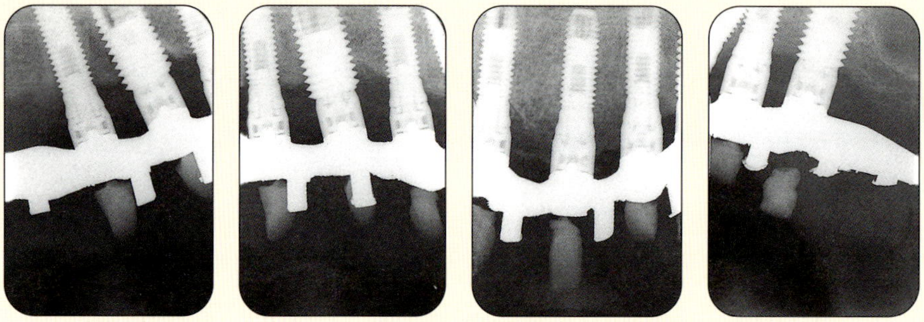

Fig 5-14 Intraoral view at the 8-year follow-up after conclusion of the study (1999).

Patient 4 (Unusual Group)

Background

This male patient was born in 1922. The mandibular dentition was dysfunctional and should have been reinforced prior to surgery in the maxilla.

Preoperative comments

The patient had a sinus that was extremely expanded bilaterally, almost bordering the midline. The available bone for fixture support was approximately 3 mm bilaterally. The patient exhibited a resorption pattern equivalent to type II and a sinus configuration equivalent to type E (see Figs 2-1 and 2-2).

Surgical procedure

In January 1986, an onlay graft was taken from the left lateral ilium and secured to the maxillary base with six conical self-tapping fixtures ranging in length from 10 to 15 mm. The two distal fixtures on the right penetrated the maxillary sinus, which had a wall resembling an eggshell. The medial fixtures penetrated the bottom of the nasal cavity. A small fracture in the graft (region 14) was corrected with spongious tissue from the donor site.

Complications

At the recall visit 1 month later, a small cyst, probably a liquified hematoma, was emptied of its content. The mucosa was not resutured because of the poor tissue quality.

In October 1986, the two distal fixtures on the left side were removed because of mobility. In preparation for a second fixture installation procedure, the dentition in the mandible was reinforced and adapted to the maxillary situation, a procedure that should have been done prior to the initial grafting procedure.

Additional surgery

In March 1987, the two distal fixtures on the right were removed. Large portions of the graft had resorbed and extensive amounts of granulation tissue and bone sequestra were removed. The resorption was extreme at this point, and the remaining bone was osteoporotic. However, two self-tapping 10-mm fixtures (the anterior fixture was 3 mm in diameter) could be installed on the right side. Acceptable primary stability was achieved. The anatomy of the left side did not offer any support for new fixtures. Abutment connection was performed on the two existing and well-integrated fixtures close to the midline.

Restoration and follow-up

The patient initially carried a provisional fixed prosthesis for the first year. The final fixed prosthesis was designed with utmost attention to occlusion and loading conditions. The prosthetic design was challenging, as only one anterior fixture was available for support on the left side.

At the 5-year follow-up visit in 1993, the bone level was located between the second and fourth thread of the R3, R1, and L1 fixtures. The marginal bone was at the first thread of the R2 fixture. Since then, the patient has been followed at his home clinic. No complications have been reported despite the challenging mechanical situation on the left side. Today, bilateral zygoma fixtures would have been installed.

Patient 4 (Unusual Group)

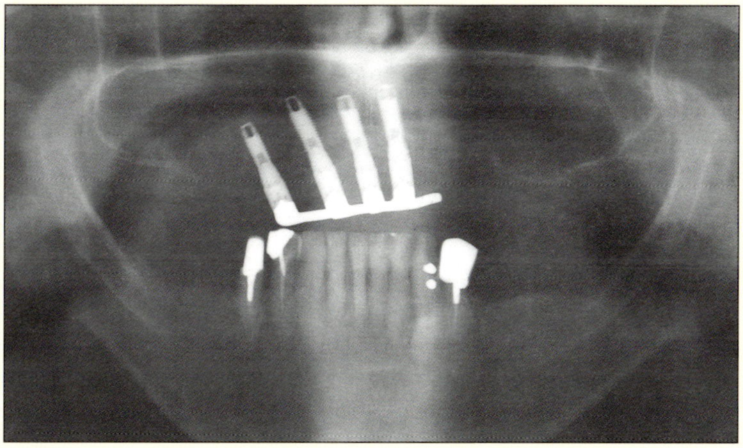

Fig 5-15 Status in February 1987. L3 and L2 were removed in October 1986.

Patient 4 (Unusual Group) continued

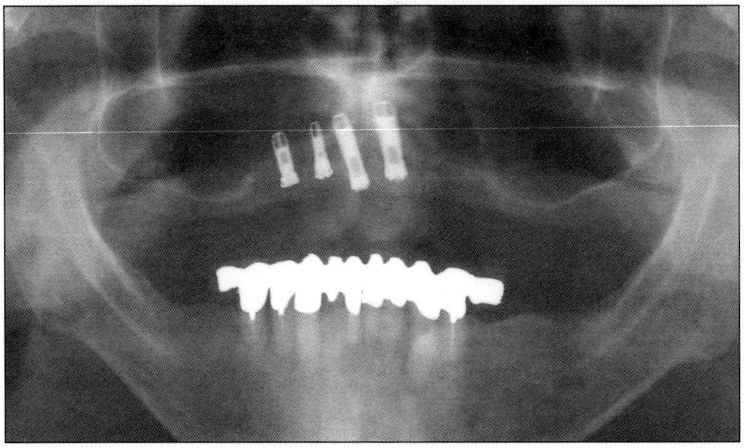

Fig 5-16 Panoramic view prior to abutment connection (September 1987). The R3 and R2 fixtures had been replaced in March 1987.

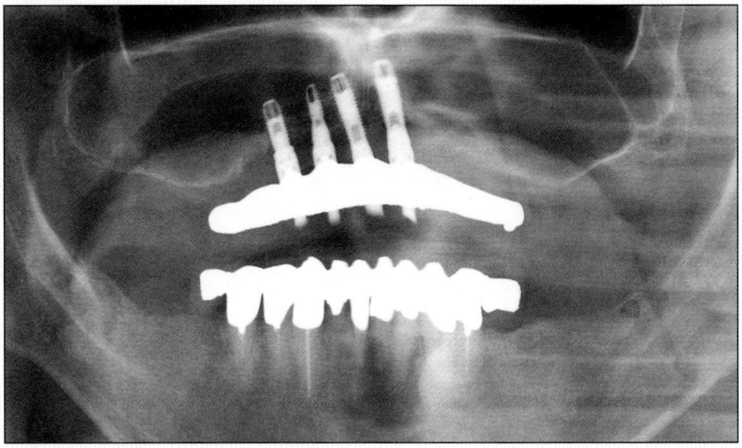

Fig 5-17 Five-year follow-up (1993).

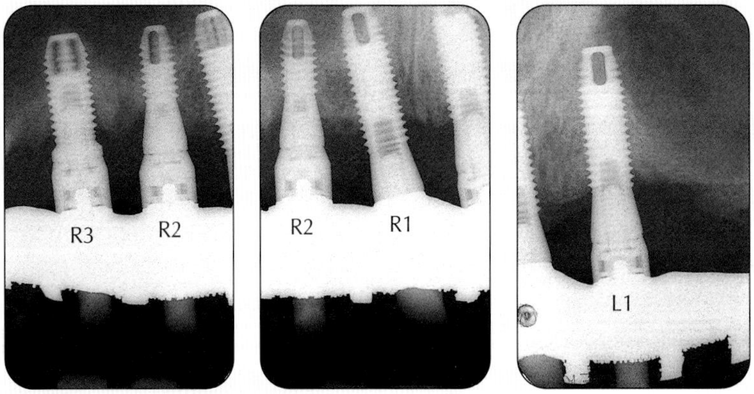

Fig 5-18 Five-year follow-up (1993).

Patient 4 (Unusual Group) continued

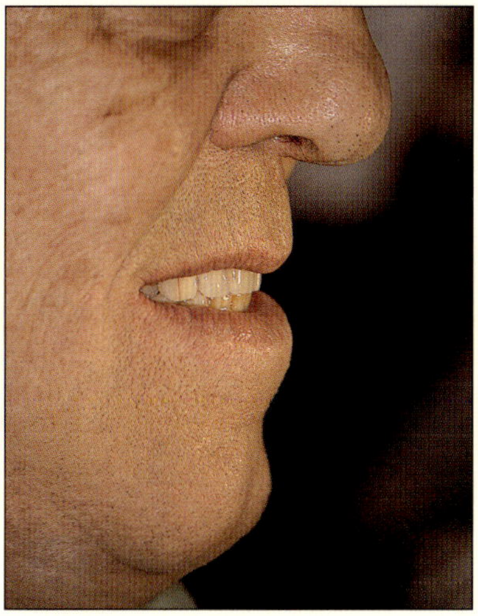

Fig 5-19 Clinical profile.

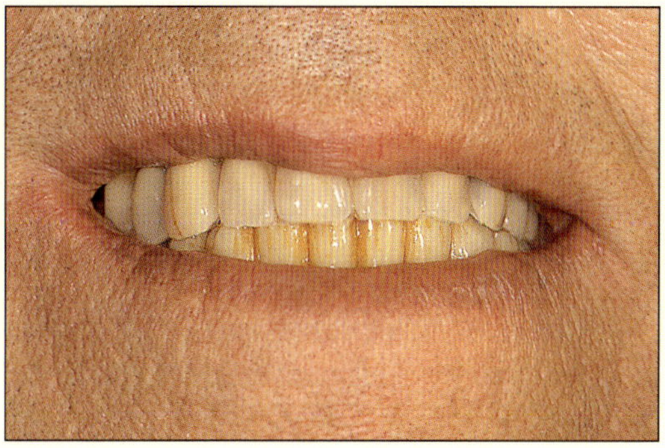

Fig 5-20 Clinical result.

Patient 5 (Unusual Group)

Background

This female patient was born in 1920. She had been edentulous since the age of 51 (1971). Her mandibular dentition required some endodontic work, but no preoperative reinforcement was needed.

Preoperative comments

The maxillary jaw was almost completely resorbed. The patient exhibited a resorption pattern equivalent to type IV and a sinus configuration equivalent to type B (see Figs 2-1 and 2-2).

Surgical procedure

In June 1986, an onlay graft was taken from the left lateral ilium. It was attached to the maxillary base with five standard fixtures. Adequate primary stability was achieved.

Complications and additional surgery

The fixed prosthesis was connected in 1987. Two years after surgery, the patient was temporarily struck by epilepsy. This occurred in association with treatment for a meningioma. She damaged both the maxillary and mandibular fixed prostheses during a seizure. After completion of the meningioma treatment, the epilepsy subsided. The R2 fixture was then removed because of mobility. It was replaced with two new fixtures (7 and 8 mm). The 7-mm swan-neck fixture was 5 mm in diameter and installed in the site previously occupied by the lost R2 fixture. The other fixture was placed in region R3. Excellent primary stability was obtained.

Follow-up

Upon completion of the medical treatment for the meningioma, the mandibular dentition was reconstructed by the patient's local dentist.

The clinical and radiographic evaluations at the 3-year follow-up visit demonstrated a stable and well-functioning maxillary situation, including good marginal bone support. The maxillary status remained unchanged at the 9-year follow-up in 1999 (after conclusion of the study).

Patient 5 (Unusual Group)

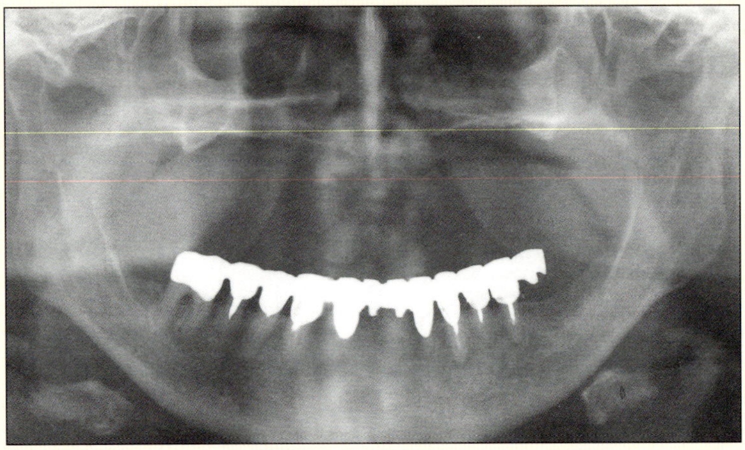

Fig 5-21 Preoperative panoramic view (1986).

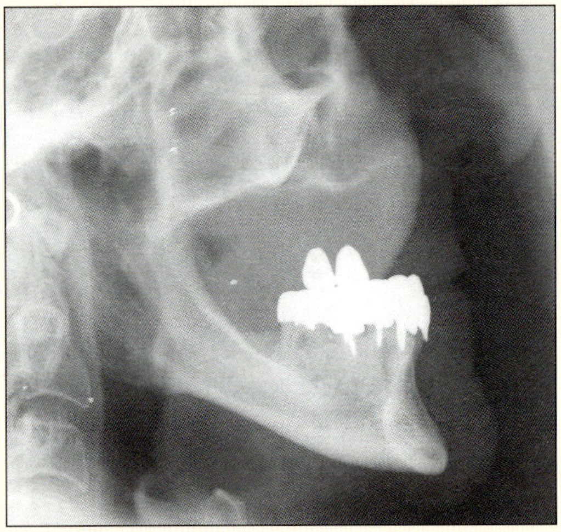

Fig 5-22 Preoperative profile.

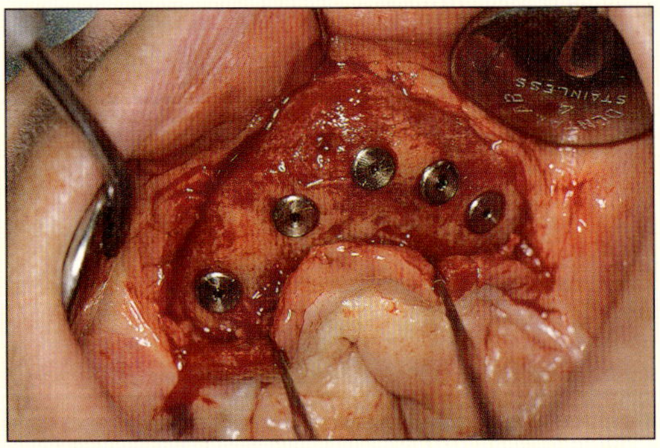

Fig 5-23 Fixtures placed through the graft.

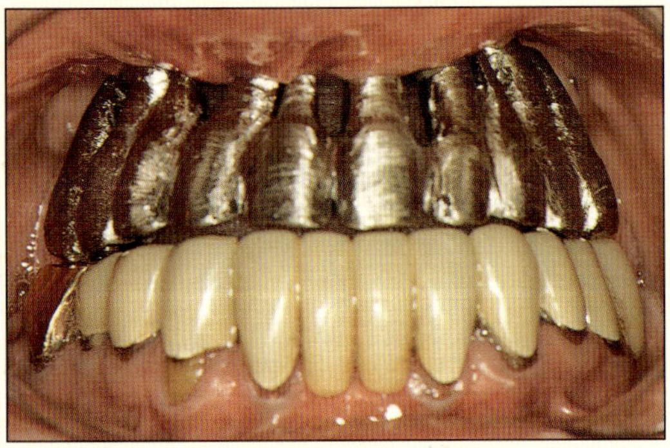

Fig 5-24 Trial of the framework of the fixed prosthesis.

Patient 5 (Unusual Group) continued

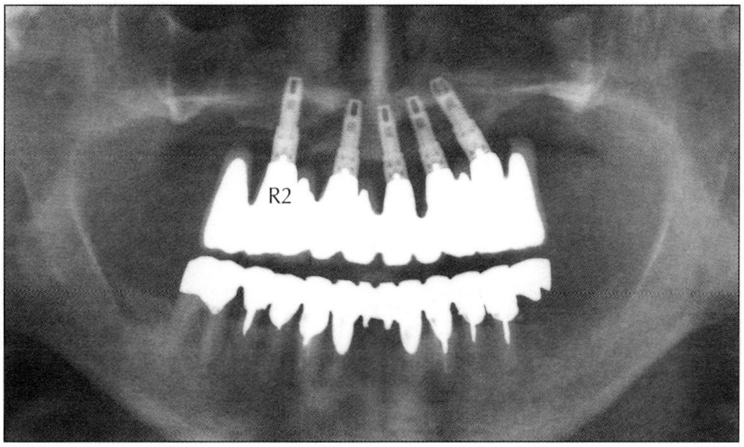

Fig 5-25 Connection of the fixed prosthesis (1987).

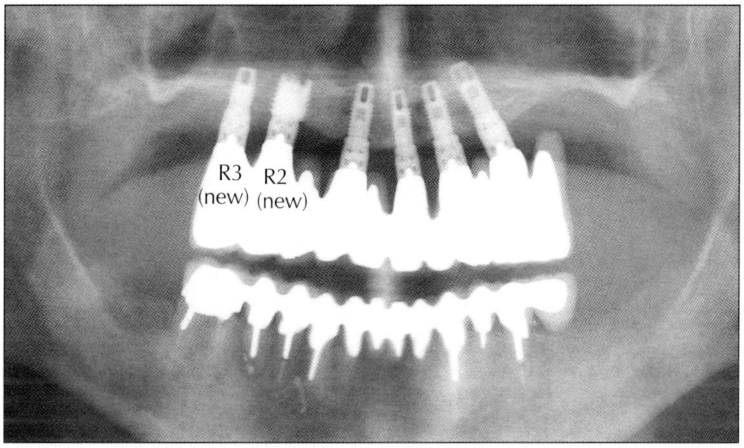

Fig 5-26 After damage to the maxillary and mandibular fixed prosthesis associated with a seizure in 1989. R2 became mobile and was replaced. Additional support was provided by a new fixture in the R3 region. The adjusted prosthesis was connected in early 1991.

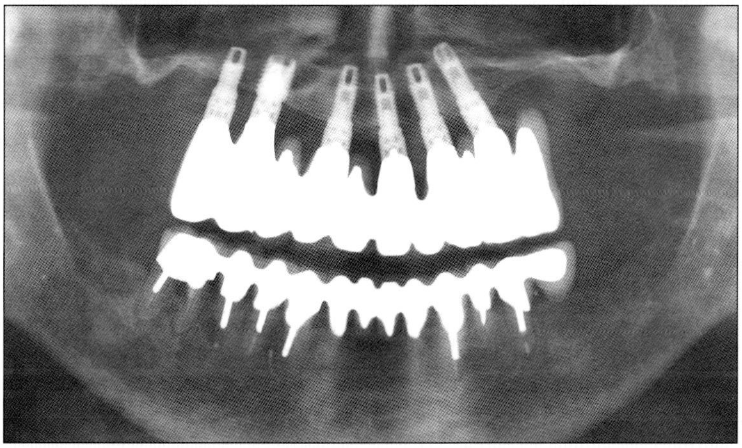

Fig 5-27 Nine-year follow-up after conclusion of the study (1999).

Patient 5 (Unusual Group) continued

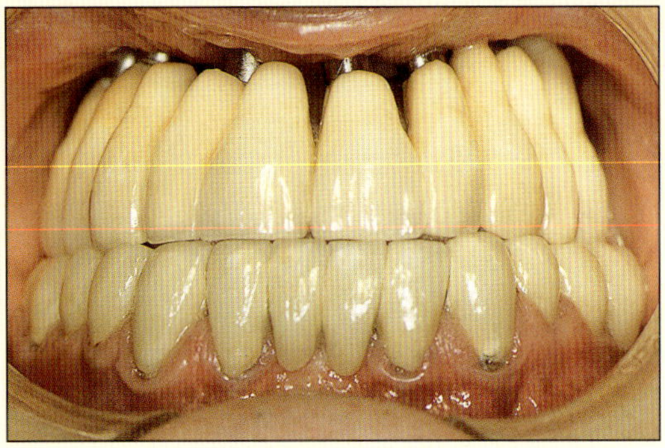

Fig 5-28 Clinical result.

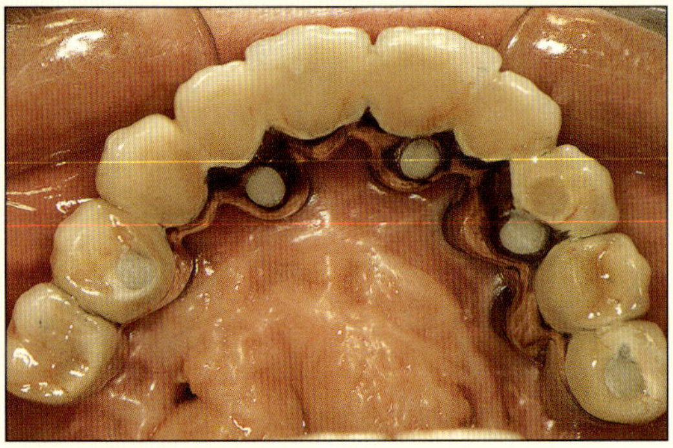

Fig 5-29 Intraoral view.

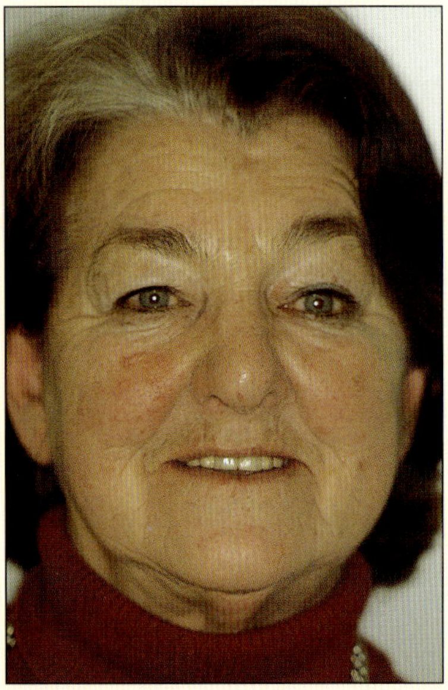

Fig 5-30 Facial view.

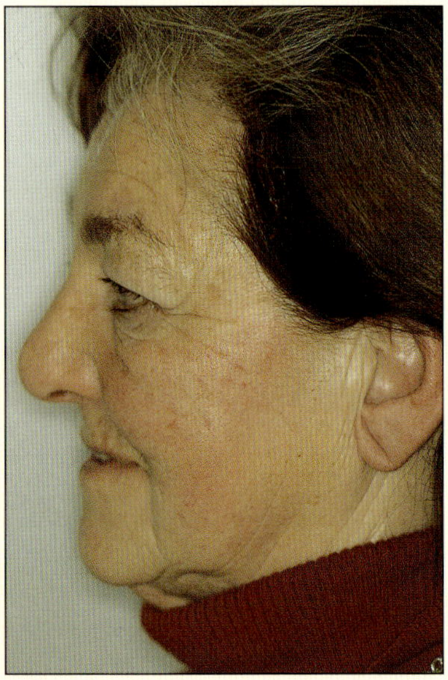

Fig 5-31 Facial profile.

Patient 6 (Unusual Group)

Background

This female patient was referred from the United States. She had been edentulous in the maxilla for decades and had been augmented with hydroxyapatite (HA) several times to enhance maxillary overdenture support. The treatment had failed each time and the patient was left with remnants of hard HA. Complete removal of the compact HA-particles was impossible. Such a procedure would have created direct communication with the sinus.

Preoperative comments

The maxillary bone height was 2 mm in the interior region and 1 mm at the base of the sinus region. The patient exhibited a resorption pattern equivalent to type IV and a sinus configuration equivalent to type B (see Figs 2-1 and 2-2).

Surgical procedure

At fixture surgery in January 1990, minimum bone was available distal to the piriform aperture. After removal of as much HA as possible (it was encapsulated in two distinct areas), an onlay graft of good strength and vascularity was taken from the left medial ilium. The graft was secured with five fixtures (13 and 18 mm). Good primary stability was achieved. The abutments were connected in early August 1990, at which time the graft was vital and all fixtures were stable.

Restoration and follow-up

The patient received her fixed prosthesis in late August 1990 and returned to the United States. When she came back for her first annual radiographic examination, a stable situation was noted. The clinical examination at that time revealed small amounts of granulation tissue around two of the abutments. Both abutments were therefore replaced with longer ones. The graft was well preserved and the soft tissue was healthy.

In December 1993, she returned for her 3-year follow-up visit. The fixed prosthesis was well adapted and the patient was pleased with both function and esthetics. Continued follow-up was carried out by her home clinic in the United States, but sporadic contacts (most recently in 2000) have verified that no complications have occurred and that the fixed prosthesis continues to function well. The results of the serial rehabilitation have been particularly appreciated by the patient.

Patient 6 (Unusual Group)

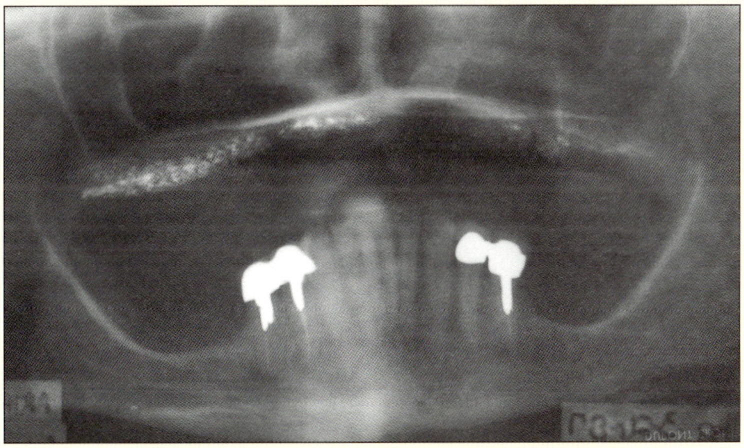

Fig 5-32 Preoperative panoramic view. Note the remaining hydroxyapatite.

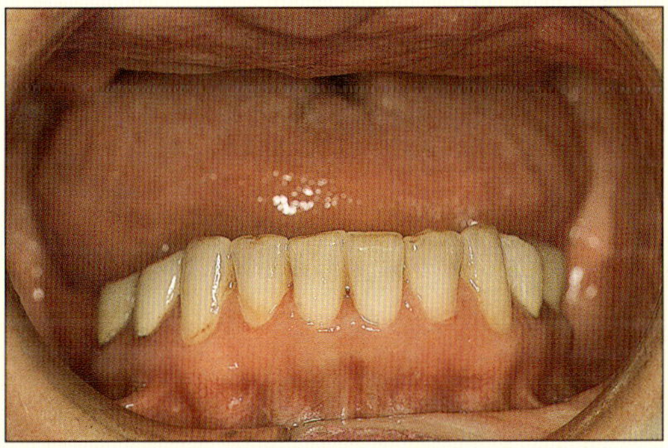

Fig 5-33 Clinical status before treatment.

Patient 6 (Unusual Group) continued

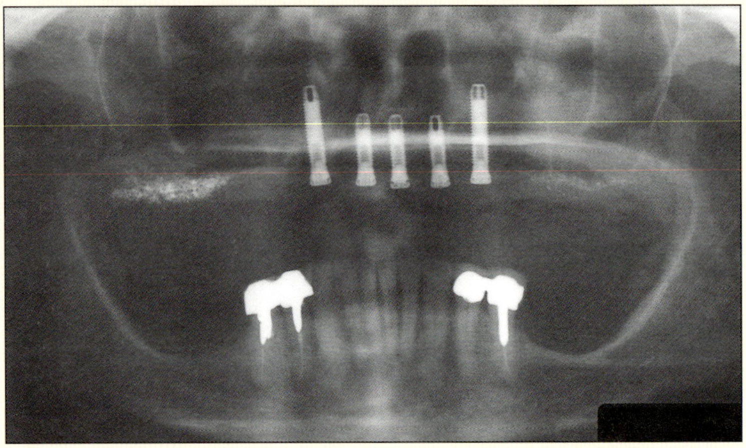

Fig 5-34 Fixture placement (1990). Only part of the encapsulated hydroxyapatite could be removed because of the risk of penetrating the palate.

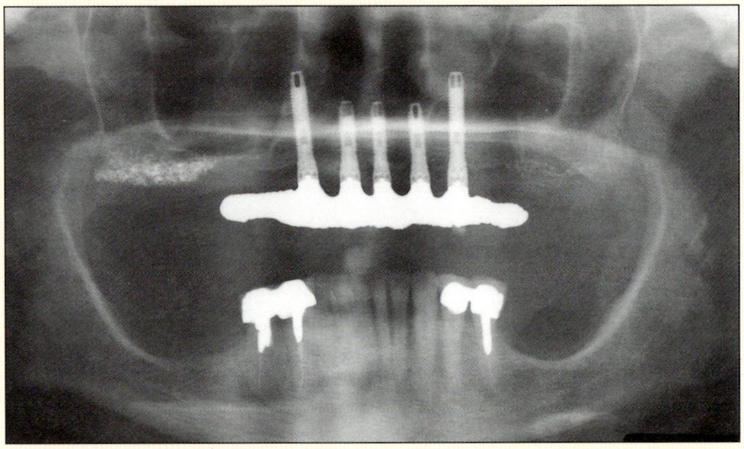

Fig 5-35 One-year follow-up (1991).

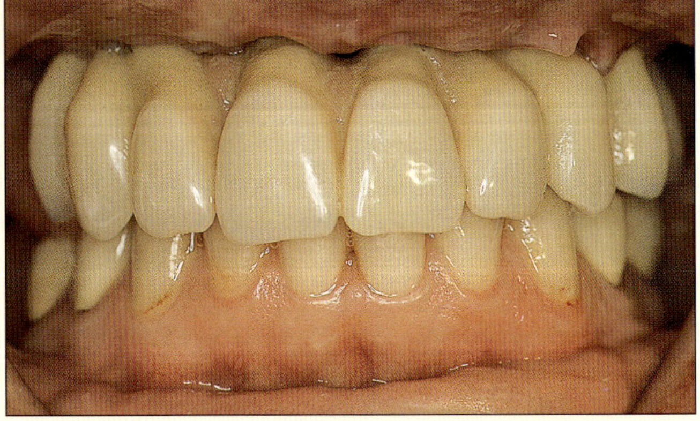

Fig 5-36 Clinical status after treatment.

Patient 6 (Unusual Group) continued

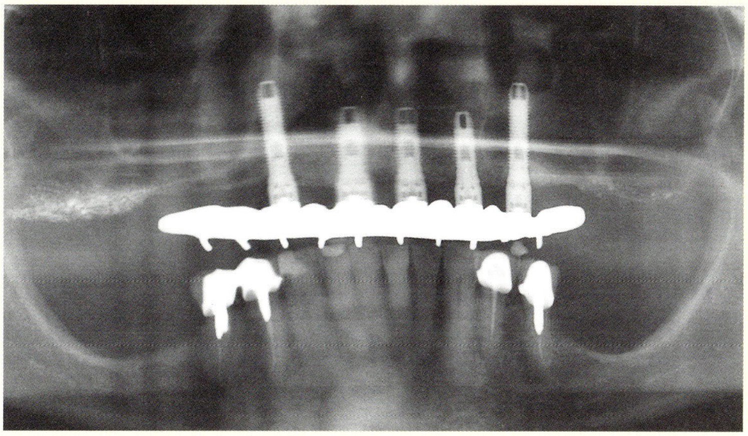

Fig 5-37 Ten-year follow-up after conclusion of the study (2000; courtesy of Dr. Thomas J. Balshi).

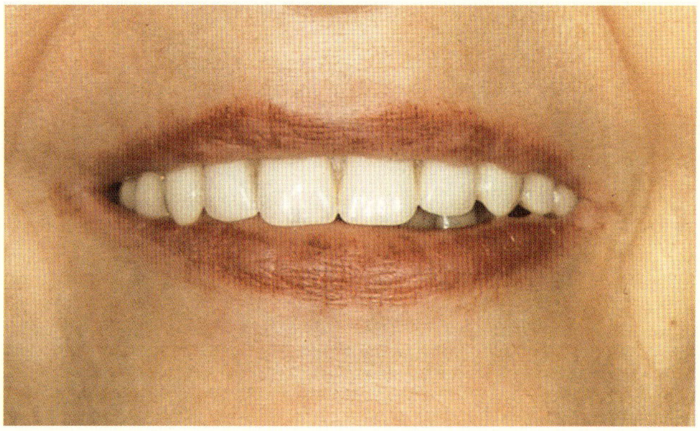

Fig 5-38 Clinical status at 10-year follow-up after conclusion of the study (2000; courtesy of Dr. Thomas J. Balshi).

CHAPTER 6

Appraisal of Restored Anatomy and Function

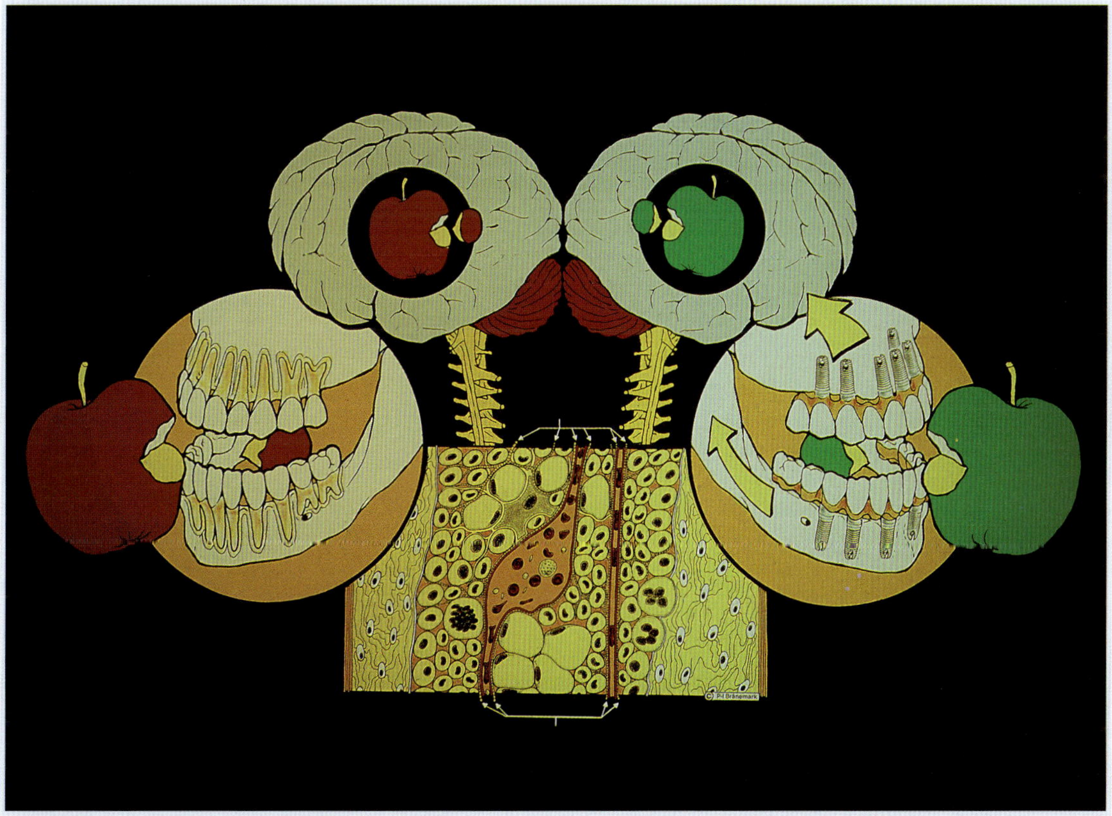

Table 6-1 Status of prosthetic rehabilitation at the end of the study*

Status of prosthetic	Development group (n = 27)	Routine group (n = 138)	All patients (N = 165)
Original bone-anchored fixed prosthesis in function	20 (12.1%)	108 (65.5%)	128 (77.6%)
Original overdenture in function	1 (0.6%)	13 (7.9%)	14 (8.5%)
Changed or altered prosthesis in function	3 (1.8%)	9 (5.5%)	12 (7.3%)
Early failure (no bone-anchored prosthesis delivered)	2 (1.2%)	2 (1.2%)	4 (2.4%)
Failure after delivery of prosthesis	1 (0.6%)	6 (3.6%)	7 (4.2%)

*Percentages are calculated using the entire patient population (N = 165).

The data is not divided into routine and development groups; rather, results are primarily reported as totals for all 165 patients–with the focus on the originally installed fixtures. Emphasis has also been placed on treatment result; that is, whether or not the patient could carry a maxillary prosthetic restoration anchored on the original fixtures installed. Individual fixture survival rates are also reported.

Restored Prosthetic Function

The study ended on December 31, 1998, at which time 154 of the 165 patients carried a functioning bone-anchored maxillary prosthesis. Eleven patients were forced to revert to wearing a conventional denture (Table 6-1). Of these, 4 patients experienced early failures and were never fitted with a fixture-supported fixed prosthesis. These 4 patients had 22 fixtures installed. All but 7 of the fixtures were lost within the first year following surgery. The other 7 patients had bone-anchored prosthetic devices in function between 2 and 6 years (mean, 4 years) prior to conversion to a conventional denture.

Continuous fixed prosthesis function

Continuous fixed prosthesis function throughout the study period was achieved by 128 (78%) of the 165 patients who wore the same fixed prostheses at the end of the study as they did in the beginning. Fourteen of 16 patients who carried an overdenture at the end of the study exhibited continuous function. Two patients converted from a fixed prosthesis to an overdenture. One patient converted from an overdenture to a fixed prosthesis.

Aspects of time

The rates of restored prosthetic function for the routine period as well as for all patients are found in Table 6-2 and Fig 6-1. The main difference between the total group of patients and those treated during the routine period was that the latter demonstrated slightly higher survival rates, for example 94% vs 93% after 10 years. Table 6-3 shows the number of patients at risk as well as failures at the different annual time intervals.

Results for patients with less than four fixtures

At the end of the study, 21 patients had their prosthetic devices anchored on less than four fixtures. This was usually because of failure of one or more fixtures. The system survival rate for these 21 patients was 81% after 3 years, 61% after 5 years, and 44% after 10 years.

Results by donor site

The treatment results by graft donor site are shown in Table 6-4. The survival rate was slightly higher for the medial vs the lateral ilium ($P = .07$): 96% after 8 years when the graft was taken from the medial ilium and 88% when it was taken from the lateral side. A contributing factor might be that the lateral ilium was primarily used in the developmental period of the study.

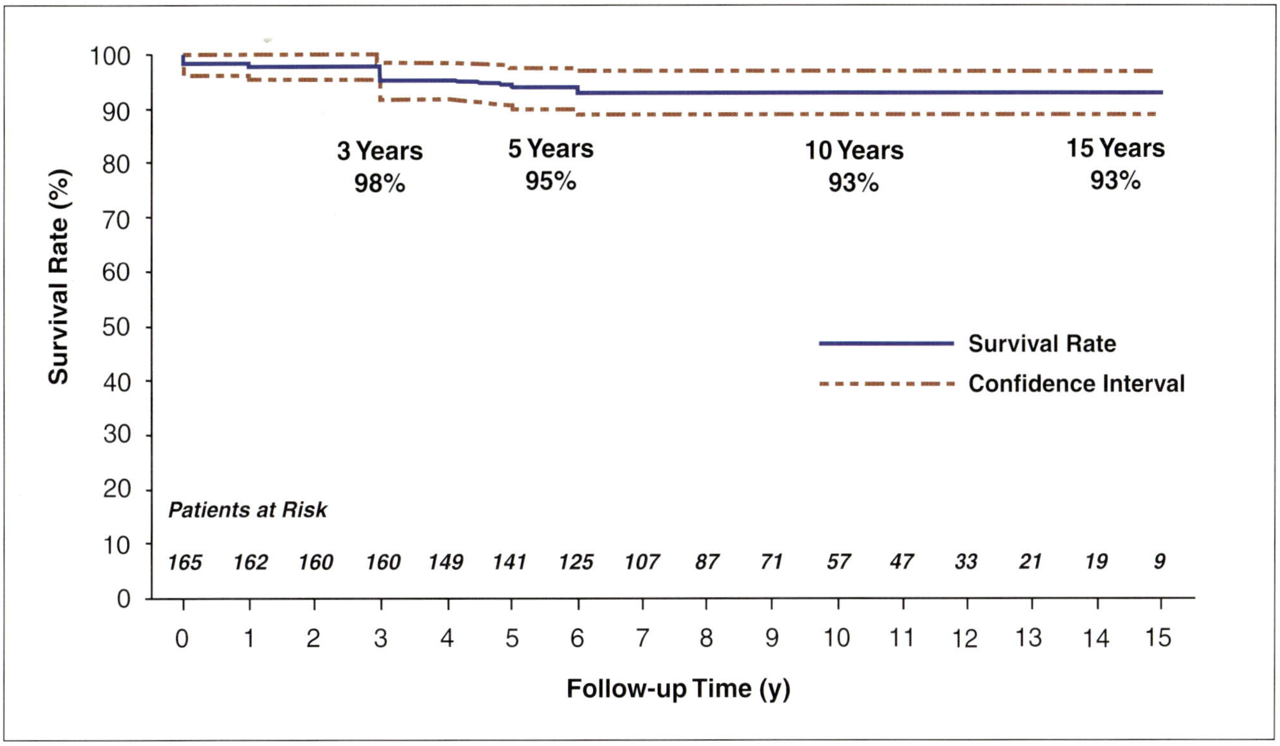

Fig 6-1 Restored prosthetic function—all patients (survival distribution function and 95% confidence interval).

Table 6-2 Prosthetic system survival

Time since surgery (y)	Routine group (%) (n = 138)	All patients (%) (N = 165)
3	98.5	97.6
5	96.3	95.0
10	93.6	92.8
15	n/a*	92.8

*No patients in the routine period were followed for 15 years.

Table 6-3 Number of patients at risk and failures by annual follow-up intervals

Follow-up time (y)	Patients at risk at start of period	Treatment failures
0–1	165	3
1–2	162	1
2–3	160	0
3–4	160	4
4–5	149	0
5–6	141	2
6–7	125	1
7–8	107	0
8–9	87	0
9–10	71	0
10–11	57	0
11–12	47	0
12–13	33	0
13–14	21	0
14–15	19	0
0–15	165	11

Table 6-4 System survival by donor site (Kaplan-Meier)

Graft donor site	Number of patients	3-year survival (patients)	5-year survival (patients)	8-year survival (patients)
Medial ilium	83	99% (82)	96% (69)	96% (39)
Lateral ilium	57	95% (54)	93% (52)	88% (47)
Medial and lateral ilium	8	100% (7)	100% (5)	n/a*
Iliac crest	17	100% (17)	94% (15)	n/a*

*Too few patients for analysis.

Table 6-5 Postoperative donor site morbidity (postoperative pain)

Donor site morbidity	Development group (n = 27)	Routine group (n = 138)	All patients (N = 165)
Pain	3 (11.1%)	8 (5.8%)	11 (6.7%)
No pain	24 (88.9%)	130 (94.2%)	154 (93.3%)

Table 6-6 Failed fixtures vs donor site morbidity (postoperative pain)*

Donor site morbidity	No fixture failure	1–4 fixtures lost	> 4 fixtures lost	Mean no. of fixtures lost	*P* value
Pain	5 (62.5%)	1 (12.5%)	2 (25.0%)	2.38	ns
No pain	72 (55.4%)	46 (35.4%)	12 (9.2%)	1.17	

*Only includes data for patients in the routine group (n = 138).

Donor Site Morbidity

Few complications occurred at the donor site during the study. The only parameter that warranted concern was related to postoperative pain, which was therefore thoroughly investigated. Pain from the hip donor site persisted longer than 2 weeks in 11 (7%) of the 165 patients. Three patients (2%) exhibited local hematoma formation. The frequency of pain is shown in Table 6-5. When the results were correlated to fixture loss, no significant statistical difference was noted between the two groups (Table 6-6).

When the graft was taken from the lateral side, a subperiosteal dissection of the external gluteal muscles was necessary to provide access to the donor area. Subsequently the postoperative morbidity could be reduced when the medial ilium constituted the donor site. The preoperative topography of the upper lateral aspect of the iliac crest was also preserved. The combination of these factors favored the procedural alteration of taking the graft from the medial ilium with the intention of preserving the external periosteum intact and attached to the muscles. This, in turn, minimized the risk for hematoma formation, postoperative pain, and other complications.

Results of multidisciplinary study on donor site morbidity

The study comprised 61 patients who were consecutively treated during the routine period. These patients were evaluated according to the multidisciplinary approach described under "Surgical and Prosthetic Procedures" in chapter 2. The patients gave their subjective appraisal of pain according to questionnaires prepared by orthopedic and physiotherapeutic experts. The pain was rated on a scale from 0 (no pain) to 10 (severe pain). The mean subjectively assessed pain was 5 within the first 1 to 7 days after surgery. It then decreased to 3 (range, 0 to 8) after one month and 0.1 (range, 0 to 2) at the last follow-up visit. At their last recall visit, 66% of the participating patients had been followed for 3 to 5 years (mean, 4 years; SD, 1.9). The detailed results are shown by baseline data in Table 6-7, and by donor site in both Table 6-7 and Fig 6-2. There was no statistical correlation between the subjective degree of pain and the donor site.[30]

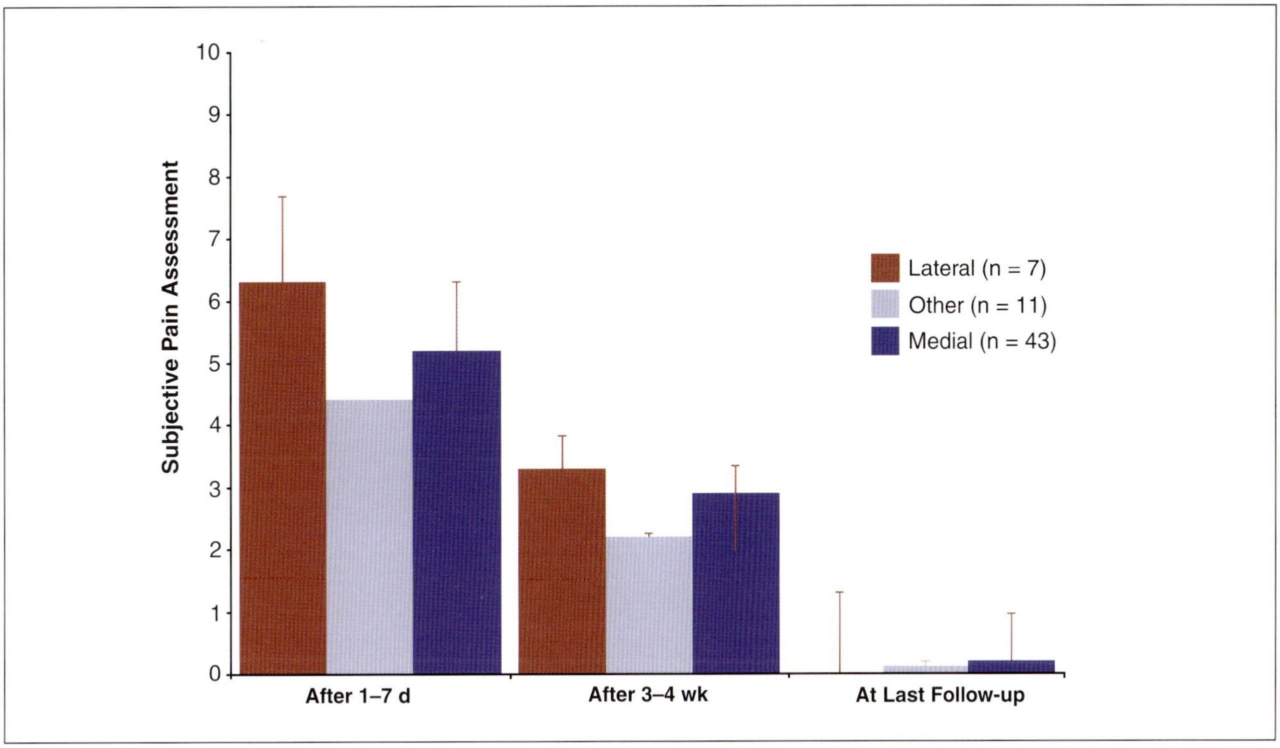

Fig 6-2 Multidisciplinary study of donor site morbidity including standard error (n=61).

Table 6-7 Result of multidisciplinary study on assessment of donor site morbidity vs baseline patient profile and donor site

Patient characteristics	Number of patients	Mean pain after 1-7 days (SD)	Mean pain after 3–4 weeks (SD)	Mean pain at last follow-up visit* (SD)
All patients	61	5.2 (3.9)	2.8 (2.8)	0.1 (0.4)
Sex				
Male	22	5.1 (3.8)	2.0 (2.6)	0.1 (0.3)
Female	39	5.2 (3.5)	3.3 (2.9)	0.2 (0.5)
Age (y)				
< 50	18	5.0 (3.2)	2.5 (2.7)	0.1 (0.3)
50–65	27	6.4 (3.2)	3.7 (2.9)	0.2 (0.5)
> 65	16	3.4 (3.9)	1.8 (2.6)	0.1 (0.3)
Donor site				
Lateral ilium	7	6.3 (3.7)	3.3 (3.0)	0.0 (0.0)
Medial ilium	43	5.2 (3.4)	2.9 (2.9)	0.2 (0.5)
Other (see Table 2-2)	11	4.4 (4.2)	2.2 (2.5)	0.1 (0.3)

*The last follow-up visit occurred after 3 to 5 years on average.

Disturbed Healing at the Recipient Site

At times dehiscences could be traced to inadequate closure of the mucoperiosteum. Lack of closure led to communication with the oral or nasal cavity and subsequent graft contamination. When such a scenario was noticed, immediate surgical intervention was initiated. This involved removal of infectious tissue followed by careful resuturing. The intervention was essential to prevent infection and subsequent fixture failure. The situation is exemplified by patients 1 and 4 (compromised group) in chapter 4.

Out of the 165 cases, there were 26 incidents (16%) of dehiscences at the recipient site (Table 6-8). The figure includes very small dehiscences. A subsequent infection was seen in 14 patients (9%). Sequestra were formed in 31 patients (19%). Five

Table 6-8 Disturbed healing at the recipient site

Disturbed healing	Development group (n = 27)	Routine group (n = 138)	All patients (N = 165)
Dehiscence			
Yes	5 (18.5%)	21 (15.2%)	26 (15.8%)
No	22 (81.5%)	117 (84.8%)	139 (84.2%)
Infection			
Yes	3 (11.1%)	11 (8.0%)	14 (8.5%)
No	24 (88.9%)	127 (92.0%)	151 (91.5%)
Sequestrum			
Yes	8 (29.6%)	23 (16.7%)	31 (18.8%)
No	19 (70.4%)	115 (83.3%)	134 (81.2%)

Table 6-9 Failed fixtures vs disturbed healing at the recipient site*

Disturbed healing	No fixture failure	1–4 fixtures lost	> 4 fixtures lost	Mean no. of fixtures lost	*P* value
Dehiscence					
Yes (n = 21)	6 (28.6%)	10 (47.6%)	5 (23.8%)	2.86	.006
No (n = 117)	71 (60.7%)	37 (31.6%)	9 (7.7%)	0.96	
Infection					
Yes (n = 11)	3 (27.3%)	2 (18.2%)	6 (54.5%)	4.27	.001
No (n = 127)	74 (58.3%)	45 (35.4%)	8 (6.3%)	0.98	
Sequestrum					
Yes (n = 23)	6 (26.1%)	12 (52.2%)	5 (21.7%)	2.56	.003
No (n = 115)	71 (61.7%)	35 (30.4%)	9 (7.8%)	0.98	

*Only includes data for patients in the routine group (n = 138).

patients (3%) experienced dehiscence, infection, and sequestrum at the recipient site, whereas 118 patients (72%) did not exhibit any of the symptoms. When the data on disturbed healing was related to fixture survival in the routine group, it was noted that all parameters were significantly correlated to fixture failure (Table 6-9).

Patients with dehiscence or local infection at the recipient site subsequently demonstrated significantly reduced system survival rates ($P < .001$). As seen in the system survival curves for these patients (Figs 6-3 and 6-4), the 5-year survival rate was 64% among patients with infection and 98% for patients without infection.

Fixture Survival

Original and additional fixtures

Table 6-10 shows the number of installed and failed original fixtures (ie, the fixtures placed at the time of grafting). The table also accounts for the same data relating to all fixtures, including additional fixtures placed later in the study. The scenario is further exemplified by Fig 6-5. The overall fixture survival rate of originally installed fixtures during the routine period was 81%. That figure remained approximately the same when the additional fixtures were included in the results.

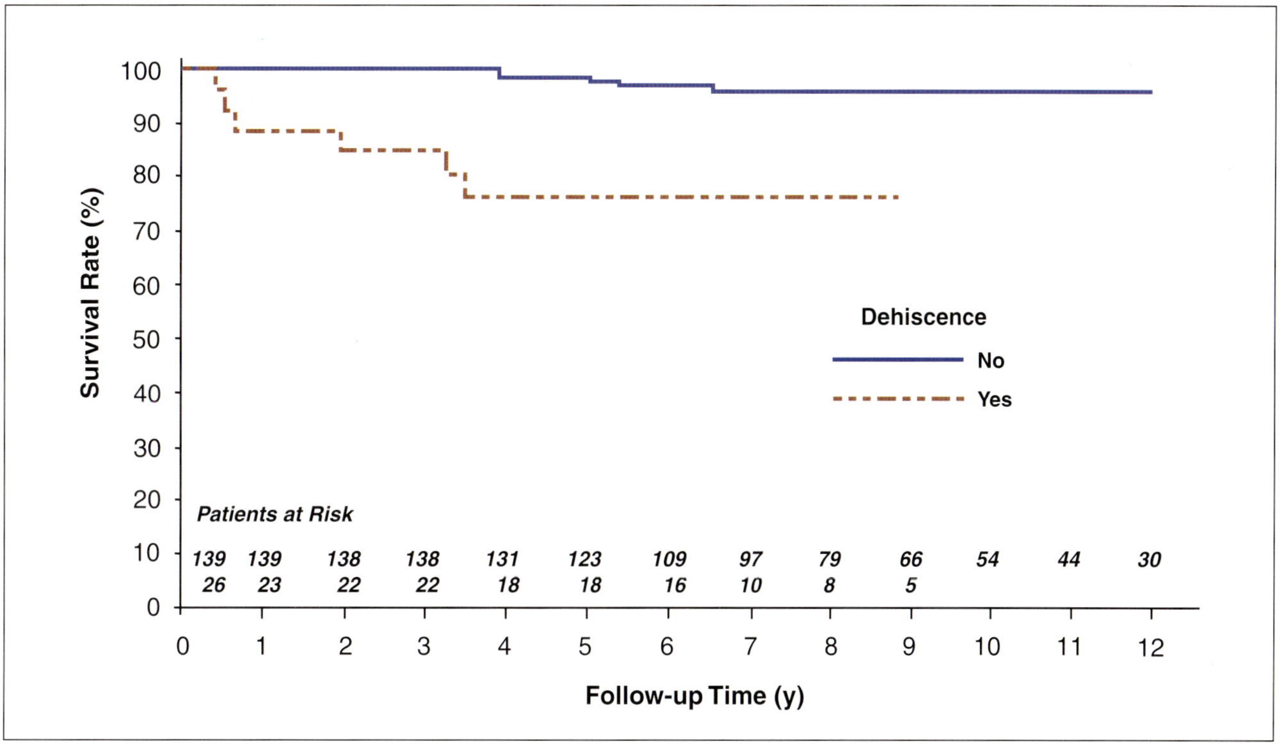

Fig 6-3 Patients with and without dehiscence at the recipient site (survival distribution function).

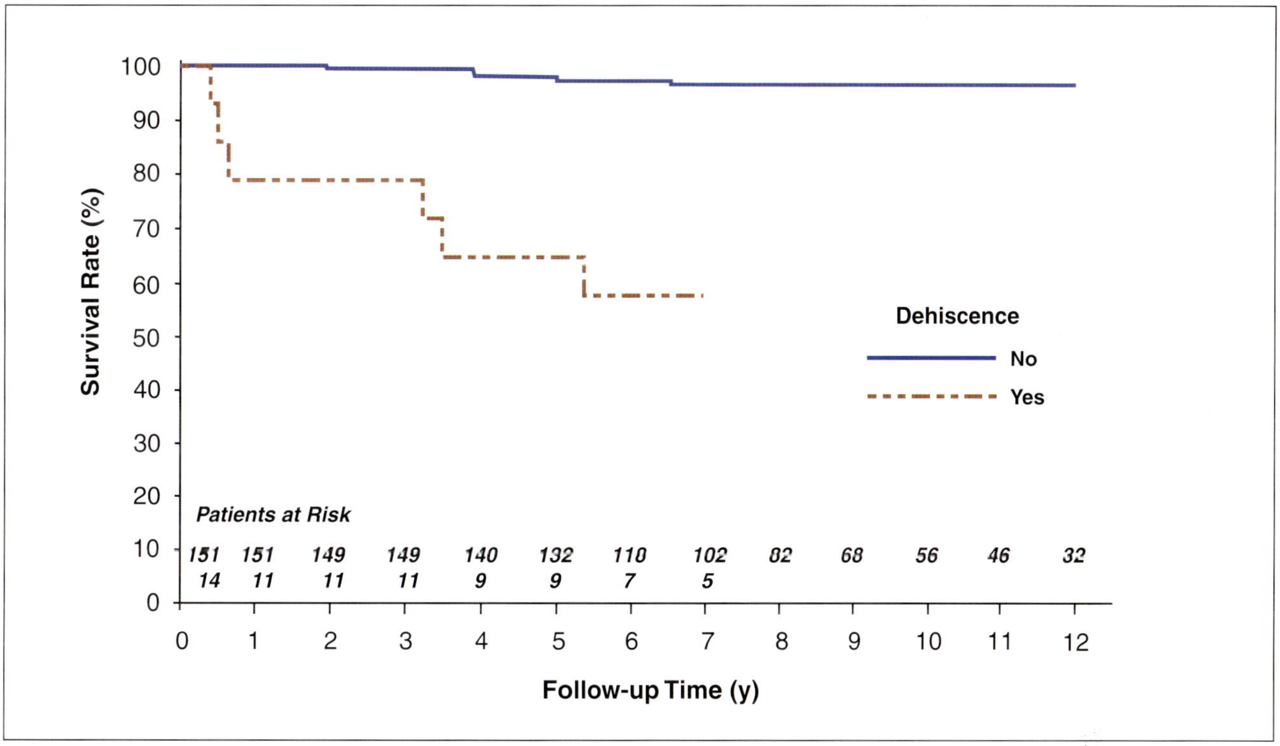

Fig 6-4 Patients with and without local infection (survival distribution function).

Table 6-10 Survival rate of original and all fixtures

	Original fixtures			All fixtures		
Patient group	**Placed**	**Failed**	**Survival rate (%)**	**Placed**	**Failed**	**Survival rate (%)**
Development	148	40	73.0	175	50	71.4
Routine	781	148	81.0	872	165	81.1
All patients	929	188	79.8	1047	215	79.5

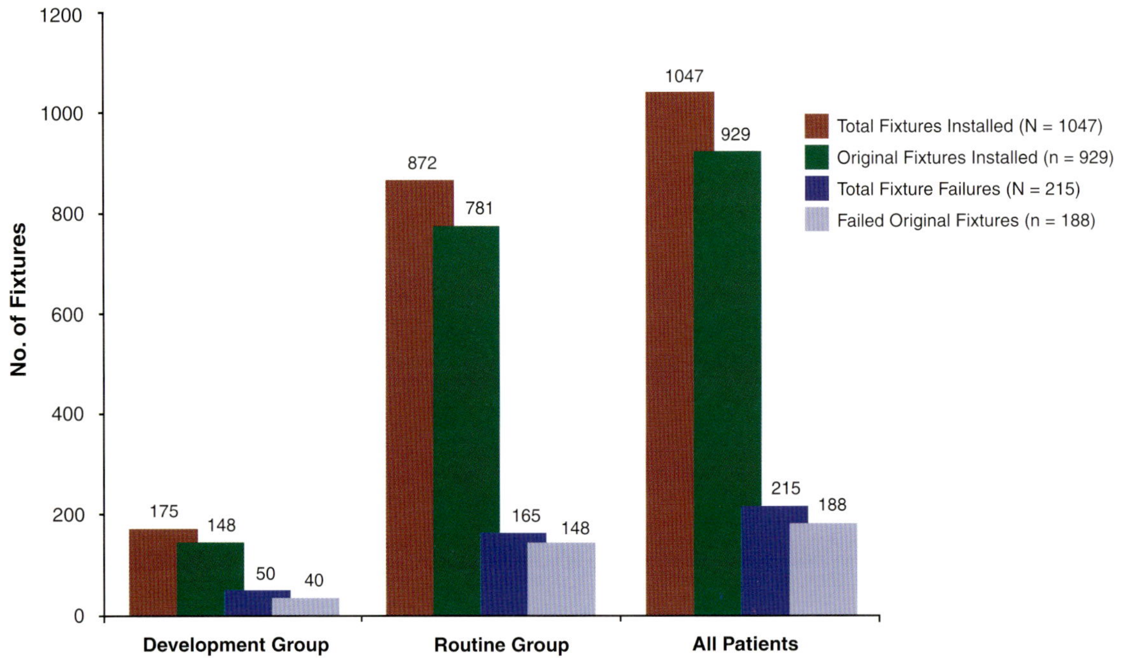

Fig 6-5 Original vs additional fixtures installed.

As shown in Fig 6-6, most patients (85%) had five or six original fixtures installed. The 30 patients with the most pronounced resorption did not have significantly more fixtures installed (mean, 5; range, 3 to 7) than the remaining 135 patients (mean, 6; range, 3 to 8).

Additional fixture placement was indicated in 23% of the patients to alleviate or prevent complications. Four or more fixtures were still functioning in 87% of the cases when the study ended (Fig 6-7). Nine percent of the patients lost more than four original fixtures, 23% lost two or more fixtures, and 35% lost between one and four fixtures (Fig 6-8).

The survival rate of additional fixtures installed in patients with complications or failures (77%) was somewhat lower than that of originally installed fixtures (81%). This is not surprising considering that patients who required additional fixture surgery usually had a risk predisposition.

Fixture survival by length, position, and design

There was a tendency toward a correlation between fixture survival and fixture length (Fig 6-9). The use of longer fixtures, however, is indicative of basal and grafted bone with high capacity and volume. These aspects are probably stronger prognostic factors than the fixture length itself.

Most fixtures were placed in the area extending from the central incisor to the first premolar. The fixture survival rates varied from 79% to 83% in these cases. The survival rates dropped when the fixtures were placed in the premolar area (Fig 6-10).

The swan-neck fixture was the most commonly used design. It also demonstrated the highest survival rate among the frequently used fixture types (Fig 6-11).

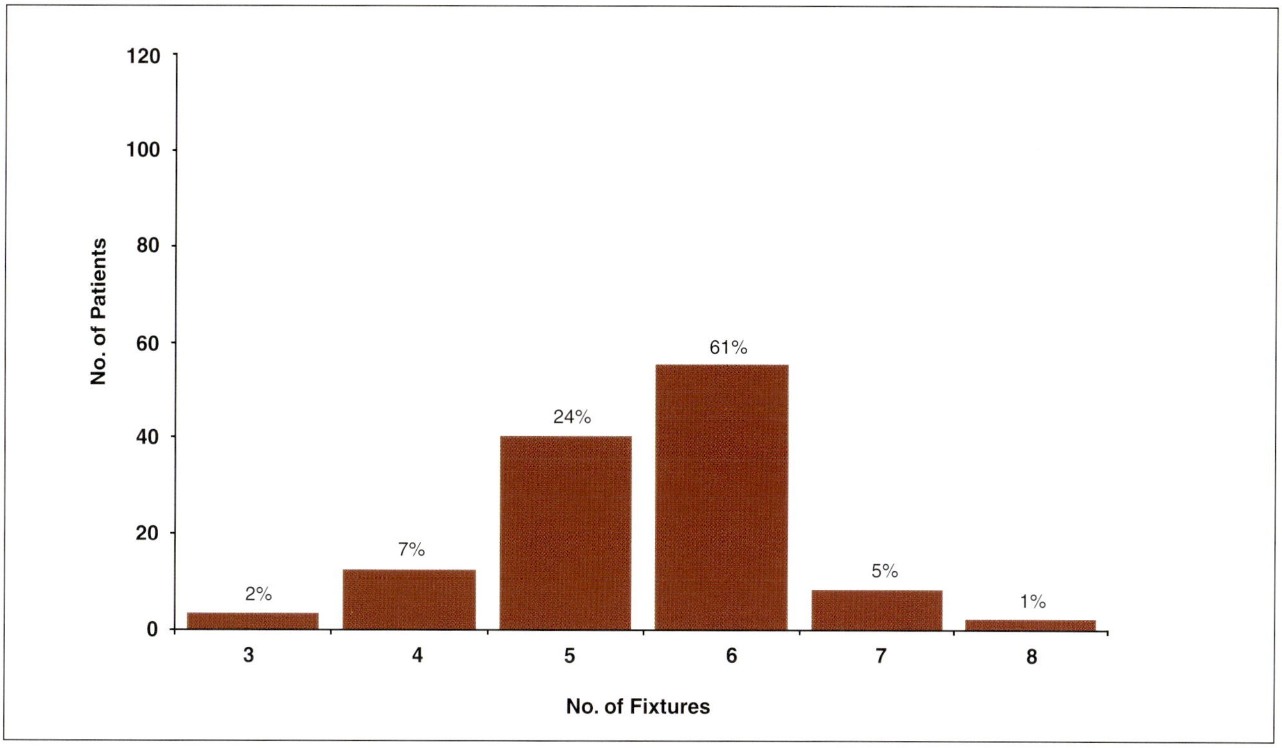

Fig 6-6 Number of original fixtures per patient (N = 165).

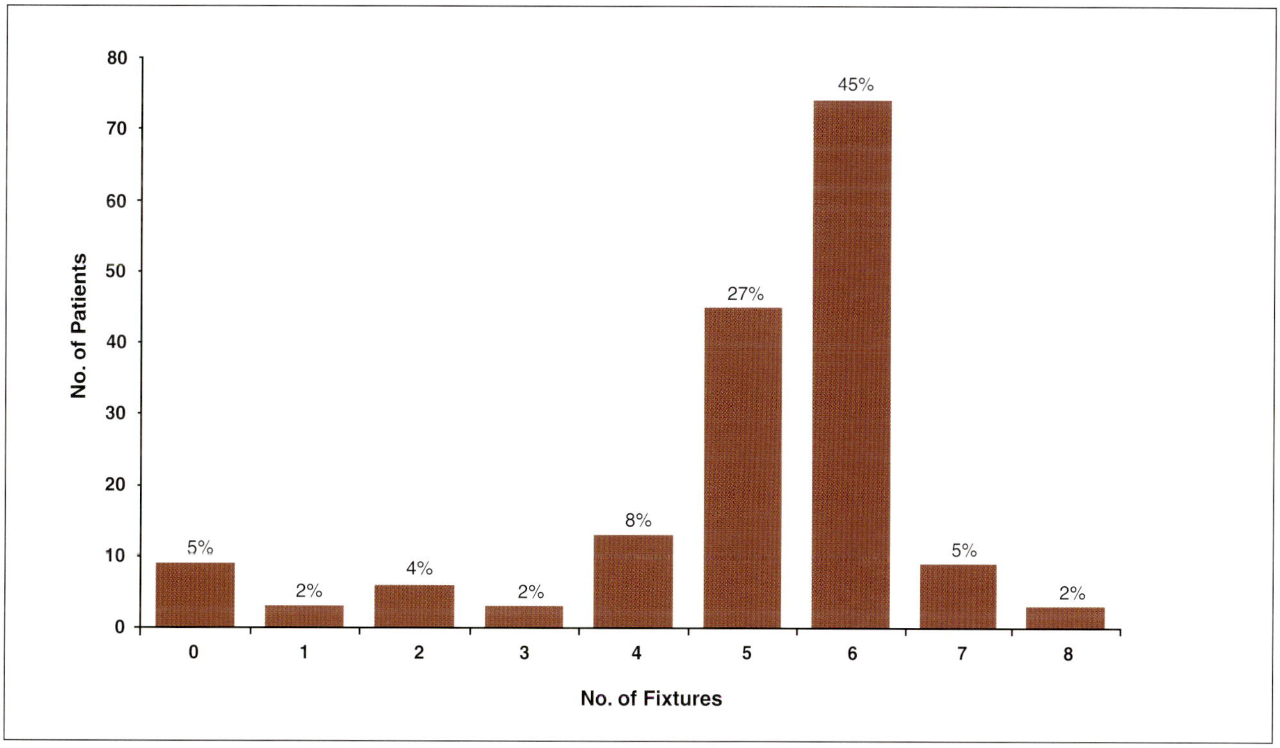

Fig 6-7 Number of original fixtures in function per patient at the end of the study (N = 165).

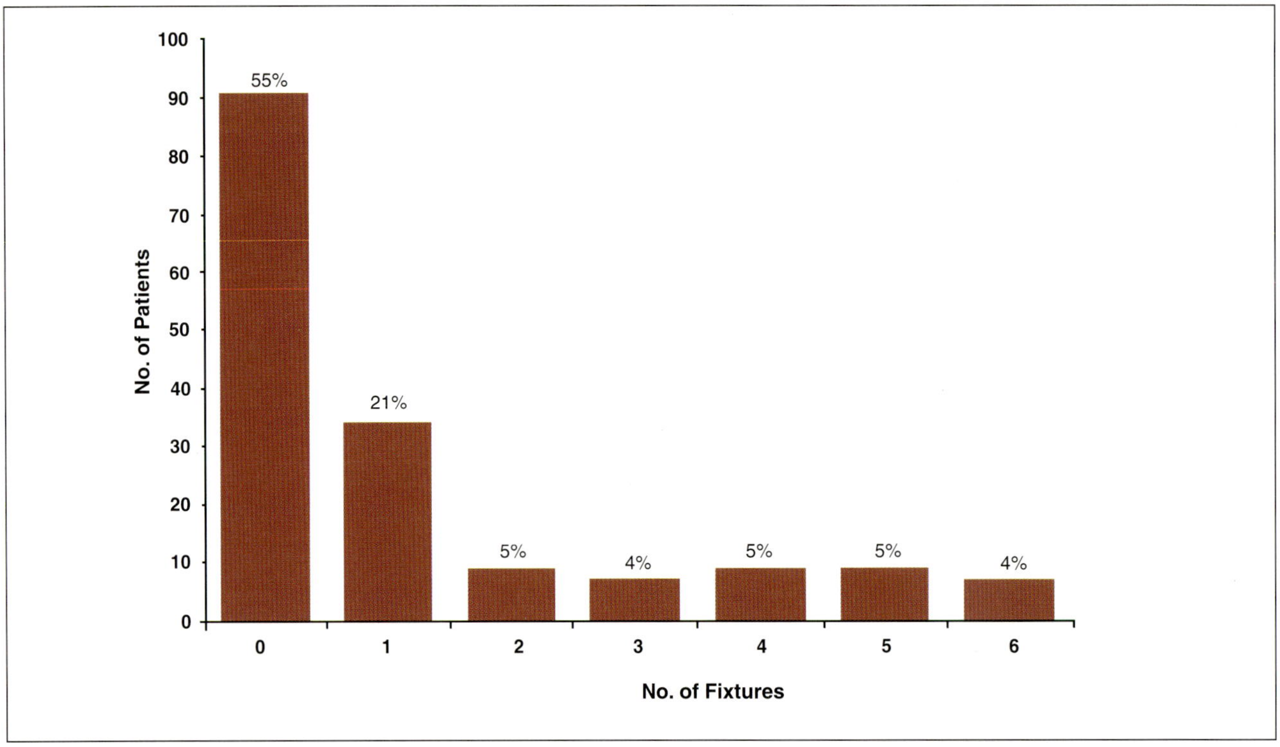

Fig 6-8 Number of lost original fixtures per patient (N =165).

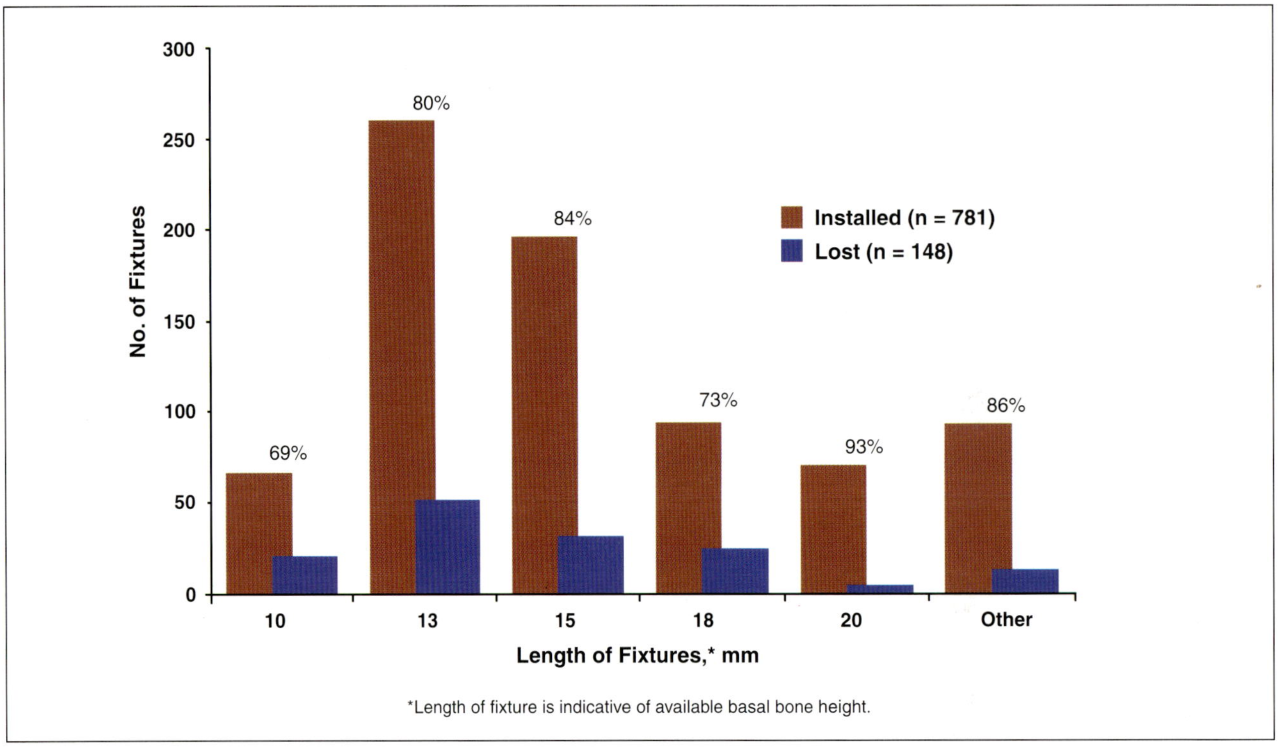

Fig 6-9 Lengths of installed and lost original fixtures. (Percentages indicate survival rate. Data include routine group only.)

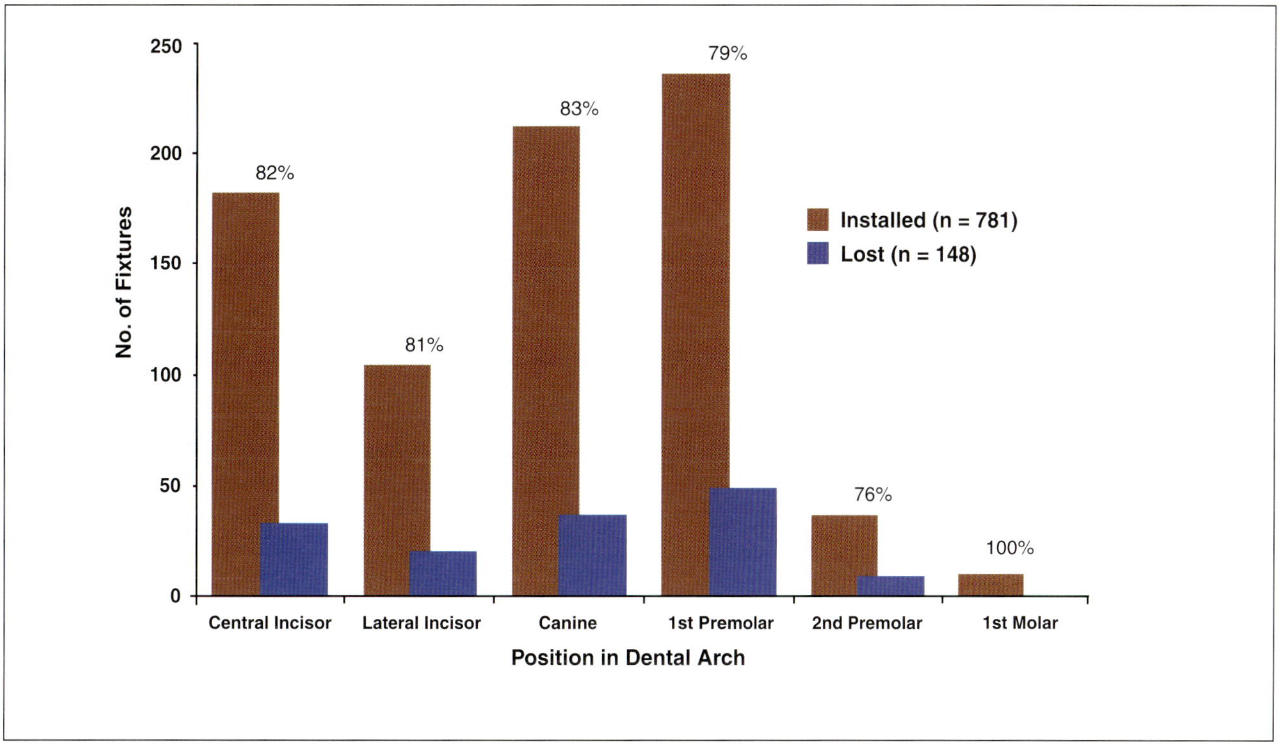

Fig 6-10 Installed and lost original fixtures by position in the dental arch. (Percentages indicate survival rate. Data include routine group only.)

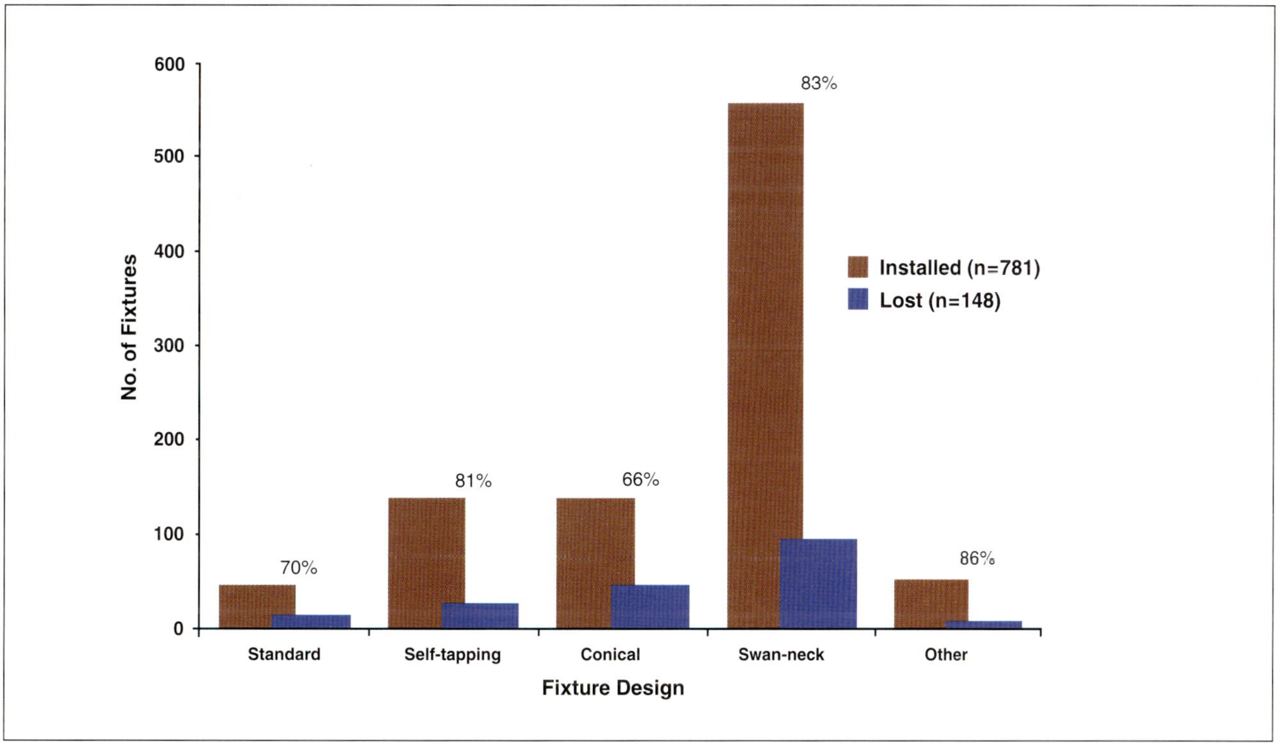

Fig 6-11 Installed and lost original fixtures by fixture design. (Percentages indicate survival rate. Data include routine group only.)

Table 6-11 Timing of fixture failure and placement of additional fixtures

Timing	Development group		Routine group		All patients	
	Original fixtures lost	Additional fixtures placed	Original fixtures lost	Additional fixtures placed	Original fixtures lost	Additional fixtures placed
Initial healing period	7	6	18	13	25	19
At AC*	7	0	30	12	37	12
Between AC and year 1	16	3	58	22	74	25
Between year 1 and year 2	2	5	12	17	14	22
Between year 2 and year 3	1	1	14	5	15	6
Between year 3 and year 4	2	0	4	11	6	11
Between year 4 and year 5	5	4	9	5	14	9
Between year 5 and year 6	0	0	3	0	3	0
Between year 6 and year 7	0	0	0	0	0	0
After more than 7 years	0	8	0	6	0	14
Total	40	27	148	91	188	118

*AC—Abutment connection.

Table 6-12 Failed fixtures by baseline patient profile*

Baseline characteristics	No failures	1–4 fixtures lost	> 4 fixtures lost	Mean no. of fixtures lost	*P* value
Age (y)					
< 50 (n = 42)	28 (66.7%)	14 (33.3%)	0	0.52	
50–65 (n = 61)	30 (49.2%)	22 (36.1%)	9 (14.8%)	1.70	.08
> 65 (n = 35)	19 (54.3%)	11 (31.4%)	5 (14.3%)	1.31	
Sex					
Male (n = 35)	16 (45.7%)	14 (40.0%)	5 (14.3%)	1.86	ns
Female (n = 103)	61 (59.2%)	33 (32.0%)	9 (8.7%)	1.04	
Clinic					
Göteborg (n = 82)	47 (57.3%)	26 (31.7%)	9 (11.0%)	1.32	ns
Other (n = 56)	30 (53.6%)	21 (37.5%)	5 (8.9%)	1.12	
Smoking					
Yes (n = 25)	9 (36.0%)	12 (48.0%)	4 (16.0%)	1.96	.03
No (n = 87)	54 (62.1%)	27 (31.0%)	6 (6.9%)	0.99	
Bruxism					
Yes (n = 11)	4 (36.4%)	3 (27.3%)	4 (36.4%)	2.63	.03
No (n = 56)	33 (58.9%)	21 (37.5%)	2 (3.6%)	0.86	
Opposing dentition					
Removable partial denture (n = 27)	10 (37.0%)	13 (48.1%)	4 (14.8%)	1.56	.04
Other (see Table 2-1) (n = 110)	67 (60.4%)	34 (30.6%)	10 (9.0%)	1.17	
Time between fixture placement and delivery of fixed prosthesis					
< 9 mo (n = 82)	51 (62.2%)	24 (29.3%)	7 (8.5%)	1.09	
9–12 mo (n = 35)	18 (51.4%)	14 (40.0%)	3 (8.6%)	1.09	.10
> 1 y (n = 19)	8 (42.1%)	8 (42.1%)	3 (15.8%)	1.89	
Time (d) between abutment connection and delivery of fixed prosthesis					
< 30 (n = 36)	20 (55.6%)	11 (30.6%)	5 (13.9%)	1.64	
30–60 (n = 59)	38 (64.4%)	17 (28.8%)	4 (6.8%)	0.93	ns
> 60 (n = 40)	19 (47.5%)	18 (45.0)	3 (7.5%)	1.05	

*Only includes data for patients in the routine group (n = 138).

Table 6-13 Univariate covariates—the influence of different parameters on system survival

Parameters	Log-rank *P* value	Hazard ratio	95% Confidence limits of hazard ratio	
			Lower	Higher
Infection	< .001	16.51	5.03	54.22
Dehiscence	< .001	7.89	2.40	25.91
Bruxism	< .001	12.77	2.48	65.89
Age classes (< 50 y; 50–65 y; > 65 y)	.03	2.54	1.05	6.11
Moderate vs extreme resorption (grades 2 and 3 vs 4 and 5)	ns	5.38	0.69	42.06
Type of fixed prosthesis construction	ns	3.94	0.72	21.57
Smoking	ns	3.34	0.84	13.36
Medial vs lateral ilium donor site	ns	3.30	0.85	12.75
Clinic	ns	2.88	0.84	9.85
Disturbed healing (sequestrum)	ns	2.59	0.76	8.85
Maxillary resorption (III–V)	ns	2.55	0.75	8.71
Sinus classification	ns	1.53	0.63	3.72
Time between abutment connection and delivery of fixed prosthesis	ns	0.99	0.96	1.02
Sex	ns	0.83	0.22	3.14
Opposing dentition (see Table 2-1)	ns	0.64	0.17	2.40
Number of original fixtures	ns	0.57	0.31	1.06
Time between fixture placement and delivery of fixed prosthesis	ns	0.18	0.00	10.59

Time of fixture failure

Most fixture failures were observed at abutment connection or during the first year in function (Table 6-11). Not all lost fixtures were replaced. Because four to six fixtures were most often installed in each patient, and four fixtures usually suffice for retention of the fixed prosthesis,[29] it was frequently possible to resolve the prosthetic requirements without additional fixture surgery.

Fixture failure vs patient profile

The lost fixture distribution in the routine period is given according to patient profile in Table 6-12. Although bruxing and smoking data were not available for all patients, it was clear that these two parameters could be significantly correlated to fixture loss. In the identified bruxer category, 36% of the patients lost more than five fixtures in spite of prosthetic prevention.

Prognostic Factors for System Survival

In an attempt to quantitatively evaluate the prognostic risk factors associated with autogenous onlay bone grafting of the severely resorbed maxilla, the various treatment parameters were correlated to fixture and system survival. Table 6-13 contains the *P* values of the log rank test for prosthetic system survival. The table includes all analyzed variables, the hazard ratio, and the 95% confidence interval for the hazard ratio.

The results exhibited the anticipated increased hazard ratios for–in order of significance–infection, dehiscence, and bruxism. The hazard of reverting to a conventional denture was 16.5 times higher for patients with a local infection than it was for patients without an infection. Among patients with bruxism, the system survival was reduced ($P <$ .001) and the hazard ratio was 13.

Differences in age also showed a positive correlation to system survival (Fig 6-12). This, in turn, can be explained by the fact that younger patients (younger than 50 years) usually have been edentulous for shorter periods than elderly patients (older than 65 years). Therefore, the capacity of their residual bone is higher and can better respond to trauma. Elderly patients also may be osteoporotic, which may have an adverse effect on long-term success. In addition, there were more smokers among the older patients (10 out of 32) than there were in the younger age group (8 out of 68). The 12-year system survival rate was 98% for younger patients and 84% for elderly patients.

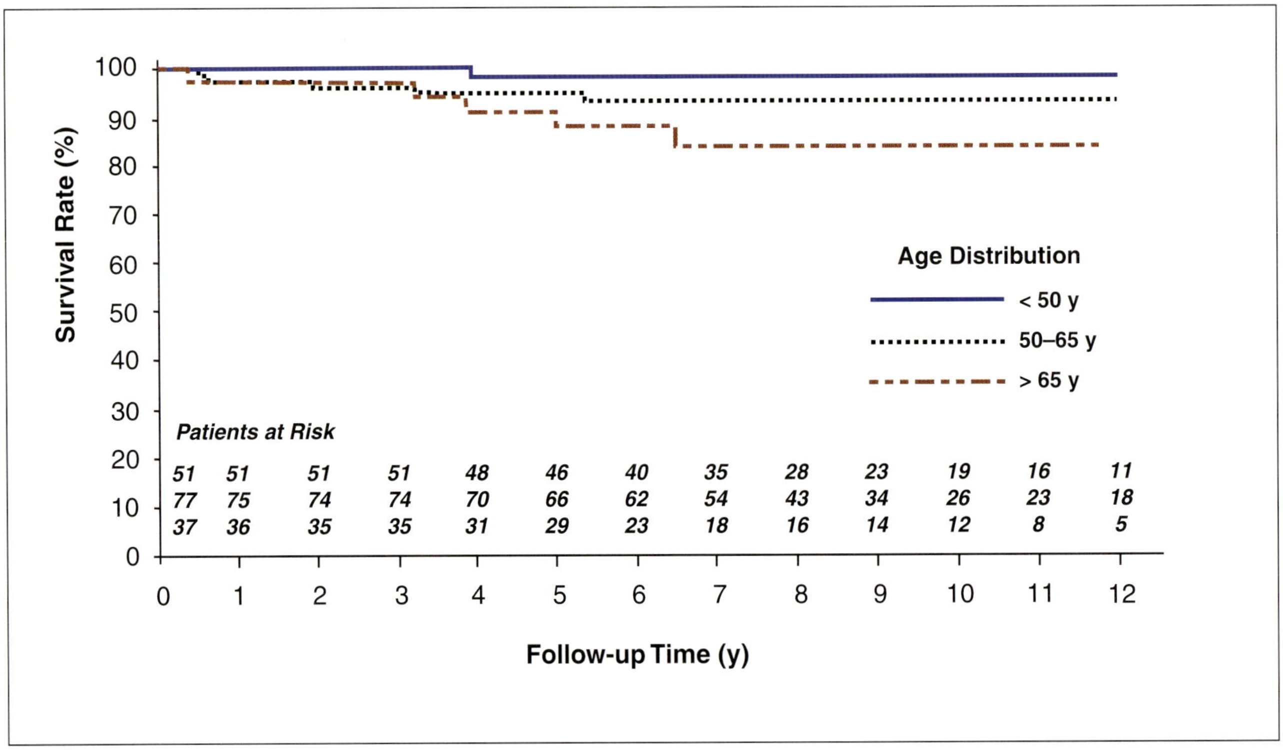

Fig 6-12 Rate of restored prosthetic function for different patient age groups (survival distribution function). Differences may also be correlated to age-related remodeling capacity of bone.

There was also a tendency for reduced system survival among identified smokers ($P = .07$); the 10-year system survival rate for smokers was 85%, compared to 96% for nonsmokers (Fig 6-13). A third of the smokers belonged to the oldest age group.

Patients with the highest resorption grades and patients with the lateral ilium as the donor site also tended to be at risk for reduced system survival.

Correlation Between Predictors

The correlation matrix of major predictors with significant influence on system survival is shown in Table 6-14. Dehiscences found at the recipient site could be significantly correlated to infection ($P <$ .001). Smoking could be correlated to dehiscence ($P = .004$) and infection at the recipient site ($P =$ .002). Eleven (39%) of 28 smokers experienced dehiscence at the recipient site compared to 11 (9%) of 93 nonsmokers. Eight smokers (29%) experienced infection at the recipient site compared to four nonsmokers (4%).

Radiographic Results

The radiographic evaluation was limited to the 77 patients treated in Göteborg, Sweden, for whom postoperative intraoral or extraoral radiographs (panoramic or dental scanograms) were available.

Preoperative bone height

Preoperative radiographs for 56 patients (73%) could be evaluated for determination of total and available bone height. In another 3 patients, panoramic radiographs were used for total bone height measurements. As was previously stated, available bone height refers to the bone between the nasal cavity and the alveolar crest that has a width of 4 mm in the buccolingual direction (see Fig 2-9).

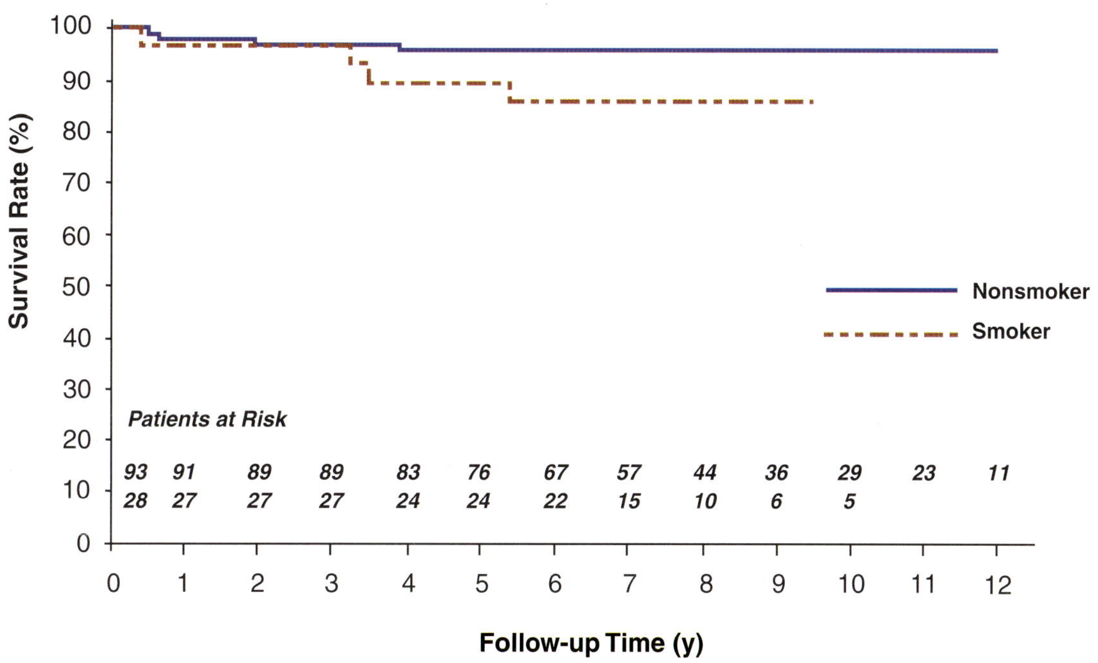

Fig 6-13 System survival rate in smoking vs nonsmoking patients (survival distribution function).

Table 6-14 Correlation matrix of selected predictors

		Age	Smoking	Bruxism	Resorption grade	Thin maxillary base	Infection at recipient site	Dehiscence at recipient site
Smoking	*P* value	.04						
	n	121						
Bruxism	*P* value	.09	.16					
	n	74	72					
Resorption grade	r*	0.18						
	P value	.27	.34	.11				
	n	165	121	74				
Thin maxillary base	*P* value	.38	.77	.24	.22			
	n	165	121	74	165			
Infection at recipient site	*P* value	.53	.002	.001	.94	.97		
	n	165	121	74	165	165		
Dehiscence at recipient site	*P* value	.45	.004	.25	.34	.93	< .001	
	n	165	121	74	165	165	165	
Number of original fixtures	r*	–0.10						
	P value	.18	.75	.74	.47	.12	.36	.005
	n	165	121	74	165	165	165	165

*r—Pearson correlation coefficient.

Table 6-15 Mean distance (SD and range) between reference point* and marginal bone level at different time intervals

Time of evaluation	Patients	Mean	SD	Minimum	Maximum
Baseline	40	1.68	1.17	0.00	4.80
Year 1	47	2.61	1.42	0.30	7.71†
Year 2	44	2.74	1.11	0.00	4.80
Year 3	38	2.91	1.30	0.31	5.15
Year 4	21	3.24	1.62	1.21	8.50‡
Year 5	24	3.44	1.14	1.25	5.22
Year 6	11	2.54	0.84	1.50	3.57
Year 7	6	3.25	0.62	2.43	4.12
Year 8	7	2.63	1.11	1.38	4.11
Year 9	5	3.02	0.99	1.40	3.97
Year 10	15	2.63	0.94	1.15	4.38
Mean year 2–3	59	2.79	1.16	0.00	4.98
Mean year 4–5	40	3.34	1.41	1.21	8.50
Mean year 6–10	26	2.80	0.90	1.15	4.38
Mean year 11–16	3	3.94	0.43	3.57	4.41

*The reference point was the coronal part of the fixture head.

†This was the first of two patients who exhibited mobility of the fixed prosthesis prior to fixture loss, resulting in extraordinary bone loss. He was a heavy smoker and a bruxer who showed unusual bone loss at delivery of the fixed prosthesis and a distance of 7.71 mm at the first annual follow-up visit.

‡The second patient was also a smoker. She was diagnosed with fibrosclerosis a few years after treatment. At the 3-year follow-up, the mean distance was 8.50 mm. She lost all but two fixtures shortly thereafter.

The mean total bone height was 8.8 mm (SD, 4.3; range, 1 to 16 mm), and the corresponding value for available bone height was 4.8 mm (SD, 2.0; range, 1 to 9 mm). The available bone height was less than 7 mm in 82% of the patients.

Postoperative bone level measurements

Radiographs were regarded as unreadable for six fixtures because of incorrect vertical projection geometry. Table 6-15 shows the distance between the reference point (coronal part of fixture head) and the marginal bone level at baseline (connection of fixed prosthesis) and at the different follow-up examinations for all patients. Patients are represented by a mean value for all of their fixtures.

Two patients with extraordinary bone loss contributed to high mean and maximum values, particularly at the year 1 and year 4 examinations. One of the patients was a bruxer who had smoked 30 cigarettes per day for the past 50 years. The other patient was also a smoker who was later diagnosed with fibrosclerosis.

In Fig 6-14, the mean distance between the reference point and the marginal bone level is shown for patients with all types of fixture designs. Because radiographs were not taken at all annual checkups, there is a discrepancy between the number of observations and the total number of patients followed at each observation point.

The mean bone loss during the first year of function was 1.1 mm (SD, 1.1) for the 27 patients examined at both delivery of the fixed prosthesis and the first annual follow-up visit (Table 6-16). The finding was statistically significant ($P < .001$).

To reach a higher level of certainty, a 2-year time interval was calculated after the first year. The average between the two mean values at each examination represented the mean for all fixtures at each given interval. The mean bone loss of 0.2 mm (SD, 0.7) between year 1 and year 3 (ie, between year 1 and year 2 to 3 follow-up examinations) was not statistically significant. The 0.3-mm bone loss (SD, 0.7) between year 3 and year 5 was, however, statistically significant ($P = .01$). As seen in Table 6-16, minimal bone loss also was noted at the later time intervals. No statistically significant differences were noted between the development and routine groups.

If it can be assumed that the measurement error amounts to 0.5 mm,[40] 60% of the patients showed some degree of mean bone loss between connection of the fixed prosthesis and the 1-year follow-up. During the same interval, 25% of the total number of evaluated patients showed an average bone loss of ≥ 2 mm. Between years 1 and 5, about 3% of the patients showed a mean bone loss of 2 mm or more.

The bone level changes over time are shown in Tables 6-17 and 6-18 for patients with only one

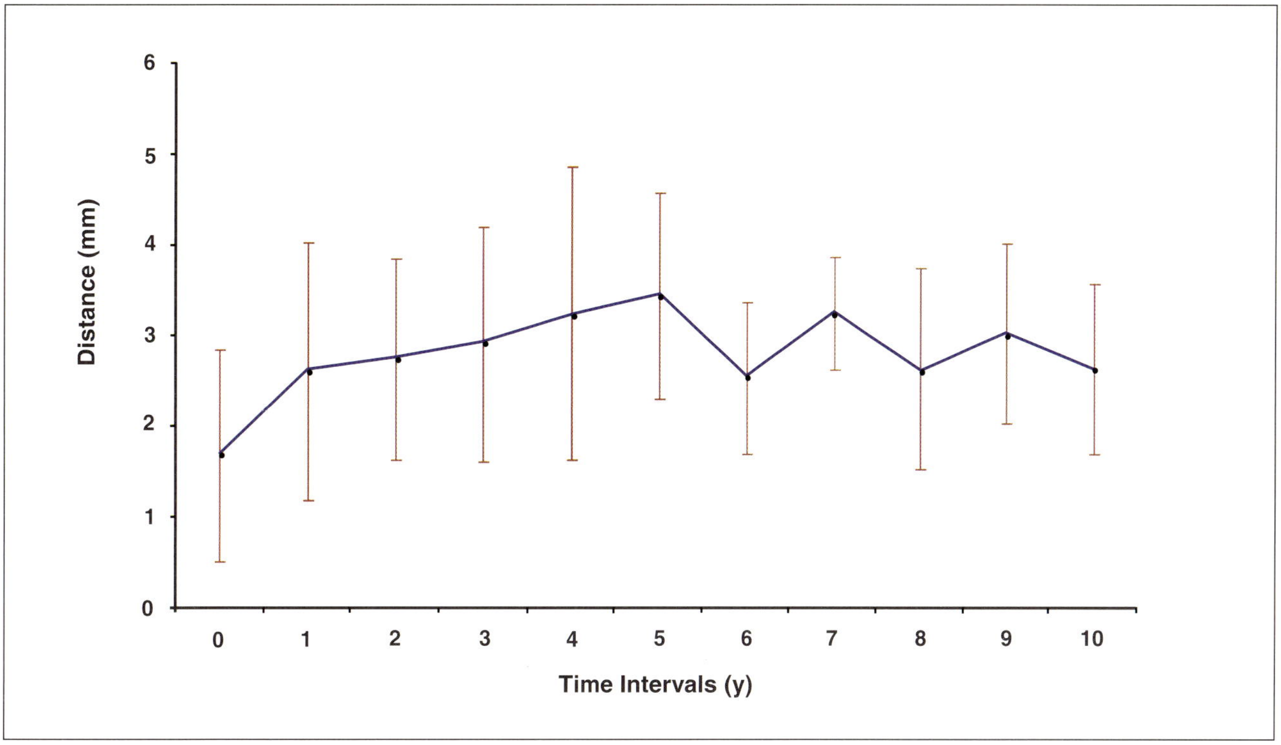

Fig 6-14 Mean distance (SD) between reference point and marginal bone level for all fixture types.

Table 6-16 Bone loss at different time intervals for all patients expressed as mean values (SD, range) and *P* values

Time interval	Patients	Mean	SD	Minimum	Maximum	*P* value
Baseline to year 1	27	1.13	1.06	-0.42	3.96	< .001
Year 1–3	37	0.19	0.69	-1.83	2.21	ns
Year 3–5	34	0.29	0.71	-0.61	3.83	.01
Year 5–10	20	0.00	0.43	-0.82	1.03	ns

fixture design (conical, standard/self-tapping, or swan-neck fixtures). When comparing the different fixture designs, a statistically significant difference ($P = .03$) was noted in the mean values of year 4 to 5 for swan-neck vs standard/self-tapping fixtures. The same comparison also revealed a statistically significant difference ($P = .004$) during the first year in function (year 0 to 1). In addition, a statistically significant difference ($P = .006$) was noted when bone loss between connection of the fixed prosthesis and year 3 for conical fixtures was compared to that of self-tapping fixtures. No statistically significant differences could be found for any of the other parameter combinations (eg, fixture design and time intervals). Figures 6-15 to 6-17 illustrate the mean distance between the reference points and the marginal bone levels for the swan-neck, standard/ self-tapping, and conical fixture designs. The values can be compared to the same type of curve for all fixture designs combined, as shown in Fig 6-14.

Radiographic results using the fixture as the measurement unit

In most follow-up studies aimed at evaluating implant treatment efficacy, single fixtures have been used as the unit when determining bone level changes over time. Such an approach neglects the interdependency among implants placed in the same jaw. To allow comparison of results, however, the bone loss also is presented here with the fixture as the measurement unit. Table 6-19 shows the bone level for all individual fixtures (development and routine groups) at different time intervals.

Table 6-17 Mean distance between reference point and marginal bone level for different fixture types

	Conical			Standard/self-tapping			Swan-neck		
Time interval	**Patients**	**Mean**	**SD**	**Patients**	**Mean**	**SD**	**Patients**	**Mean**	**SD**
Baseline	6	1.60	1.70	9	1.81	0.88	16	1.69	1.32
Year 1	3	2.65	1.65	8	1.89	0.49	22	2.60	1.74
Year 3	7	2.98	0.89	11	2.63	1.06	27	2.63	1.34
Year 5	6	3.39	0.94	8	2.53	1.06	16	3.76	1.71
Year 10	5	3.21	0.36	9	2.69	1.05	5	2.60	0.74

Table 6-18 Bone loss adjacent to different fixture types

	Conical			Standard/self-tapping			Swan-neck		
Time interval	**Patients**	**Mean**	**SD**	**Patients**	**Mean**	**SD**	**Patients**	**Mean**	**SD**
Baseline to year 1	2	1.36	1.46	7	0.26	0.63	9	1.66	1.15
Year 1–3	3	0.83	1.22	8	0.23	0.16	14	0.21	0.90
Year 3–5	5	0.09	0.56	8	0.12	0.36	11	0.57	1.13

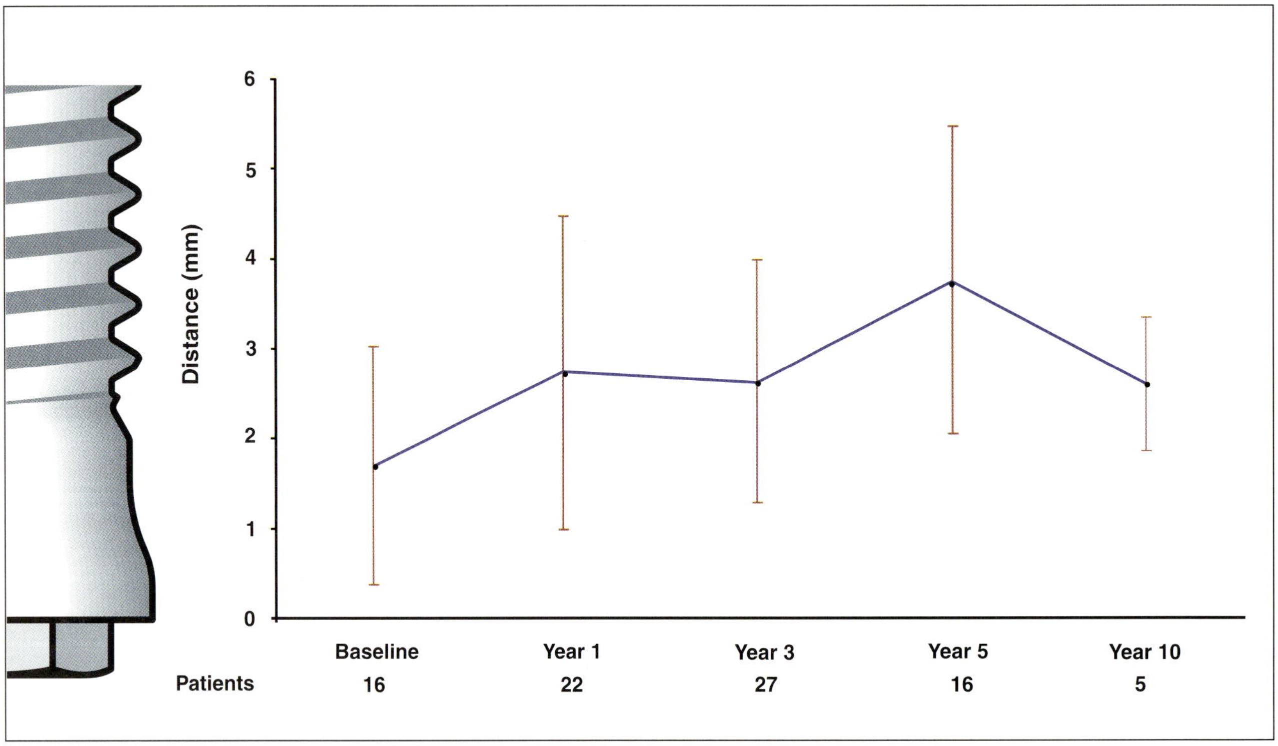

Fig 6-15 Mean distance (SD) between reference point and marginal bone level for swan-neck fixtures.

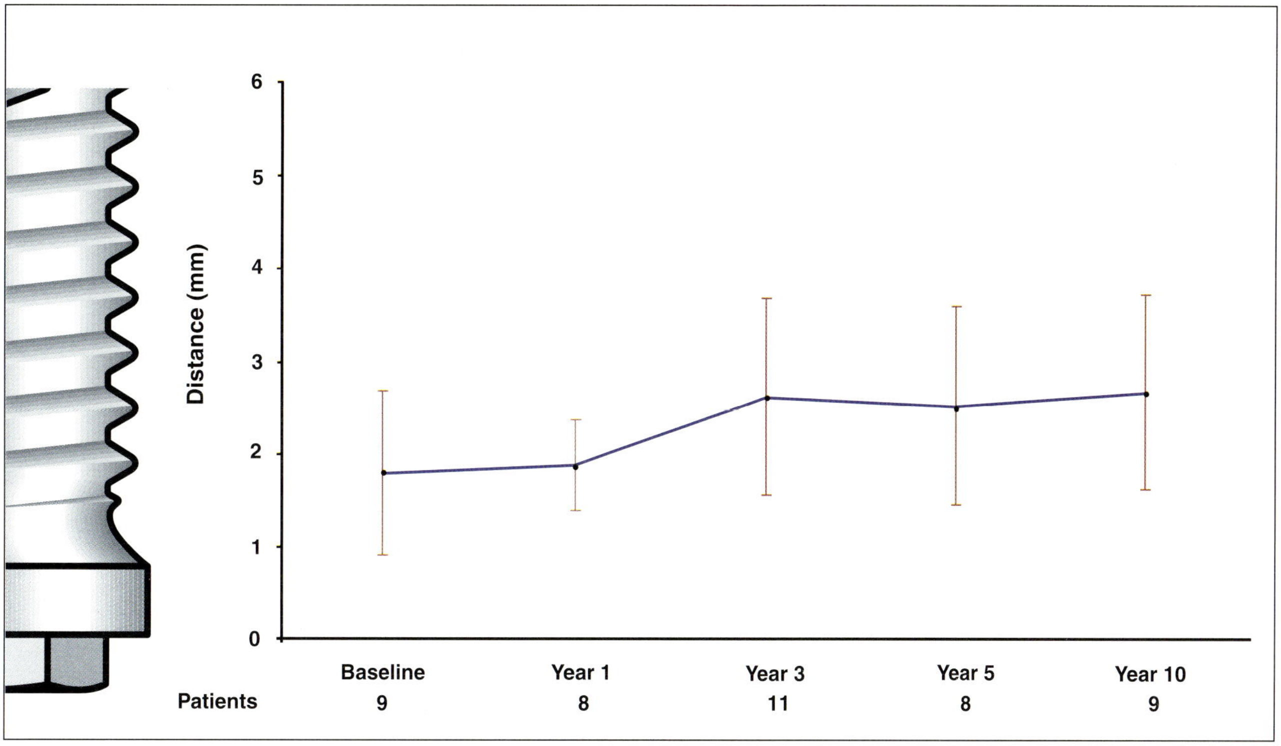

Fig 6-16 Mean distance (SD) between reference point and marginal bone level for standard and self-tapping fixtures.

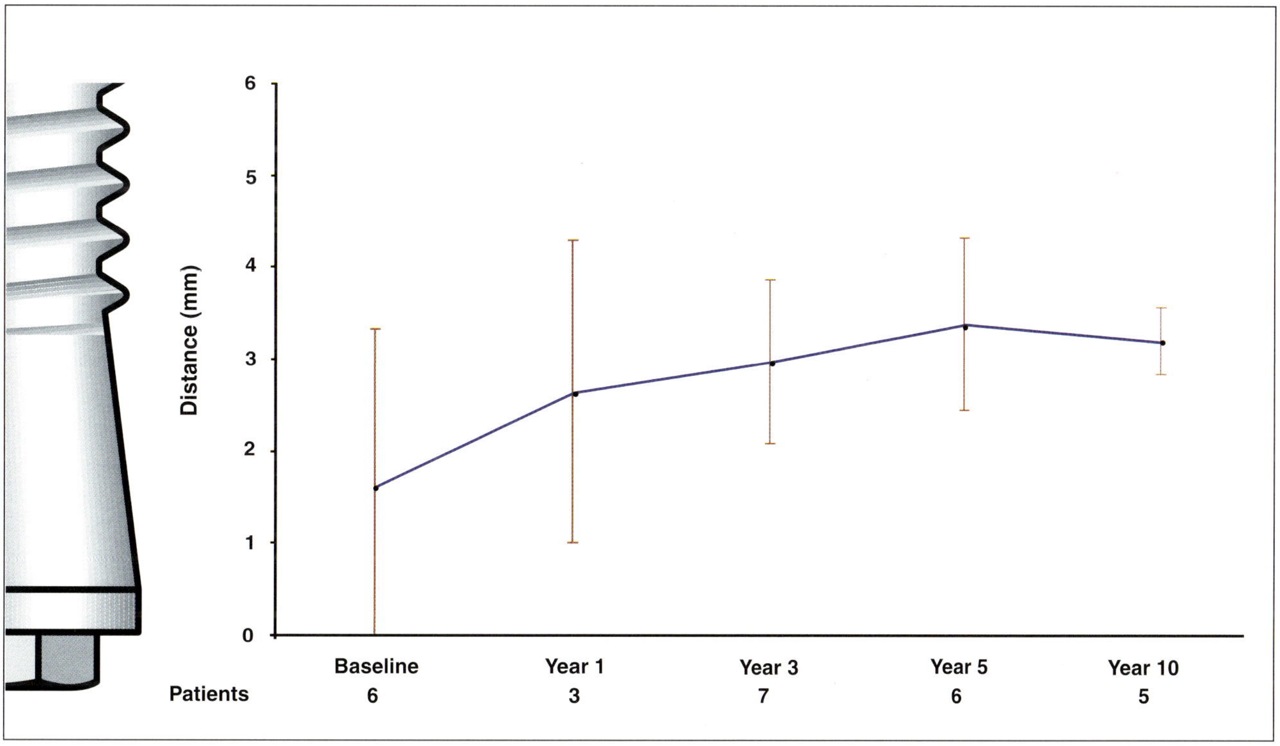

Fig 6-17 Mean distance (SD) between reference point and marginal bone level for conical fixtures.

Table 6-19 Mean distance between reference point and marginal bone level for all individual fixtures

Time of evaluation	Fixtures	Mean	SD
Baseline	206	1.59	1.40
Year 1	241	2.55	1.77
Year 2	208	2.70	1.49
Year 3	184	2.87	1.51
Year 4	97	3.06	1.69
Year 5	112	3.35	1.64
Year 6	52	2.51	1.27
Year 7	27	3.12	1.07
Year 8	30	2.43	1.49
Year 9	22	3.03	1.43
Year 10	75	2.51	1.23

Indications of lost osseointegration were seen around 27 fixtures distributed among 14 patients. Eight patients showed loss of osseointegration of a single fixture, 3 patients demonstrated such signs around 2 fixtures, and 1 patient showed loss of 3 fixtures. All fixtures failed in 2 patients. One standard fixture was found fractured at the 4-year follow-up. Otherwise, failures were detected for the most part at the 1-year control.

Seventeen of the failures affected swan-neck fixtures, the type of fixture most commonly used among the patients included in the radiographic examinations. Most fixtures that demonstrated signs of lost osseointegration were removed in association with the radiographic diagnosis and are included in the statistics as lost fixtures.

Radiographic correlation analyses between predictors

The influence of various factors on the marginal bone level over time was analyzed (Table 6-20). The evaluated parameters were age, sex, smoking habits, resorption pattern, dehiscence, postoperative infection, and sequestrum. The time intervals between fixture placement and abutment connection and between abutment connection and delivery of the fixed prosthesis were also evaluated. The grade of resorption (index I–V) did not have a significant influence on the bone level. Presence of dehiscence followed by postoperative infection influenced the bone level at year 1 ($P = .03$). Patients with infection had significantly more bone loss (mean, 4.6 mm; SD, 2.8) than did patients without infection (mean, 2.5 mm; SD, 1.2).

Smokers tended to have higher mean marginal bone loss; a significant influence was seen at installation of the fixed prosthesis (mean, 3.2 mm; SD, 0.8; $P = .002$), at year 1 (mean, 4.4 mm; SD, 1.8; $P = .01$), and at year 5 (mean, 4.8 mm; SD, 2.2; $P < .05$). The same figures for nonsmoking patients were 1.3 mm (SD 0.9) at installation of the fixed prosthesis, 2.6 mm (SD 1.3) at year 1, and 3.2 mm (SD 1.1) at year 5.

Patients with a shorter healing time between abutment connection and prosthetic loading demonstrated less bone level changes after one year ($P = .04$). This finding corresponds with the clinical results and indicates that the bone anatomy responds favorably to early prosthetic loading as long as it does not apply to individual fixtures.

In summary, all parameters that had a statistically significant impact on the marginal bone level could be prevented to some extent; for example, the patient could stop smoking, proper suturing technique could be applied, and it could be assured that the postoperative care was carried out in a fashion that minimized the risk for dehiscence formation or infection. Early loading of the prosthetic device also proved to be beneficial when evaluating the marginal bone levels. Functional loading for remodeling should be applied no later than 12 to 18 months after fixture installation, preferably within 8 months.

Table 6-20 The influence of various factors on the marginal bone level related to the reference point, expressed as r (Pearson correlation coefficient), *P* value (Pitman nonparametric permutation test), and n (number of patients).

Time of evaluation	Age	Sex	Resorption	Dehiscence	Infection	Sequestrum	Smoking	Initial healing period (y)	Time (d) from AC[*] to FP[†] delivery
FP[†] delivery	r = 0.20 *P* = ns n = 49	r = 0.01 *P* = ns n = 49	r = –0.12 *P* = ns n = 40	r = 0.38 *P* = .02 n = 40	r = 0.31 *P* = 0.4 n = 40	r = 0.28 *P* = ns n = 40	r = –0.67 *P* = .002 n = 21	r = 0.03 *P* = ns n = 40	r = 0.31 *P* = .04 n = 40
Year 1	r = 0.19 *P* = ns n = 47	r = 0.02 *P* = ns n = 47	r = –0.14 *P* = ns n = 47	r = 0.43 *P* = .003 n = 47	r = 0.37 *P* = 0.03 n = 47	r = 0.28 *P* = .04 n = 47	r = 0.50 *P* = .007 n = 26	r = 0.10 *P* = ns n = 47	r = 0.32 *P* = .02 n = 47
Year 2–3	r = 0.02 *P* = ns n = 59	r = 0.01 *P* = ns n = 59	r = –0.16 *P* = ns n = 59	r = 0.21 *P* = ns n = 59	r = –0.08 *P* = ns n = 59	r = –0.28 *P* = .02 n = 59	r = –0.19 *P* = ns n = 32	r = –0.24 *P* = .04 n = 59	r = –0.13 *P* = ns n = 59
Year 4–5	r = 0.12 *P* = ns n = 40	r = 0.31 *P* = .03 n = 40	r = –0.04 *P* = ns n = 40	r = 0.16 *P* = ns n = 40	r = 0.24 *P* =ns n = 40	r = 0.03 *P* = ns n = 40	r = 0.46 *P* = .02 n = 21	r = 0.42 *P* = ns n = 40	r = 0.10 *P* = ns n = 40
Year 6–10	r = 0.06 *P* = ns n = 26	r = 0.11 *P* = ns n = 26	r = –0.10 *P* = ns n = 26			r = –0.03 *P* = ns n = 26	r = –0.17 *P* = ns n = 9	r = –0.06 *P* = ns n = 26	r = –0.06 *P* = ns n = 26

*AC—Abutment connection.
†FP—Fixed prosthesis.

Discussion

Clinical findings

The autogenous onlay bone grafting was conducted to restore a compromised jaw anatomy. The procedure differs from sinus grafts and related procedures. In such cases, the bone is intended to provide fixture stability to the region, but the location of the graft does not provide topographical restitution.

The surgery included simultaneous placement of endosseous fixtures to anchor prosthetic restorations. The purpose of the treatment was to restore the patient's ability to masticate efficiently and speak clearly and to improve the patient's maxillofacial appearance and social confidence.

Although new approaches to handling these types of cases were developed during the course of the study, we report our findings because similar long-term studies of large patient populations are limited in the scientific literature. In addition, our learning process may provide other clinicians with ideas that will prove valuable to these types of severely orally handicapped patients.

We set out to follow a standardized study protocol, but increased clinical experience inevitably led to certain procedural modifications. Such changes are attributed to the learning curve we experienced during the developmental period. For example, we found that using the medial ilium as the graft donor site minimized postoperative donor site morbidity; as a result, the medial ilium, rather than the lateral ilium, became the preferred donor site.

We also found that the risk for failure could be reduced by filling the fixture site and all crevices and peripheral spaces at the grafted recipient site with particulated autogenous bone and marrow. If voids were allowed to persist between the graft and the recipient maxilla, bone was less likely to form. There was also a risk for disturbed healing symptoms, such as dehiscences and subsequent infections.

Dehiscences that progressed into infections increased the risk for communication between the oral cavity and sinus or nasal cavity. Such infections caused severe complications and fixture loss. Therefore, if an existent communication to the sinus or oral cavity was noted, it was essential to conduct a surgical intervention immediately (ie, the same day) to remove deranged tissue. The surgical flap had to be resutured without tension in two layers; first the periosteum and then the submucosa and mucosa. Complete closure at the initial surgery reduced the risk for these types of serious complications.

Careful prosthetic design was also essential. Focus was placed on minimizing torque and bending forces. In addition, the mandibular dentition had to be carefully evaluated to minimize occlusal disharmony and reduce the risk for overloading any of the fixtures in the graft.

Most failed fixtures were caused by lost integration rather than excessive marginal bone loss. As presented earlier in this chapter, efforts were made to establish risk factors by evaluating whether fixture or prosthetic failures could be correlated to other parameters. The main risk factor turned out to be dehiscence formation with subsequent infection.

In the aforementioned literature review,[23] Tolman concluded that wound dehiscence seemed to have the most deleterious effect on implant survival rate. In the long-term study by Keller et al,[24] nicotine use, history of sinusitis, molar site implant placement, and limited bone height (shorter implant lengths) had the most significant influence on implant failure.

In this study, we also found a declining fixture survival rate in the smoker category and an even sharper decline among patients with extreme bruxism. It was noted that 50% of the smokers, compared to 17% of the nonsmokers, experienced dehiscence at the recipient site.

There was little variation in the survival rates of the different fixture designs. Most fixtures ranged in length from 10 to 18 mm. Within this range, there was a slightly discernible trend toward increased survival for longer fixtures. This is not surprising, since a longer fixture implies a greater amount of available bone for anchorage. It also implies that the surgeon has been able to engage cortical bone of the maxilla at a high level, which enhances the stability and load-bearing capacity of the fixture.

Relatively few fixtures were placed in the second premolar or first molar regions. As expected, the highest survival rates were associated with fixtures in the canine region, where fixture anchorage can be found in the bony septum between the anterior aspect of the sinus and the lateral nasal wall. A recent long-term study on single tooth replacement reported that the majority of the failed fixtures (8 out of 14) were placed in the upper central incisor region.[41] A possible explanation for the reduced integration in this region was that soft tissue from the neurovascular bundle in the incisive canal contaminated the fixture surface during the placement procedure. Consequently, efforts were made in the current study to clean out the incisive canal thoroughly before filling it with particulated autogenous bone, which would enhance the stability of fixtures placed in the region.

As shown in several of the case presentations, the new maxillary reconstructions could survive the increased mechanical forces originating from mandibular bone-anchored restorations. The potential overload may have been prevented by osseoperception–the restored sensory perception associated with an osseointegrated device[42] (Fig 6-18).

Most fixture failures occurred before or at the time of abutment connection. The failure rate declined after the first year following abutment connection, possibly because of adequate bone remodeling. A likely explanation for the early losses is that many of the patients demonstrated an extremely compromised anatomy with respect to the volume and density of the residual bone. This was also reflected in the number of recipient site dehiscences where tissue of questionable quality proved inadequate to cover the graft.

Radiographic findings

The registered bone loss was similar to what has previously been reported for Brånemark fixtures in nongrafted cases.[43] After the first year of function, the mean bone loss was approximately 1 mm. Thereafter it was about 0.1 to 0.2 mm annually. Usually the fixtures were positioned at an adequate depth that allowed the cover screws to be placed flush with the bony surface of the alveolar crest. Subsequently the bone loss for the initial healing period was calculated as the increased distance between the reference point (at the coronal part of the fixture head) and the bone level. The mean distance between the reference point and the bone level at connection of the fixed prosthesis was 1.7 mm (SD, 1.2), which is comparable to results described elsewhere.[44]

It was also shown that bone responded favorably to a minimal delay of time between abutment connection to fixture and subsequent application of prosthesis. This is demonstrated in several of the case presentations in this book, as well as in the overall results.

It should also be considered that patients who were subjected to radiographic evaluations between scheduled recalls usually were afflicted with some type of complication and therefore required additional analysis.

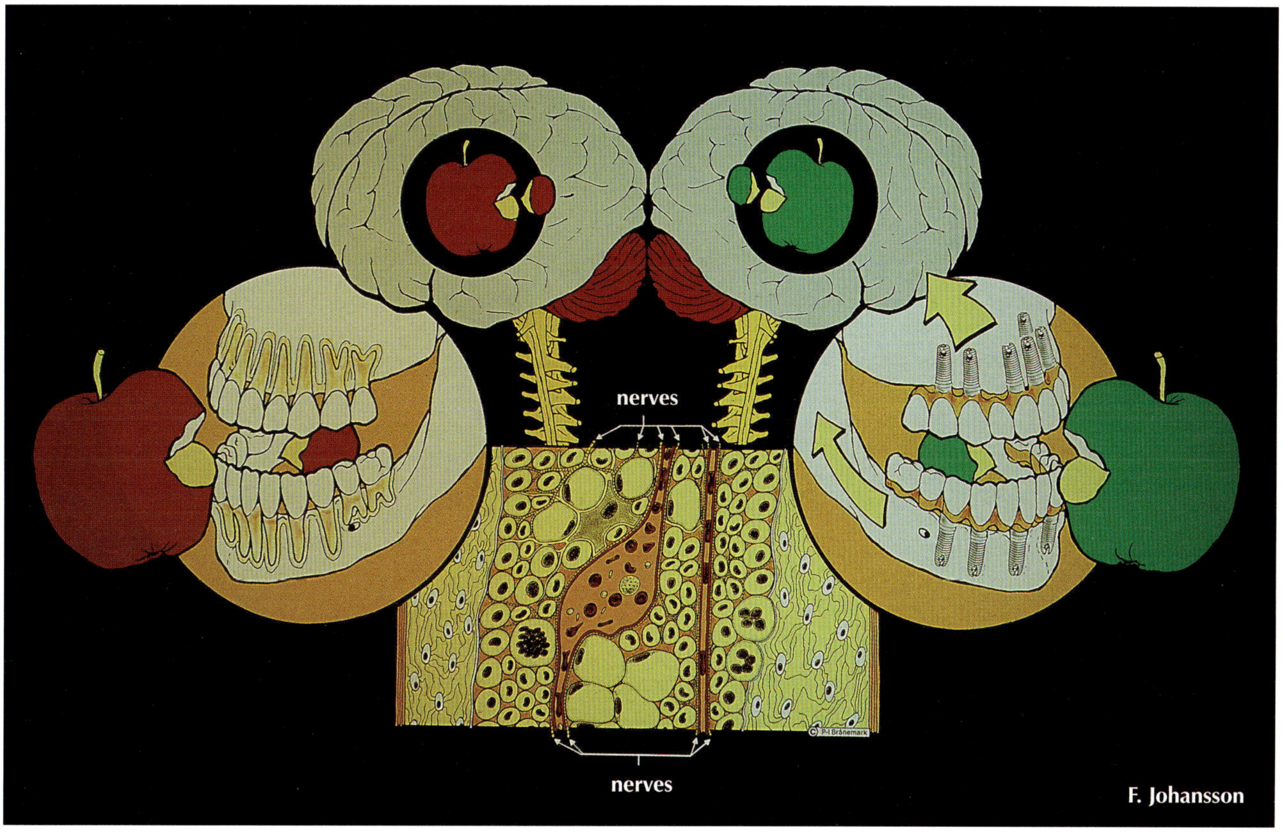

Fig 6-18 Osseoperception.

The grade of resorption (index I–V) did not have a significant influence on the bone level. This lack of significance indicates revitalized and fully incorporated grafts.

Summary of clinical and radiographic results

Both radiographic and clinical results clarified the following facts.

- Simultaneous treatment of the opposite jaw was an important preoperative consideration because it helped to avoid biomechanical overload of the maxillary reconstruction.
- Proper suturing in two layers was essential to avoid dehiscence and subsequent infection.
- Four to six fixtures were usually adequate to support a bone-anchored prosthetic restoration.
- Heavy smoking and bruxism adversely affected the results.
- The grafted bone could remineralize under optimal dynamic functional loading.
- "Early" loading of the prosthetic device had a favorable impact on the bone tissue.

The learning curve and time

The technique was new when the study began. It is therefore not surprising that initial failures occurred, both in terms of fixture integration and occasionally in system survival–all clinicians are familiar with the "learning curve" that occurs when new techniques are introduced and refined. A contributing factor to the limited overall success rate of the fixtures may have been the pressure put upon the surgeon to accept and treat patients with an extremely compromised anatomy. Yet the results are similar or compare favorably with reports on related procedures in the scientific literature.[16,24–26,44–47]

On a more subjective note, it became obvious during the course of the study that there are no magical shortcuts to clinical success. As always, skills were enhanced with experience. Meditative surgery that focused on the biological conditions at hand was the most important success factor. The grafted bone is not homogenous. The study offered many examples of how reduced tissue injury enhanced the likelihood of treatment success.

Development of the zygoma option

The study led to increased surgical and biomechanical experience. This, in turn, led to the development of the zygoma option.[27] The new fixture was a direct response to the acknowledged need for improvements in onlay bone grafting procedures, specifically for enhanced fixture stability and minimized surgery. The zygoma fixture was available for use during the latter part of the study and spared several patients from reverting to a denture.

The zygoma fixture is now routinely used to enhance load-bearing capacity and minimize the need for grafting. It offers an opportunity to treat the severely resorbed maxilla with reduced invasiveness and tissue injury.

Typical examples of the value of the zygoma fixture were shown in chapter 4 in the presentation of five of the most compromised patients in the study. Some of these patients would have been extremely difficult, perhaps even impossible, to treat without the zygoma option. Therefore the use of such fixtures is now a natural alternative when doing a treatment plan for a severely resorbed maxilla.

The Future of Onlay Grafting

With an overall prosthetic rehabilitation rate of 95% after 5 years and 93% after 10 years, onlay grafting with simultaneous placement of endosseous fixtures is a valuable approach to managing the resorbed edentulous maxilla. The results of this study compare well with similar reports in the literature. Many of our patients had no other realistic alternative to the despair they associated with the dysfunction of their removable prostheses.

In the future, alternative approaches may supersede the onlay grafting procedure. Potential examples involve bone conditioning by cyclic loading and/or the use of stem cells, growth factors, and other bone promoting agents.

New fixture designs will also prove beneficial. This can be said with certainty because our documented long-term clinical experiences with the zygoma fixture have so far demonstrated increased system survival, retained anatomy, and adequate lip support when treating patients with severely resorbed maxillae.[27,48] The need for grafting has been significantly reduced to the degree that sometimes it is no longer required at all, particularly when careful presurgical prosthetic planning is respected and performed.

CHAPTER 7

Patients with Discontinuous Maxillae

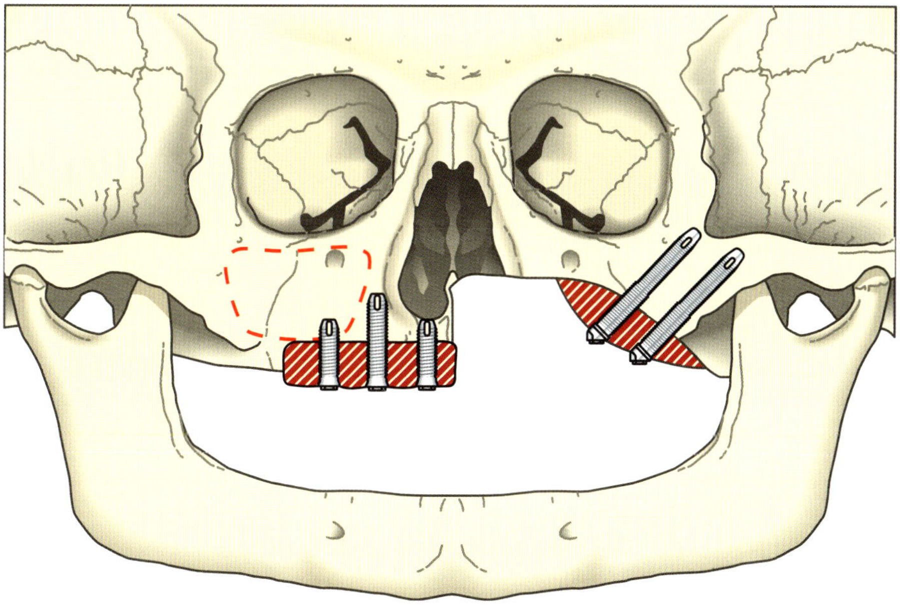

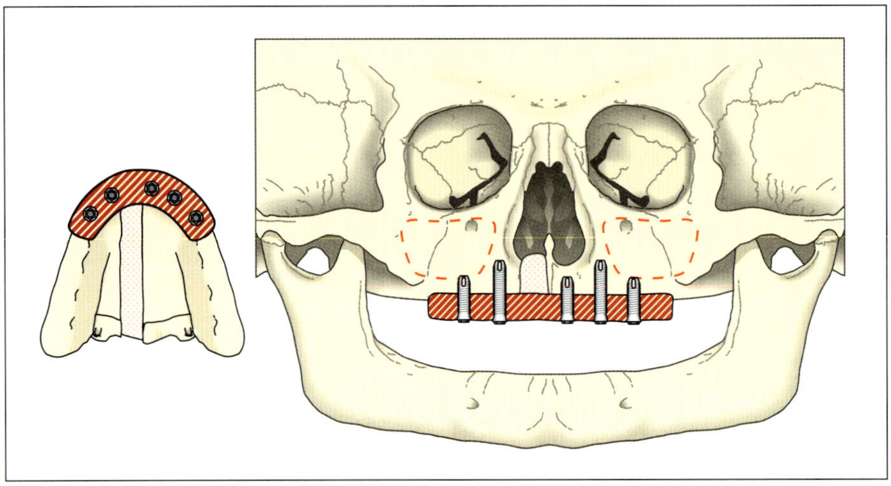

Fig 7-1 Schematic of typical cleft treatment.

Table 7-1 Baseline patient profile and fixture data for patients with cleft defects

Baseline characteristics	Patients (n = 25)	Mean observation time (y)	Total fixtures placed (n = 131)	Failed fixtures (n = 47)	Fixture survival rate (%)
Age (y)					
< 50	17	5.9	83	28	66.3
50–65	6	9.9	36	13	63.9
> 65	2	5.6	12	6	50.0
Sex					
Male	11	5.8	50	20	60.0
Female	14	7.6	81	27	66.7
Surgical clinic					
Göteborg	7	7.6	38	16	57.9
Other	18	6.5	93	31	66.7
Opposing dentition					
Complete denture	2	5.8	9	4	55.6
Natural teeth	12	7.3	63	23	63.5
Partial fixed prosthesis	1	6.4	7	1	85.7
Removable partial denture	7	6.0	34	13	61.8
Fixed prosthesis	3	8.0	18	6	66.7

Patients with Cleft Defects

Study design

During the autogenous onlay bone grafting study that took place between 1978 and 1998, a consecutive series of 25 patients with maxillary cleft defects underwent oral rehabilitation. The procedure (Fig 7-1) has been thoroughly described elsewhere.[49] The treatment included simultaneous placement of endosseous fixtures. These patients are not included among the 165 patients previously reported in this text.

Only one patient received an onlay bone graft before 1986; the remaining 24 patients were treated between 1986 and 1996. Eleven (44%) of the 25 patients were men and 14 (56%) were women. The mean age at the time of surgery was 34 years (range, 20 to 56) for men and 49 years (range, 20 to 74) for women.

All patients were followed until the end of 1998. The mean follow-up time in the cleft group was 6.9 years and the entire material comprised 171 follow-up years. The baseline patient profile is included in Table 7-1.

Table 7-2 Survival rate of fixtures by position in the dental arch

Fixture position	Original fixtures (n = 106)	Failed fixtures (n = 44)	Survival rate (%)
Central incisor	13	8	38.5
Lateral incisor	17	11	35.3
Canine	28	13	53.6
First premolar	33	8	75.8
Second premolar	15	4	73.3

Table 7-3 Survival rate of fixtures by fixture design

Fixture designs	Original fixtures (n = 106)	Failed fixtures (n = 44)	Survival rate (%)
Standard	0	0	n/a*
Self-tapping	20	8	60.0
Conical	2	0	n/a*
Swan-neck	76	30	60.5
Other	8	6	n/a*

*Population too small for analysis.

In total, 131 fixtures were placed. Of these, 106 (81%) were installed at the time of grafting. The additional 25 fixtures (mean, 1 fixture/patient; range, 0 to 4) were placed when needed during the course of the study to prevent or alleviate complications. The number of installed fixtures per patient ranged from 2 to 9. The mean number of originally installed fixtures per patient was 4.0 (range, 2 to 7).

The original fixtures usually varied in length between 10 and 20 mm. Most fixtures were placed in the anterior region (Table 7-2). The fixture designs included 20 self-tapping, 2 conical, and 76 swan-neck fixtures (Table 7-3; see also Fig 2-6). Eight fixtures were custom designed.

A bone-anchored fixed prosthesis was delivered to 13 patients (52%), while 9 patients (36%) received a fixture-supported overdenture. Three patients (12%) with 11 fixtures were unable to undergo the prosthetic part of the rehabilitation. One of these patients was a heavy smoker and alcohol consumer. She died in 1990 at the age of 74. She was withdrawn from the study at the time of her death. Since she had previously lost all 5 of her fixtures, she was also registered as a system failure when calculating the survival data.

System survival curves were calculated using a product-limit estimate (the Kaplan-Meier survival curve).[32]

Results

The 3-year survival rate of the prosthetic reconstructions was 88%. It then remained unchanged throughout the follow-up period (Fig 7-2). At the end of 1998, 22 patients (88%) carried a bone-anchored fixed prosthesis or overdenture. As stated, the rehabilitation failed in 3 patients (12%) who subsequently continued to wear a conventional denture (Table 7-4). With the exception of 1 patient who converted from an overdenture to a fixed prosthesis, there were no reports of discontinued prosthetic use among the patients with bone-anchored prosthetic devices.

In total, 47 fixtures (36%) were lost. Of these, 44 were installed at the time of grafting. The mean number of functioning fixtures per patient at the end of the study was 3.4 (range, 0 to 9). The mean number of lost fixtures per patient was 1.9 (range, 0 to 5). One patient lost 5 fixtures while 19 patients lost between 1 and 4 fixtures. The time of original fixture loss is given in Table 7-5, where it can be noted that no failures occurred after the first year of follow-up. Too few fixtures were installed in each region of the dental arch to draw any definite conclusions, but in accordance with previous experiences,[49] there was a clear tendency for reduced survival rates in the cleft region (see Table 7-2).

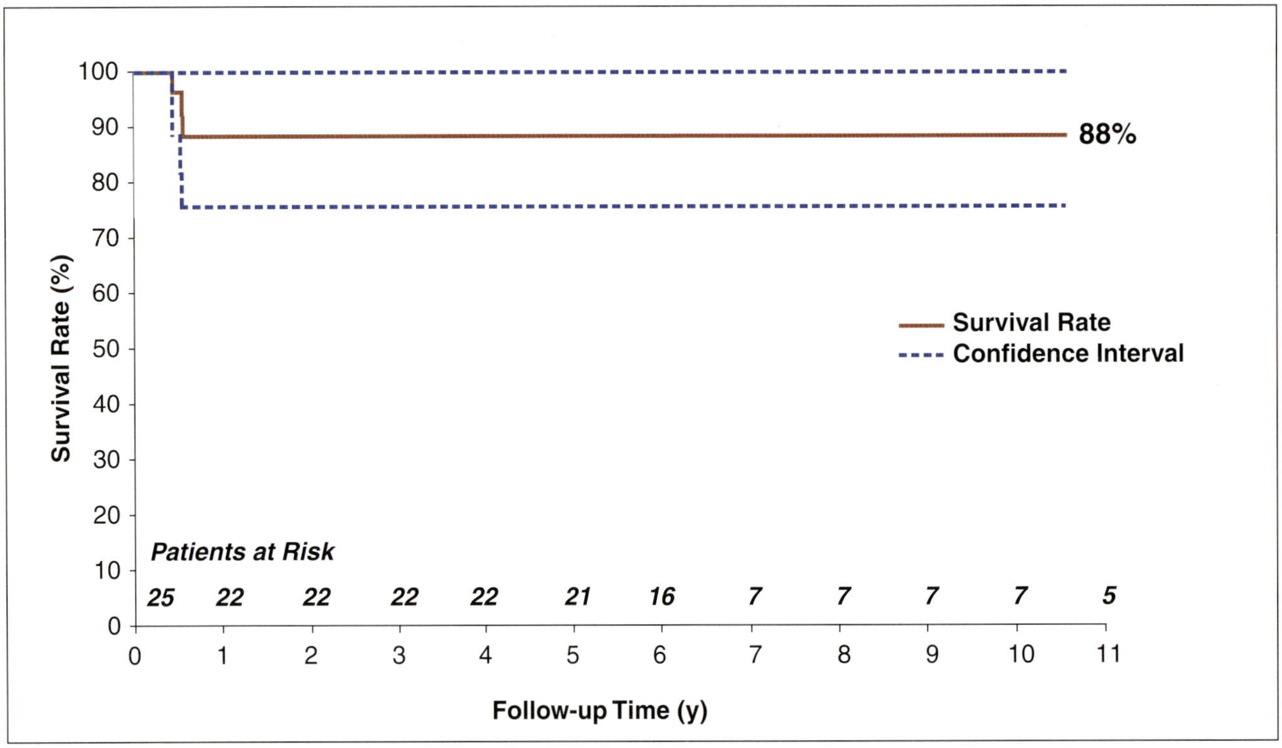

Fig 7-2 System survival (retained prosthesis)—patients with cleft defects (survival distribution function and 95% confidence interval).

Table 7-4 Prosthetic status at end of study

Status	No. of patients
Original bone-anchored fixed prosthesis in use	13
Original bone-anchored overdenture in use	8
Change of prosthesis during study period	1
Failure/death/withdrawal	3
Original bone-anchored prostheses in function at end of study	21

Table 7-5 Timing of fixture failure and placement of additional fixtures

Timing	Original fixtures lost (n = 44)	Additional fixtures placed (n = 24)
During initial healing	23	11
At AC*	8	10
Between AC and year 1	13	3
Between year 1 and year 2	0	0
Between year 2 and year 3	0	0
Between year 3 and year 4	0	0
Between year 4 and year 5	0	0
Between year 5 and year 6	0	0
Between year 6 and year 7	0	0
After more than 7 years	0	0

*AC—Abutment connection.

Table 7-6 Survival rate of fixtures by grafting procedure

Grafting procedure	Patients (n = 25)	Mean observation time (y)	Total fixtures placed (n = 131)	Failed fixtures (n = 47)	Fixture survival rate (%)
Nasal inlay					
Yes	1	4.1	2	0	n/a*
No	24	6.9	129	47	63.6
Sinus floor graft					
Unilateral	5	4.9	31	15	51.6
No sinus graft	20	7.3	100	32	68.0
Onlay graft donor sites					
Medial ilium	14	6.4	79	30	62.0
Lateral ilium	4	9.3	18	7	61.1
Medial and lateral ilium	2	6.1	9	4	55.6
Iliac crest only	5	6.5	25	6	76.0

*Population too small for analysis.

Table 7-7 Survival rate of fixtures by disturbed healing at the recipient site

Disturbed healing	Patients (n = 25)	Mean observation time (y)	Total fixtures placed (n = 131)	Failed fixtures (n = 47)	Fixture survival rate (%)
Dehiscence					
Yes	14	8.1	83	36	56.6
No	11	5.3	48	11	77.1
Infection					
Yes	10	7.4	57	25	56.1
No	15	6.5	74	22	70.3
Sequestrum					
Yes	18	6.8	95	41	56.8
No	7	6.9	36	6	83.3
Exposed threads					
Yes	3	7.4	17	8	52.9
No	22	6.8	114	39	65.8

The patients with cleft defects did not exhibit any complications at the donor site. There were no reports on increased morbidity in terms of pain or hematoma. When the fixture survival rates were correlated to the different parameters related to grafting procedures and donor sites, no statistically significant differences were noted (Table 7-6).

Table 7-7 describes the frequency of disturbed healing at the graft recipient site. Dehiscences were noted in 14 patients (56%) and infection in 10 patients (40%). Sequestra were formed in 18 patients (72%). Fixture failure was significantly more frequent when sequestra were noted ($P = .05$).

The treatment aspects related to cleft patients are exemplified by the following two case presentations.

Patient 1 (cleft group)

Background

This Irish man was born in 1966. He suffered from a major congenital palatal defect that had not been closed initially. Severe functional and social problems resulted from the handicap.

Surgical procedure

When the patient was aged 26, surgical closure of the hard and soft tissue defects was performed using a full bone graft from the left iliac crest. Two fixtures, obliquely placed, secured the graft after it had been tightly positioned into the defect. Mucoperiosteal coverage was obtained by rotating mucoperiosteal flaps. (This patient was treated in collaboration with D. Harris and K.W. Higuchi.)

Additional surgery

In February 1993, the patient returned for abutment connection and additional fixture surgery. Two small perforations were noted in the midline. Epithelialized tissue found in the perforation areas were removed. The two fixtures were well integrated and the bone graft in the palatal area was in excellent condition. A resorbed area, devitalized by vital compact bone, was noted in the anterior portion of the graft. The grafted bone located anterior to and between the two fixtures exhibited less vitality than the rest of the graft. A 10-mm long flange fixture was placed in that area. Acceptable stability was achieved. Angular abutments were connected to the two existing fixtures.

Complications

In June 1993, the patient was complaining of bad odor and taste. He also experienced an unpleasant postnasal drip. A surgical exploration of the anterior part of the graft was performed in August 1993. A small sequestrum containing the 10-mm fixture was removed and adjacent bone was curetted. Healing was uneventful and full closure of the soft tissues occurred.

The patient had complained of some difficulty in breathing through his nose. In March 1996, he underwent a septorhinoplasty. A considerable deviation of his septum was corrected. His overall facial expression improved and breathing became easier.

Restoration and follow-up

A well-adapted, rigid bar was attached when the mucosa had healed. The bar was used during the bone remodeling phase to support a provisional prosthesis, which was not placed in occlusion.

The final prosthesis, a removable overdenture, was delivered in November 1996. The patient has attended annual follow-up visits. Both fixtures have remained stable and the integrity of the bone graft and soft tissue closure has been maintained. No further complications have been recorded.

At the follow-up in 1999, adequate restitution of structure and function was noted. A letter from his clinician in Ireland dated September 2000 states: "The patient is entirely satisfied with his reconstruction. He reports that it has made a major improvement in the quality of his life as he can function well, speak clearly and socialize with confidence. The increase in confidence level is very noticeable and in dramatic contrast to the introspective, shy individual who originally presented for treatment."

Patient 1 (Cleft Group)

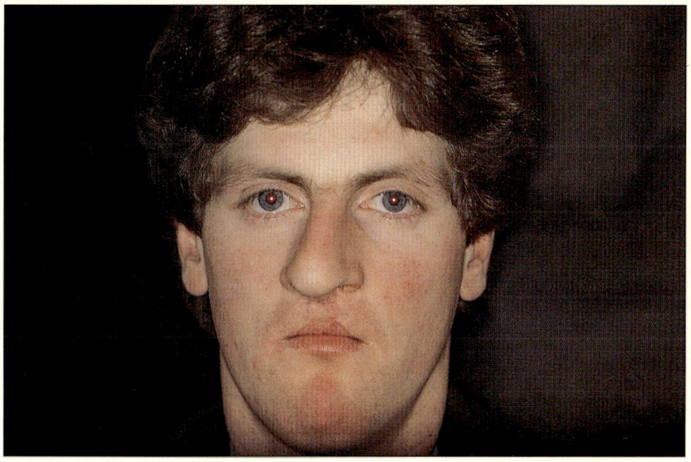

Fig 7-3 Preoperative facial view.

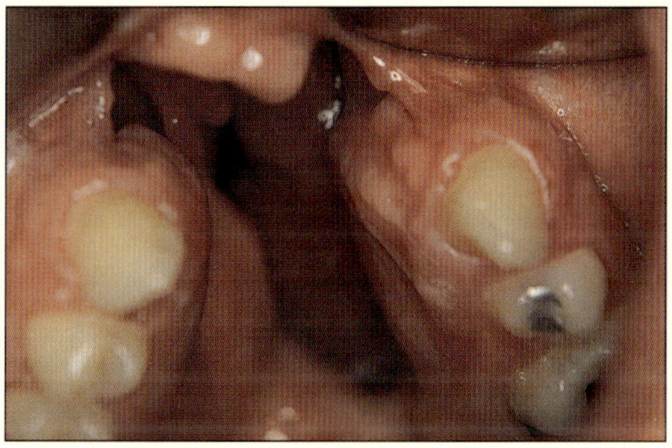

Fig 7-4 Intraoral preoperative status.

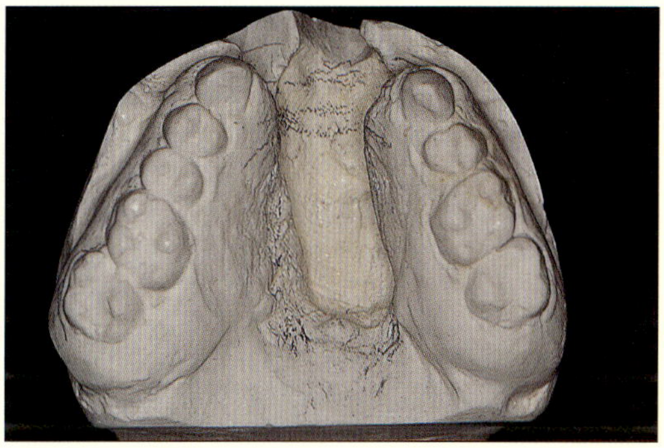

Fig 7-5 Cast of the cleft defect.

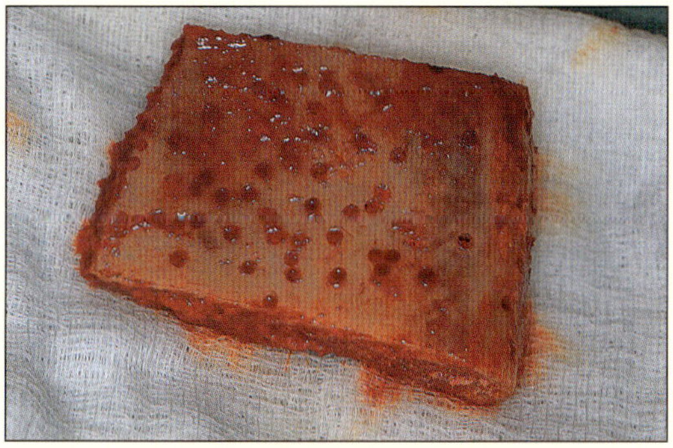

Fig 7-6 The graft. Small penetrations in the graft allowed for revascularization.

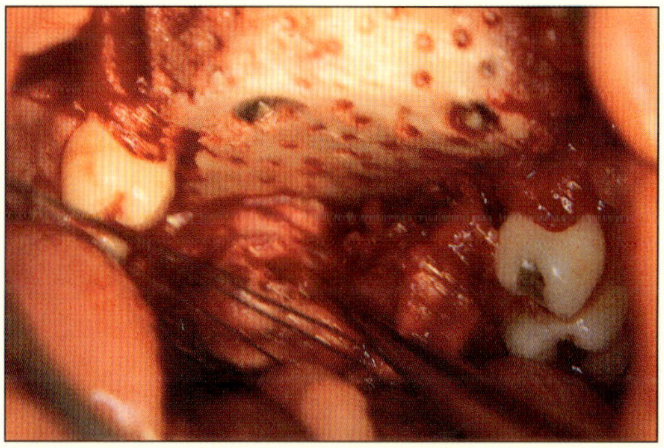

Fig 7-7 The graft in place.

Patient 1 (Cleft Group) continued

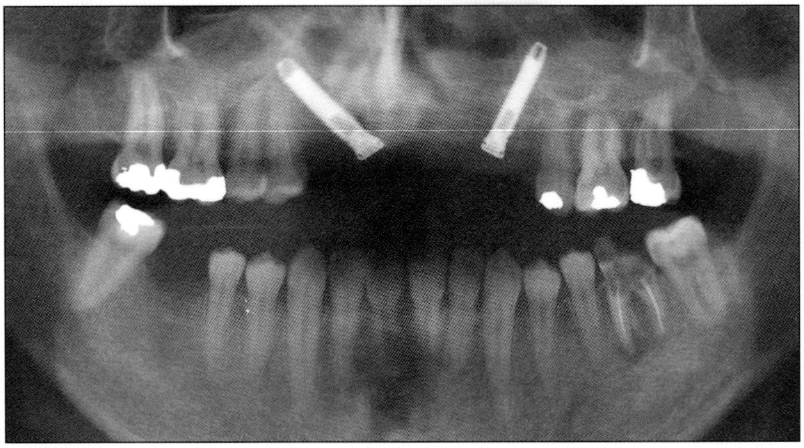

Fig 7-8 Panoramic view after fixture surgery (1993).

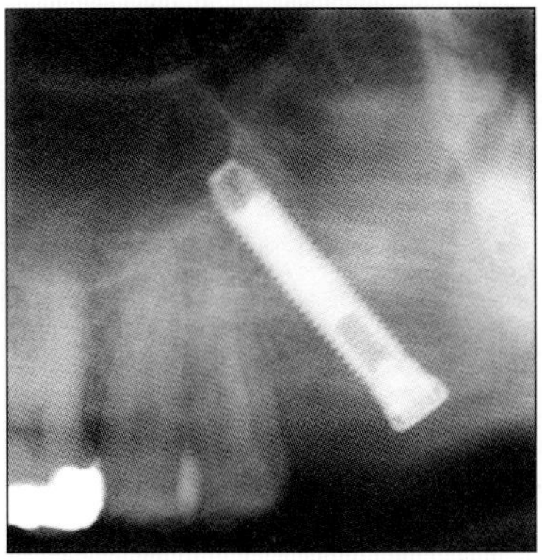

Fig 7-9 Right dental scanogram after fixture surgery (1993).

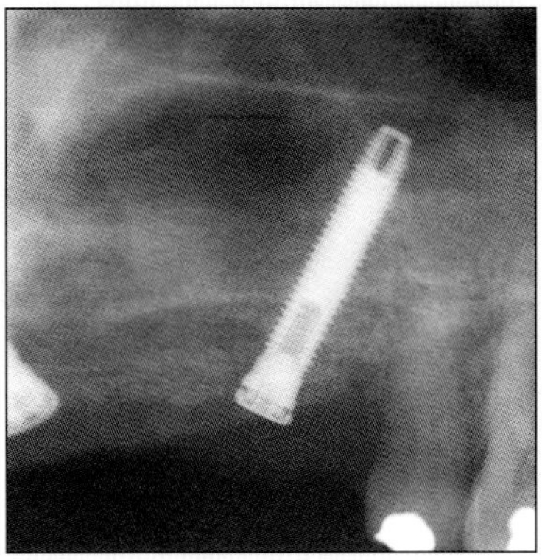

Fig 7-10 Left dental scanogram after fixture surgery (1993).

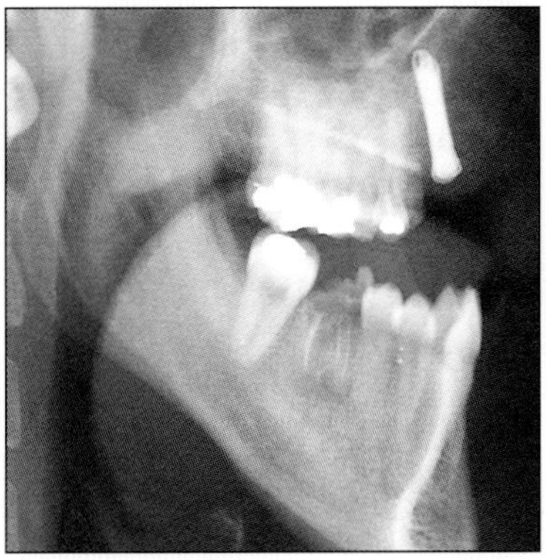

Fig 7-11 Profile after fixture surgery (1993).

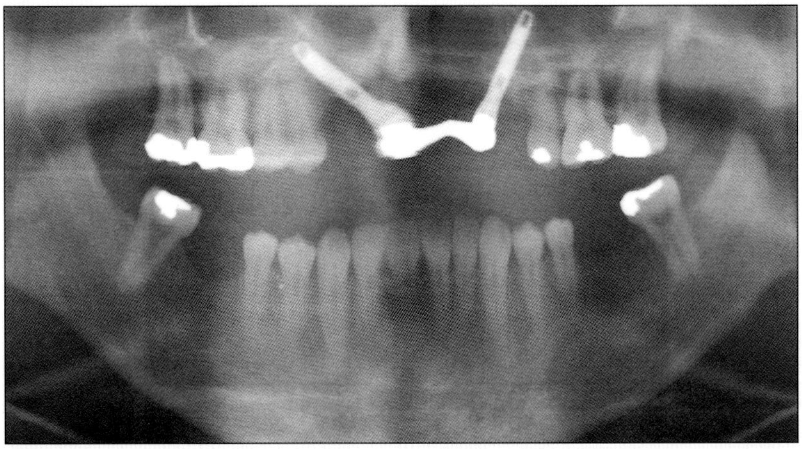

Fig 7-12 Panoramic view after bar attachment (1994).

Patient 1 (Cleft Group) continued

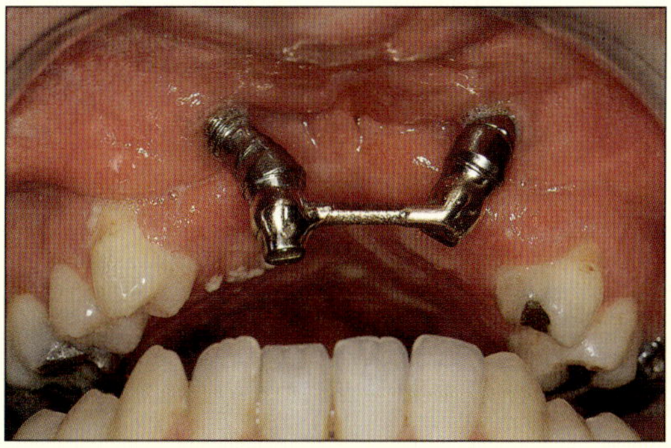

Fig 7-13 The bar construction.

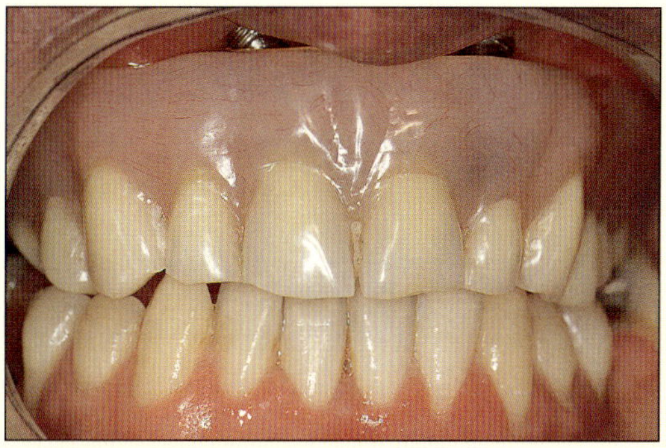

Fig 7-14 The prosthesis in place.

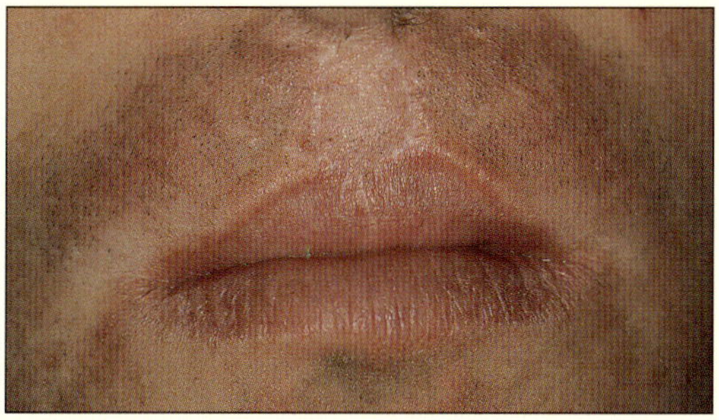

Fig 7-15 Postoperative view of improved facial anatomy.

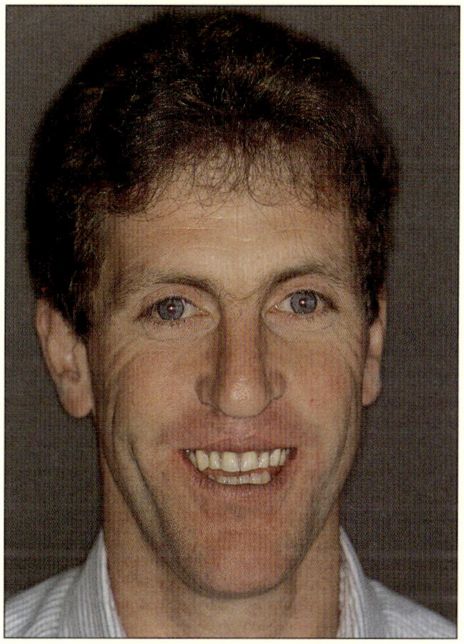

Fig 7-16 Postoperative facial view. The patient has attended annual follow-up visits in Ireland, where his attending clinician has commented on his notably increased social confidence (1998).

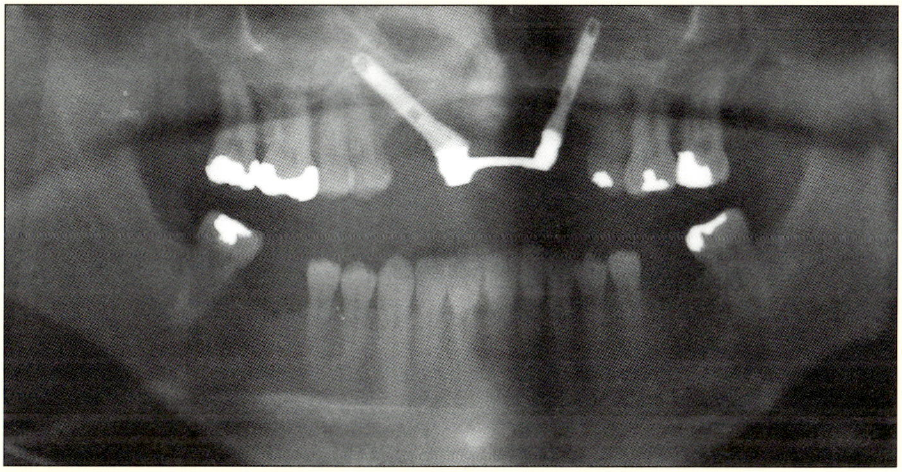

Fig 7-17 Panoramic view at 8-year follow-up after conclusion of the study (2001).

Patient 2 (cleft group)

Background

This 20-year-old French man was born in 1973 with bilateral congenital cheilognathopalatoschisis. After several surgical sessions (lip revision and Le Fort I osteotomy) and orthodontic treatment in France, the mucosa was almost closed. A bone defect remained in the anterior maxilla.

Preoperative comments

Three surgical sessions were planned:

1. Osteotomy followed by orthodontic treatment to adjust the maxillary position
2. Closure of the oronasal fistula
3. Closure of remaining defects with an autologous bone graft secured with fixtures

The fixtures would later support a bone-anchored prosthetic reconstruction.

Surgical procedure

The first surgery was performed in May 1993. A previous osteotomy on the right side had healed properly, but on the left side the posterior half of the osteotomy was infiltrated by cartilage, which left the anatomy in the anterior portion severely deranged. Three osteosutures were removed–two on the left side and one on the right side. A horizontal osteotomy was made from the nasal aperture to the pterygoid bone. The septum between the nasal and sinus cavities was separated, as was the tuber maxillae from the pterygoid bone on the right.

After the maxilla was completely mobilized, the planned down-fracture could not be performed because of resistance in the cleft region. Instead an osteotomy was made after the scarred tissue had been undermined. The postoperative period was uneventful. After orthodontic treatment, the patient returned to France until the next surgical session.

The second surgery was performed in August 1993. The anterior oronasal fistula was closed with sutures while the posterior fissure was left unaltered. The anterior mucosa was mobilized through incisions at the gingival border. Adequate closure against the oral cavity was achieved.

The final surgery was performed in October 1993. The mucosa was in good condition. The remaining fistula was closed. A bone graft taken from the left ilium was secured with two fixtures on the right side. A shorter fixture was placed in the premaxilla slightly to the left of the midline. The mucosa was carefully adapted and released prior to suturing.

No postoperative complications occurred. The patient returned to France after 2 weeks of uneventful healing.

Abutment connection and fixture replacement

Abutment connection and fixture replacement were performed in May 1994. A palatal fistula with hyperplasia required reopening of the cleft area. The graft and two osseointegrated fixtures were well incorporated on the right side of the midline. On the left side, a partially necrotic portion of the graft and a mobile fixture were removed. The area was then carefully curetted until only healthy vascularized tissue remained.

A 13-mm fixture was installed in premaxillary and grafted bone on the left side. Abutments were connected to the two integrated fixtures on the right side. The mucosa was readjusted prior to suturing to enable vestibuloplasty at a later date. Adequate closure was obtained; there was no remaining communication between the nasal and the oral cavities. In November 1994 the left fixture was found to be well integrated and a 5-mm angulated abutment was connected.

Plastic surgery

In November 1994 the patient underwent bilateral lip revision and corrections of diastasis of the musculus orbicularis oris, asymmetric nares, and the unbalanced crest height. The patient returned home after 7 days of uneventful healing.

Follow-up

At the first annual follow-up visit in December 1995, the patient had not experienced any discomfort and expressed satisfaction with the esthetic results. The upper lip and the nose had healed well. The provisional fixed prosthesis was therefore replaced with a permanent reconstruction.

At the 4-year follow-up visit in August 1998, the patient remained pleased. The situation was stable also from clinical and radiographic points of view.

Patient 2 (Cleft Group)

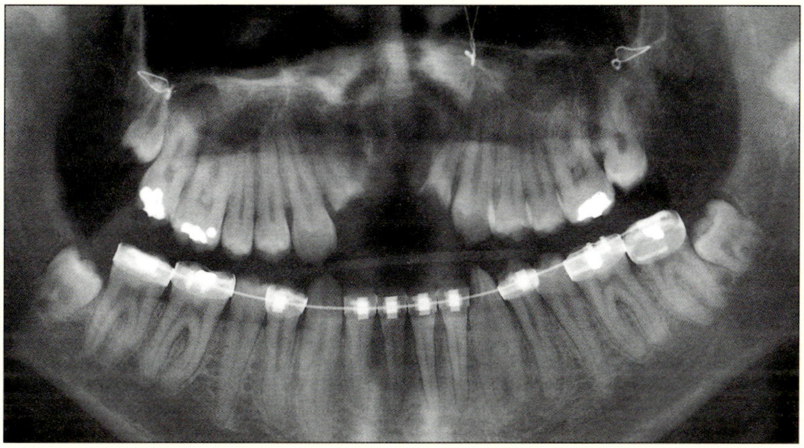

Fig 7-18 Preoperative panoramic view (1992).

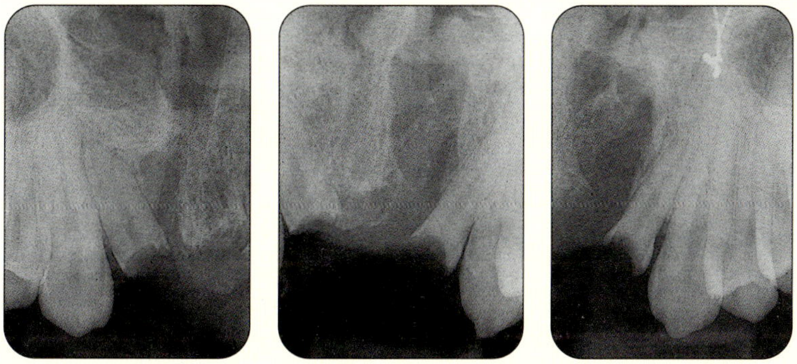

Fig 7-19 Preoperative intraoral radiographs (1992).

Patient 2 (Cleft Group) continued

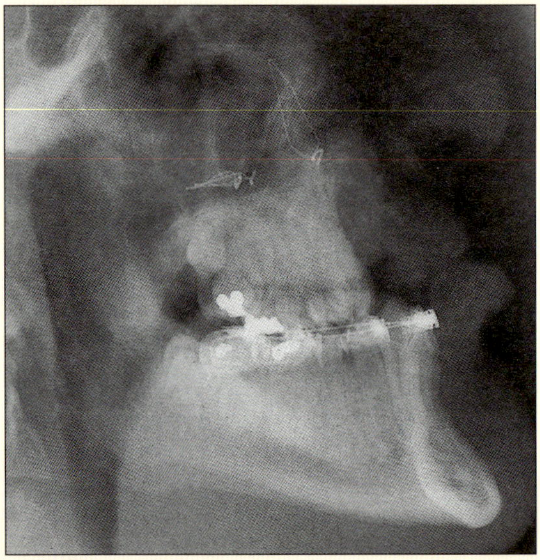

Fig 7-20 Preoperative profile (1992).

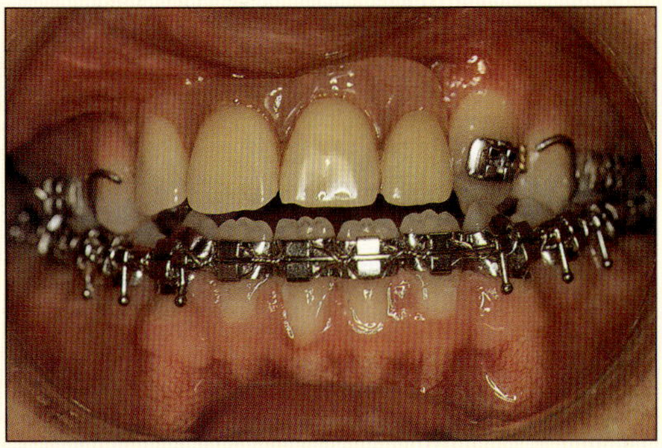

Fig 7-21 Preoperative view of partial denture covering the cleft defect (1992).

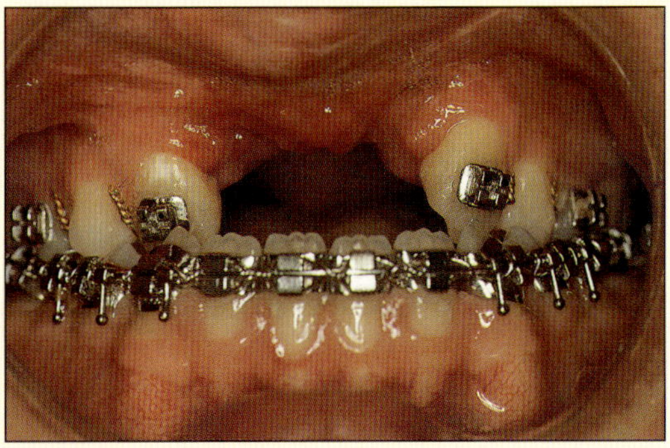

Fig 7-22 Cleft defect.

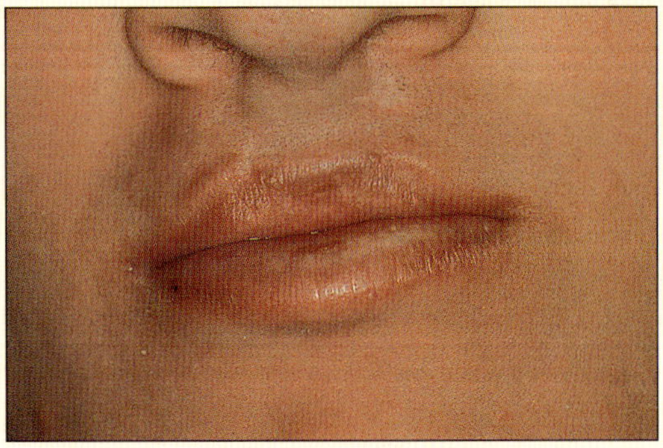

Fig 7-23 Preoperative facial anatomy.

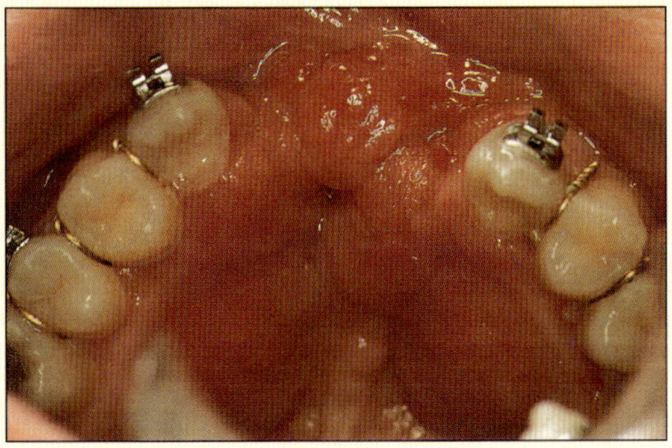

Fig 7-24 Intraoral status (1993).

Patient 2 (Cleft Group) continued

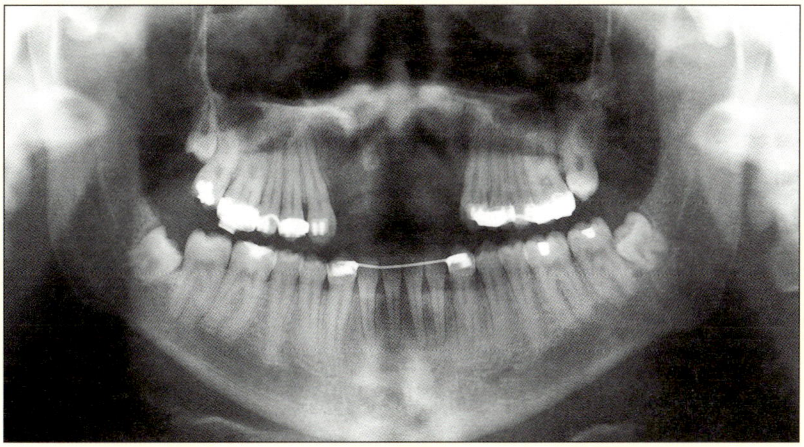

Fig 7-25 Panoramic view after closure of the oronasal fistula (August 1993).

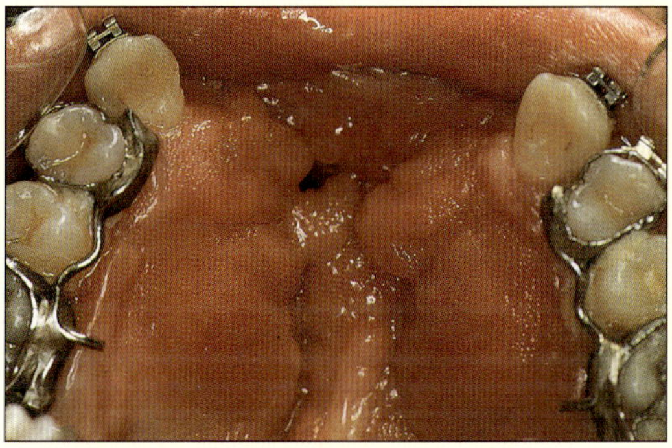

Fig 7-26 Preoperative view (October 1993).

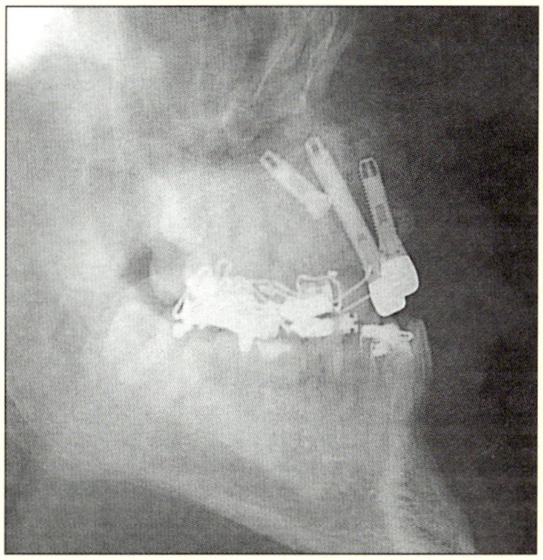

Fig 7-27 Profile (September 1994).

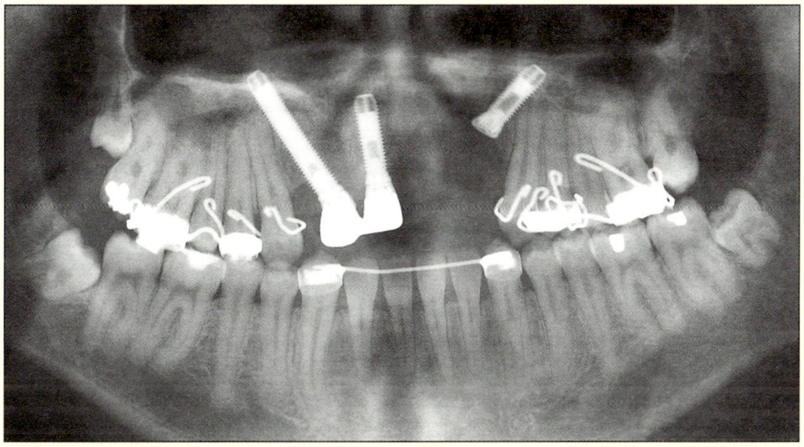

Fig 7-28 Panoramic view after abutment connection and additional fixture installation (November 1994).

Patient 2 (Cleft Group) continued

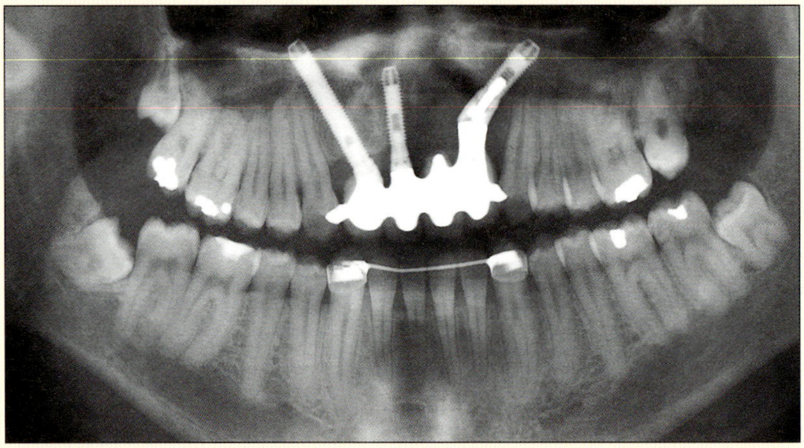

Fig 7-29 Panoramic view at 1-year follow-up (1995).

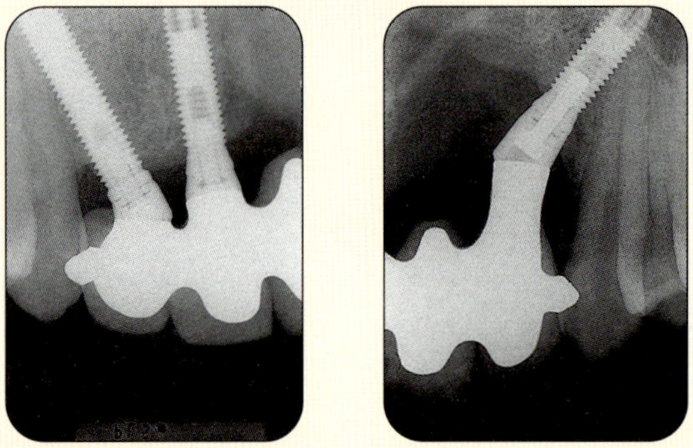

Fig 7-30 One-year follow-up (1995).

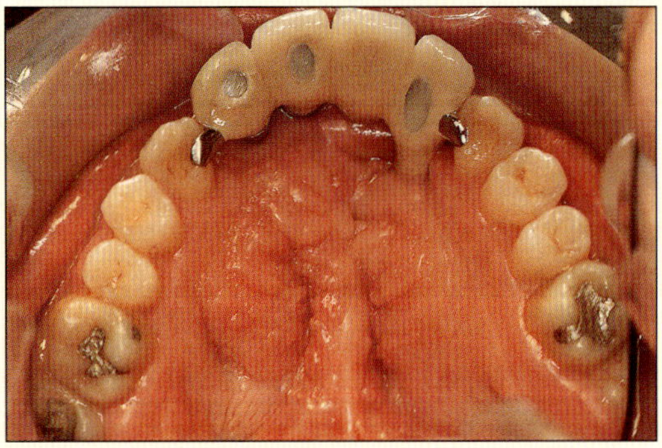

Fig 7-31 Intraoral status at 1-year follow-up (1995).

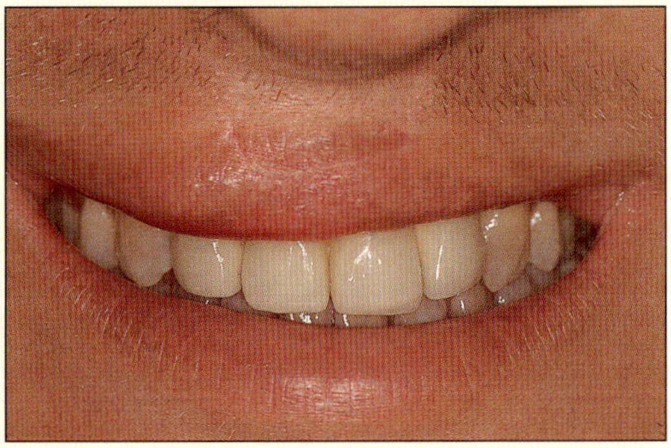

Fig 7-32 Facial anatomy at 1-year follow-up (1995).

Patient 2 (Cleft Group) continued

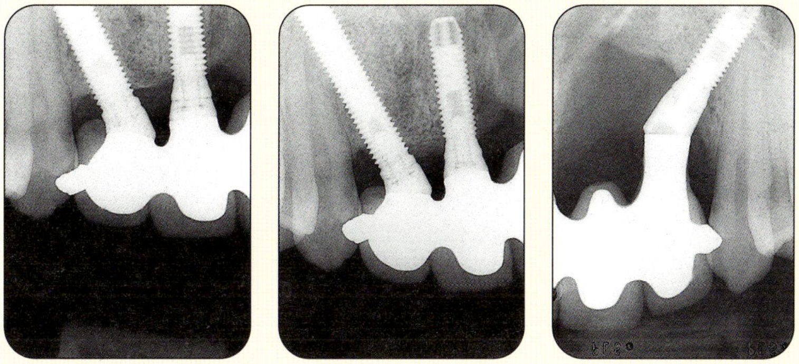

Fig 7-33 Four-year follow-up (1998).

Patients After Maxillectomy

Study design

During the autogenous onlay bone grafting study between 1978 and 1998, a consecutive series of 25 patients with maxillary defects after maxillectomy (mainly hemimaxillectomy) underwent oral rehabilitation.[49] Autogenous onlay bone grafting, with simultaneous placement of endosseous fixtures, was carried out in each case (Figs 7-34 and 7-35). These patients are not included among the 165 patients previously reported in this publication.

One patient underwent operation before 1985 while the remaining 24 patients were treated between 1986 and 1996. Many of the patients had previously undergone irradiation and/or chemotherapy. As described elsewhere, this was not considered an absolute contraindication for osseointegration. If hyperbaric oxygen therapy was available, it was prescribed before and after surgery.[50]

Eleven (44%) of the 25 patients were men and 14 (56%) were women. The mean age at the time of surgery was 47 years (range, 19 to 68) for men and 43 years (range, 16 to 75) for women. All patients were followed until the end of 1998. The mean follow-up time was 6 years and the entire material comprised 155 follow-up years. Ten patients (40%) had a fixture-supported prosthesis in the mandible. The baseline patient profile is included in the data shown in Table 7-8.

In addition to the autogenous onlay bone grafting procedure performed on all patients, a unilateral sinus graft was conducted in two patients and a nasal inlay graft was conducted in four patients. The remaining patients only received onlay bone grafts. The iliac crest constituted the donor site for the majority of the patients (n=14).

In total, 129 fixtures were placed. Of these, 123 (95%) were installed at the time of grafting. Six fixtures (mean, 0.2 per patient; range, 0 to 2) were placed when required during the course of the study. The mean number of originally installed fixtures per patient was 4.9 (range, 2 to 9). Seven patients (28%) received 4 fixtures each.

Most fixtures were placed in the posterior region of the dental arch; 72 fixtures were placed in premolar or molar positions, whereas 51 were placed in the incisor or canine regions (Table 7-9). The original fixtures varied in length from 7 to 20 mm and were mainly of the swan-neck design (Table 7-10). Forty-five fixtures were custom designed. Four patients (16%) received a fixed prosthesis and 21 patients (84%) received a fixture-retained overdenture. System survival curves were calculated using the Kaplan-Meier survival curve, a product-limit estimate.[32]

One patient was withdrawn when she died in 1996 at the age of 58. She had worn a functioning fixture-supported overdenture for 4 years.

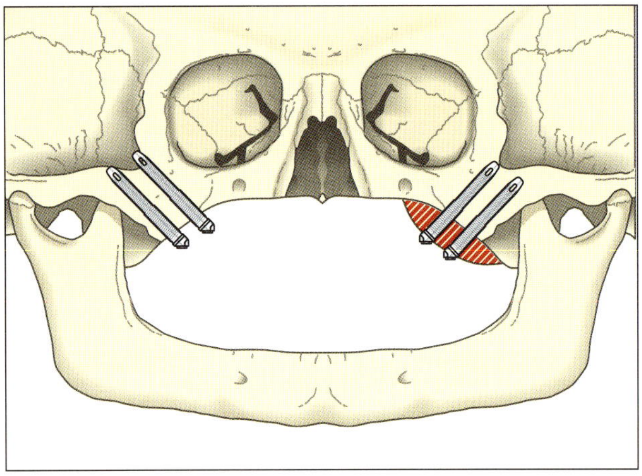

Fig 7-34 Schematic illustration of typical total maxillectomy treatment. Zygoma fixtures can be used after a total maxillectomy, thereby reducing the need for grafting.

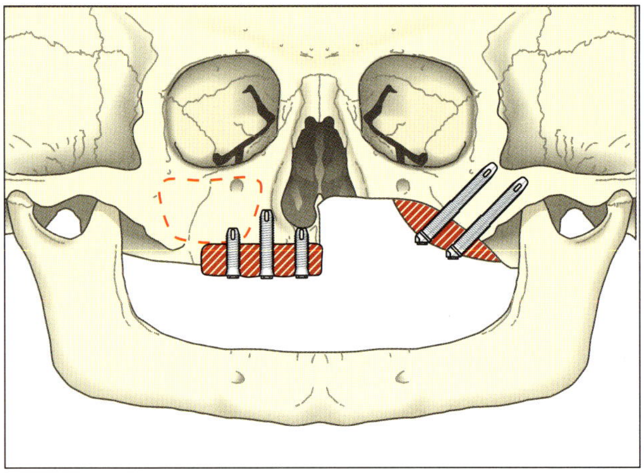

Fig 7-35 Schematic illustration of typical hemimaxillectomy treatment.

Table 7-8 Baseline patient profile and fixture data for patient with maxillectomy

Baseline characteristics	Patients (n = 25)	Mean observation time (y)	Total fixtures placed (n = 129)	Failed fixtures (n = 13)	Fixture survival rate (%)
Age (y)					
< 50	13	5.5	58	5	91.4
50–65	7	6.3	38	5	86.8
> 65	5	7.9	33	3	90.9
Sex					
Male	11	7.5	58	9	84.5
Female	14	5.2	71	4	94.4
Surgical clinic					
Göteborg	9	8.5	49	4	91.8
Other	16	4.9	80	9	88.8
Opposing dentition					
Natural teeth	11	4.2	51	6	88.2
Partial dentition	4	8.5	25	4	84.0
Fixture-supported fixed prosthesis	10	7.5	53	3	94.3

Table 7-9 Survival rate of fixtures by position in the dental arch

Fixture position	Original fixtures (n = 123)	Failed fixtures (n = 13)	Survival rate (%)
Central incisor	16	2	87.5
Lateral incisor	14	2	85.7
Canine	21	2	90.5
First premolar	26	1	96.2
Second premolar	25	3	88.0
First molar	21	3	85.7

Table 7-10 Survival rate of fixtures by fixture design

Fixture design	Original fixtures (n = 123)	Failed fixtures (n = 13)	Survival rate (%)
Standard	5	0	n/a*
Self-tapping	16	2	87.5
Conical	7	1	n/a*
Swan-neck	50	7	86.0
Other	45	3	93.3

*Population too small for analysis.

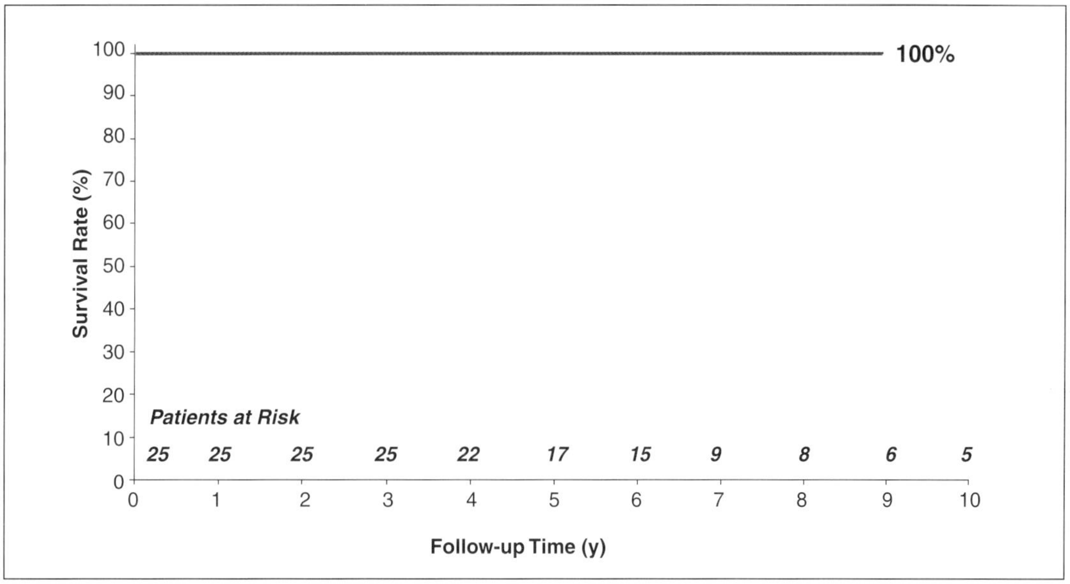

Fig 7-36 System survival (retained prosthesis)—patients subjected to maxillectomy (survival distribution function).

Table 7-11 Prosthetic status at end of study

Status	No. of patients
Original bone-anchored fixed prosthesis in use	4
Original bone-anchored overdenture in use	20
Change of prosthesis during study period	0
Failure/death/withdrawal	1
Original bone-anchored prostheses in function at end of study	24

Results

There were no prosthetic failures and no discontinuance in the use of the original prosthesis during the follow-up period. Consequently, the system survival rate was 100% (Fig 7-36; Table 7-11).

Thirteen fixtures (10%) failed and all were originally installed at the time of grafting. The time intervals for fixture loss and placement of additional fixtures are shown in Table 7-12. All fixture failures occurred within the first 2 years of follow-up. The survival rate was higher for fixtures placed in the canine or premolar regions (90% and 96%, respectively; see Table 7-9). The survival rates were comparable for the different fixture designs, albeit slightly higher for those in the "other" category, which included several zygoma fixtures (see Table 7-10).

The mean number of lost fixtures per patient was 0.5 (range, 0 to 4). Fourteen patients (56%) did not lose any fixtures, nine patients (36%) lost one fixture, and two patients (8%) lost two fixtures.

No complications were noted at the donor site. When relating the graft donor and recipient site data to fixture failure, no statistically significant differences were found (Table 7-13).

Table 7-12 Timing of fixture failure and placement of additional fixtures

Timing	Original fixtures lost (n = 13)	Additional fixtures placed (n = 6)
Before AC*	2	2
At AC	5	1
Between AC and year 1	3	1
Between year 1 and year 2	3	2
Between year 2 and year 3	0	0
Between year 3 and year 4	0	0
Between year 4 and year 5	0	0
Between year 5 and year 6	0	0
Between year 6 and year 7	0	0
After more than 7 years	0	0

*AC—Abutment connection.

Table 7-13 Survival rate of fixtures by grafting procedure

Grafting procedure	Patients (n = 25)	Mean observation time (y)	Total fixtures placed (n = 129)	Failed fixtures (n = 13)	Fixture survival rate (%)
Nasal bone graft					
Yes	4	4.6	18	1	94.4
No	21	6.5	111	12	89.2
Sinus inlay					
Unilateral	2	5.4	11	1	90.9
No sinus graft	23	6.3	118	12	89.8
Onlay graft donor sites					
Medial ilium	8	7.4	45	6	86.7
Lateral ilium	2	12.4	10	2	80.0
Medial and lateral ilium	1	3.1	4	0	n/a*
Iliac crest only	14	4.9	70	5	92.9

*Population too small for analysis.

Table 7-14 Survival rate of fixtures by disturbed healing at the recipient site

Disturbed healing	Patients (n = 25)	Mean observation time (y)	Total fixtures placed (n = 129)	Failed fixtures (n = 13)	Fixture survival rate (%)
Dehiscence					
Yes	5	7.2	25	4	84.0
No	20	5.9	104	9	91.3
Infection					
Yes	1	5.1	5	1	n/a*
No	24	6.3	124	12	90.3
Sequestrum					
Yes	3	6.7	15	3	80.0
No	22	6.1	114	10	91.2
Exposed threads					
Yes	1	8.9	7	1	n/a*
No	24	6.1	122	12	90.2

*Population too small for analysis.

Fixture survival rates in cases with disturbed healing at the recipient site are compared with those in cases without disturbed healing in Table 7-14. Dehiscences were seen in five patients (20%) and the occurrence progressed to infection in one patient. Sequestra were formed in three patients (12%).

The treatment is exemplified by the following patient presentation involving oral rehabilitation of a patient 14 years after he underwent a nearly complete maxillectomy.

Patient presentation (maxillectomy group)

Background

This male patient was born in 1923. In 1977, he underwent radiation and chemotherapy as well as a partial maxillectomy because of squamous cell carcinoma. The remaining defect left him unable to speak. He had great difficulty eating. Restorative treatment alleviated his discomfort to some extent, but he continued to have significant problems retaining the prosthetic device. He was a moderate smoker.

Preoperative comments

The preoperative computed tomography (CT) examination showed a large defect in the facial skeleton where most of the maxilla had been resected. On the right side, only the inferior orbital rim remained. The tuberosity and part of the lateral sinus wall remained on the left side.

Surgical procedure

The first surgical session took place in April 1991, when the patient was 68 years old. The anterior portion of the oral cavity showed defects related to the previous tumor extirpation, whereas the posterior area exhibited intact medial, lateral, and posterior walls.

Prior to the surgery, the patient received hyperbaric oxygen treatment.[50,51] An autogenous onlay graft of pyramid shape was taken from the left hip and placed in the posterior portion of the maxillary defect toward the zygoma region. Good adaptation was achieved.

Two fixtures were then placed in the left zygoma region. These were placed medially through the graft until they perforated the posterior aspect of the sinus wall into the body of the zygoma. A third fixture was placed posterior of (and almost horizontal to) the anterior base of the zygoma. The fixture apex perforated the lateral cortical bone plate. Adequate primary stability was achieved for all three fixtures.

One fixture was then placed in a similar fashion on the right side, anchored into os zygomaticum. The anterior aspect of the pterygoid bone was then exposed on the right side. A U-shaped autogenous graft was applied onto the bone and secured by two fixtures that penetrated the pterygoid plate. The mucoperiosteal flap was well vascularized and repositioned with sutures. One 7-mm fixture was placed in a vertical direction in the lower anterior rim of the orbit. Five 13-mm standard fixtures were then placed in the mandible. Postoperatively the patient was prescribed continued hyperbaric oxygen treatment.

Maxillary abutment connection was performed in November 1991. At that time, bone overgrowth was noted on one of the zygoma fixtures. All fixtures were stable. The short infraorbital fixture on the right side was stable but did not receive an abutment. In the mandible, all fixtures were stable and provided with abutments.

Additional surgery

In September 1993, the patient returned with one fractured and one mobile fixture on the left side. The mobile fixture was removed. After careful curettage, the site was prepared for a fixture 13 mm in length and 5.5 mm in diameter. Excellent stability was obtained. The fractured fixture was repaired with custom-made components.

In March 1994, abutment connection was performed on the wide-diameter fixture. Partial bone overgrowth was noted. The fixture was well osseointegrated.

Restoration and follow-up

A provisional fixture-supported overdenture with obturator construction was delivered to the patient in March 1994. Several adjustments were required to avoid leakage to the nasal cavity. The wide-diameter fixture underwent abutment connection in June 1994. The patient then received his final fixture-supported overdenture. Several adjustments needed to be made during the adaptation period to avoid leakage and soreness. The clinical and radiographic examinations at the 5-year follow-up visit in 1999 revealed a stable situation with adequate function of the prosthesis.

Patient Presentation (Maxillectomy Group)

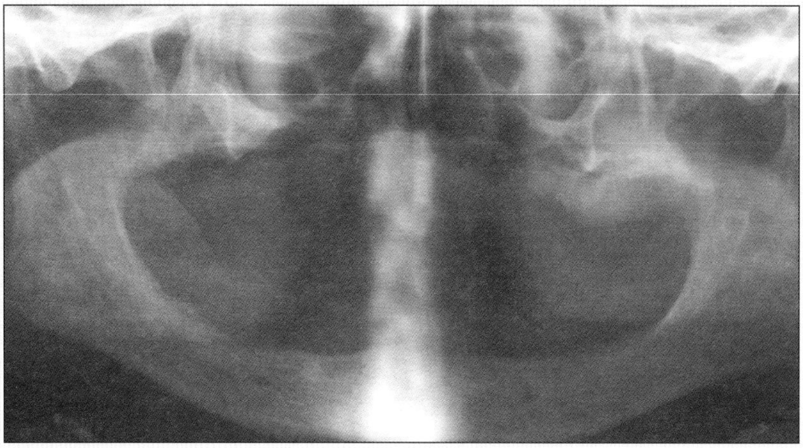

Fig 7-37 Preoperative panoramic view (1991).

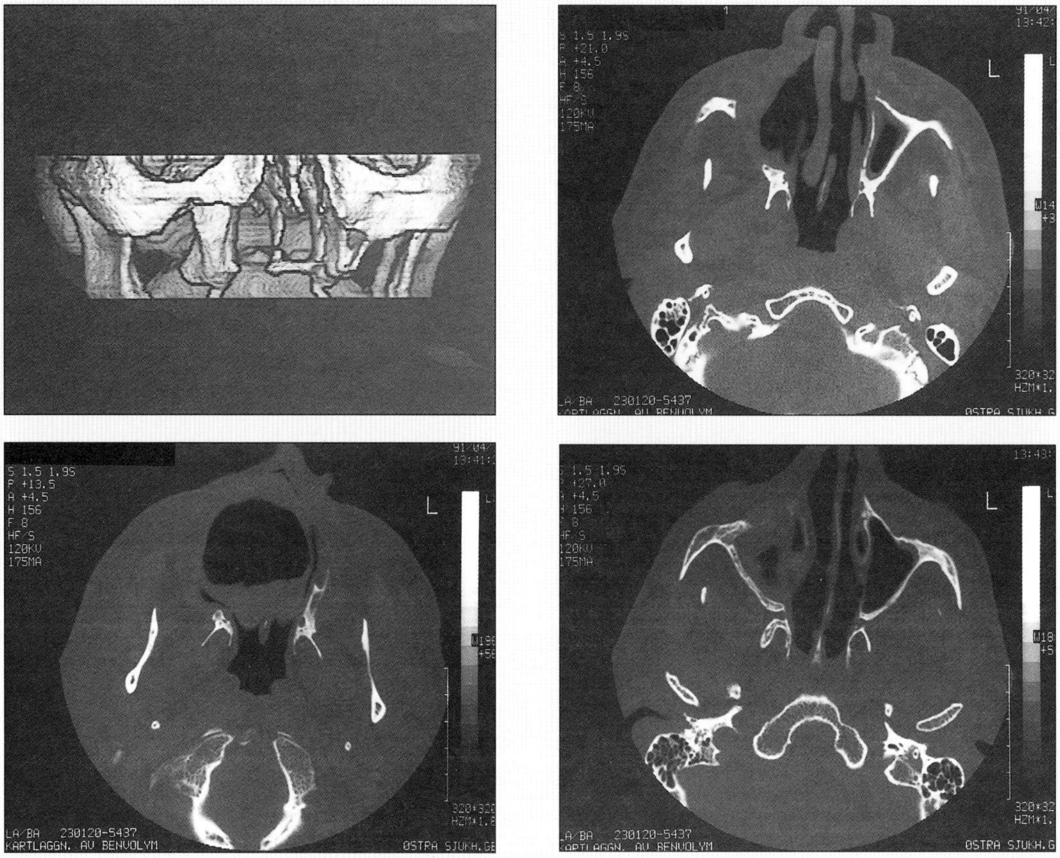

Figs 7-38a to 7-38d Preoperative CT scans (1991).

Patient Presentation (Maxillectomy Group) continued

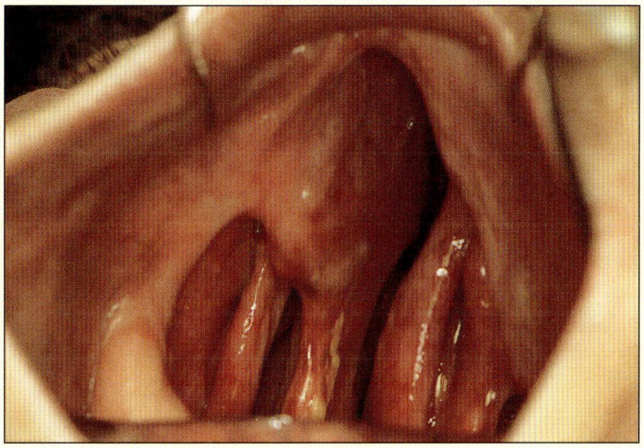

Fig 7-39 Clinical view of the defect.

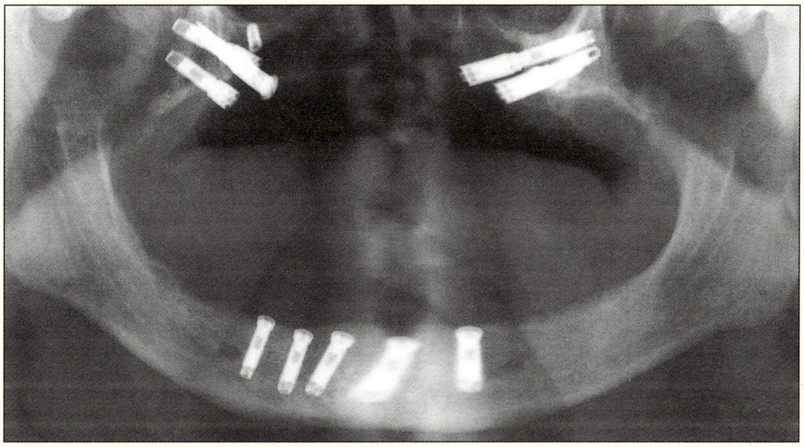

Fig 7-40 Panoramic view at abutment connection (1991).

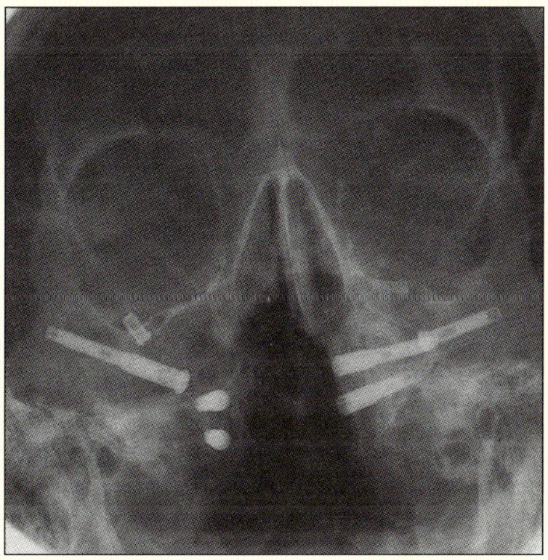

Fig 7-41 Occipitomental (Waters) view at abutment connection (1991).

Patient Presentation (Maxillectomy Group) continued

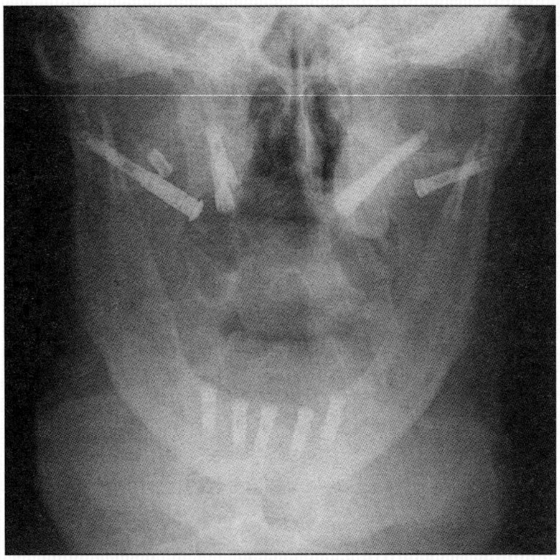

Fig 7-42 Posteroanterior view at abutment connection (1991).

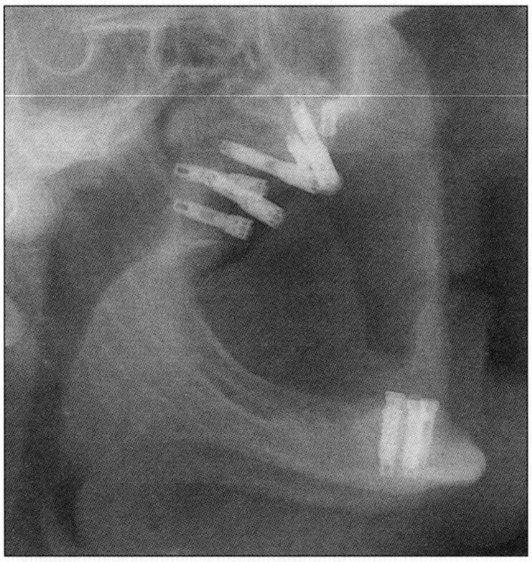

Fig 7-43 Profile at abutment connection (1991).

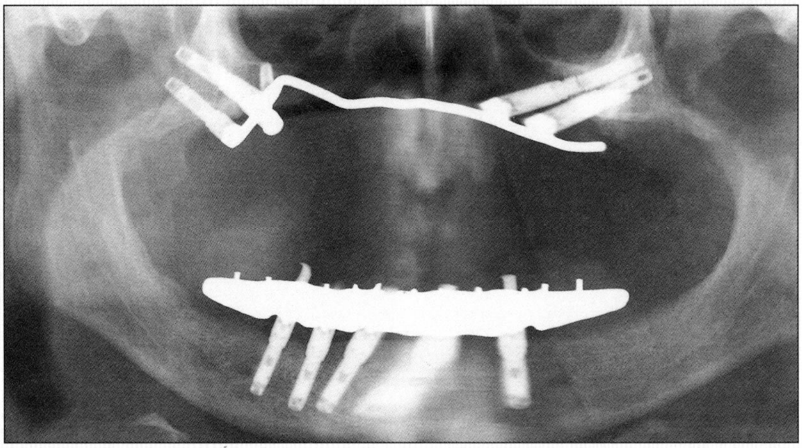

Fig 7-44 Panoramic view prior to replacement of a fractured fixture on the left side (1993).

Patient Presentation (Maxillectomy Group) continued

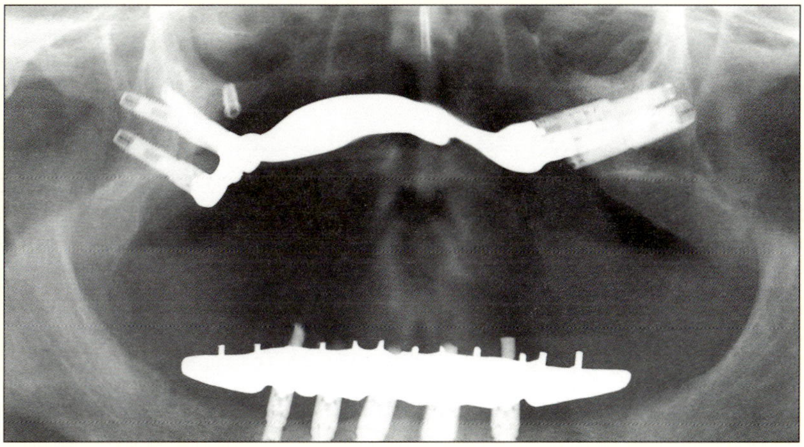

Fig 7-45 Panoramic view after revision surgery (1994).

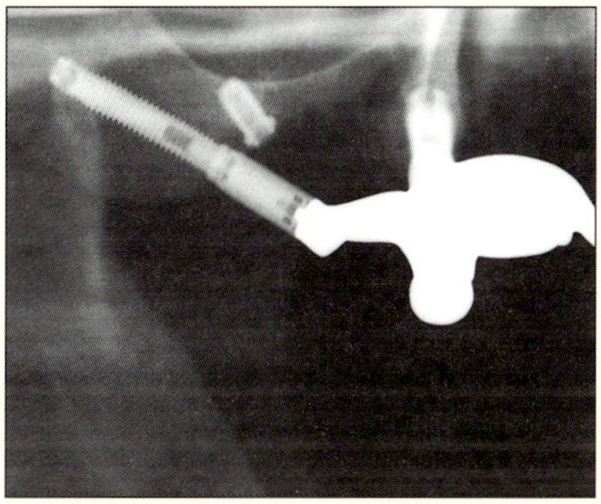

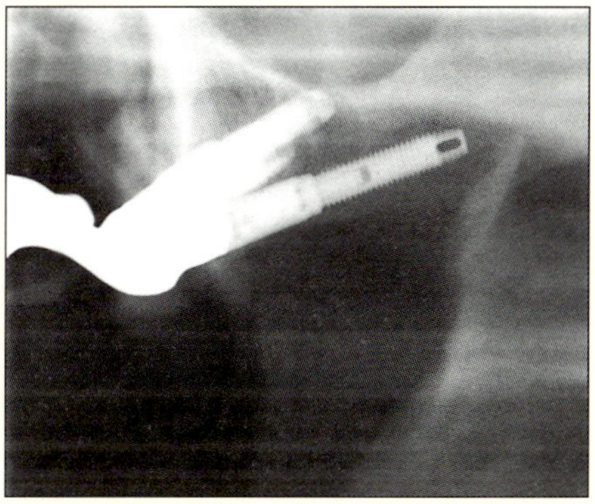

Figs 7-46a and 7-46b Sinus scanograms (frontal view; 1994).

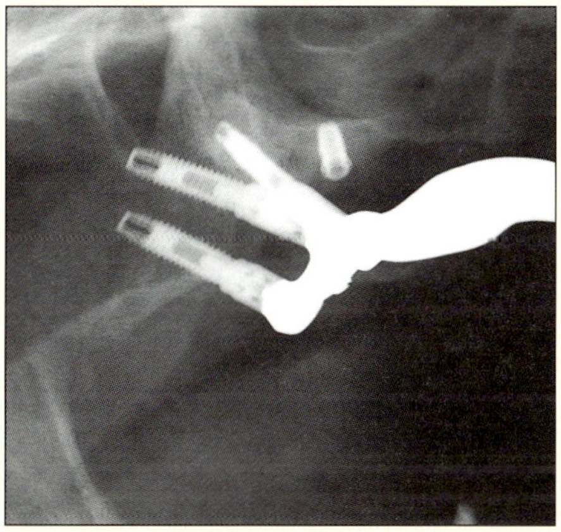

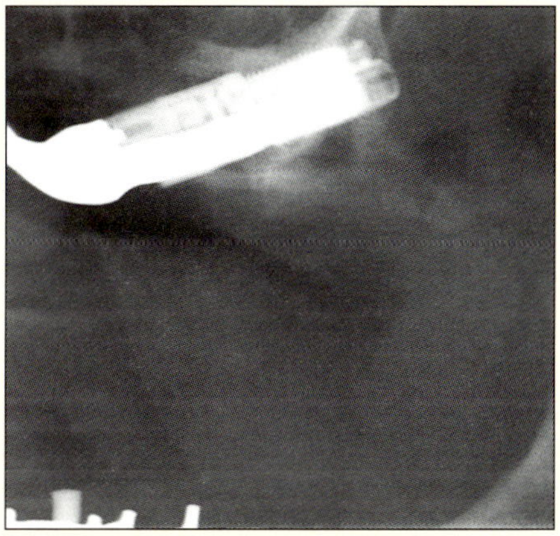

Figs 7-47a and 7-47b Sinus scanograms (lateral view; 1994).

Patient Presentation (Maxillectomy Group) continued

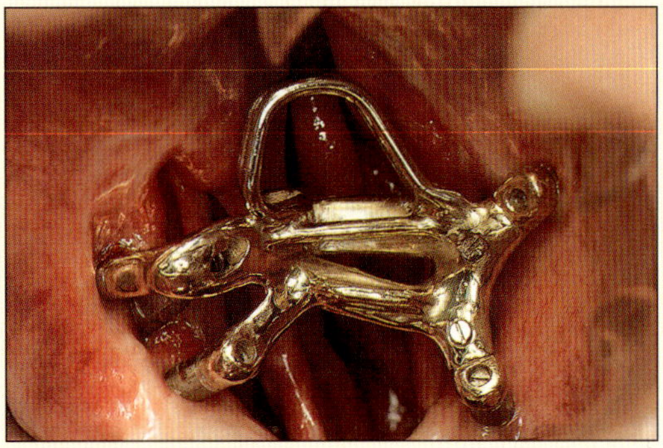

Fig 7-48 Bar construction for the fixture-supported overdenture with obturator.

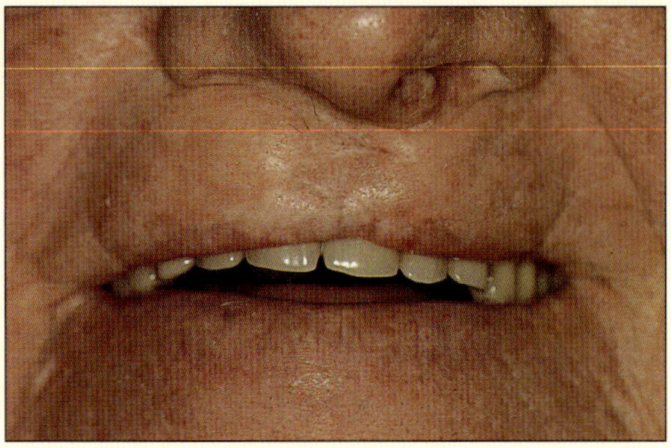

Fig 7-49 Clinical result.

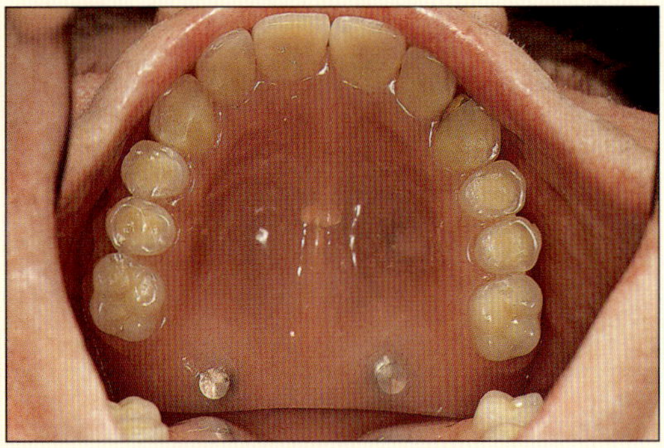

Fig 7-50 Intraoral view of prosthesis.

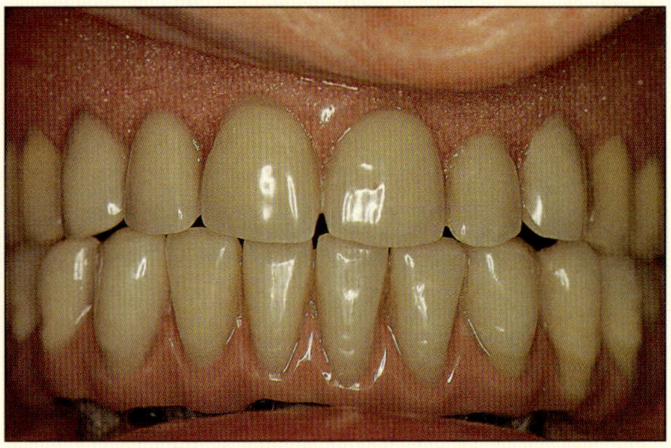

Fig 7-51 The final prosthesis.

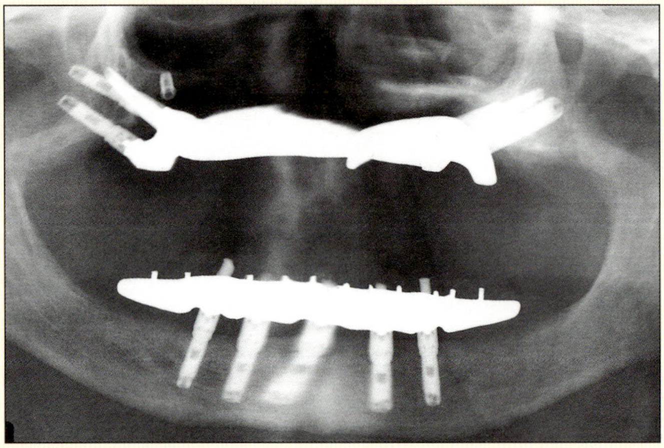

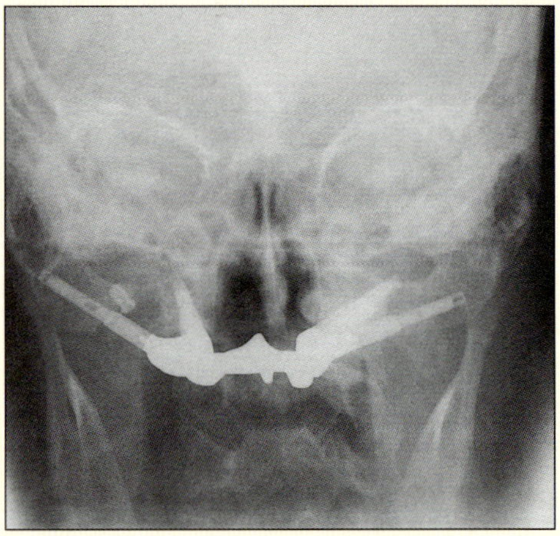

Figs 7-52a and 7-52b Stable situation shown 5 years after revision surgery (1999).

References

1. Brånemark P-I. Jaw reconstruction and intraosseous anchorage of dental prosthesis [in Swedish]. Läkartidningen 1971;68:3105–3116.
2. Brånemark P-I. Osseointegration and its experimental background. J Prosthet Dent 1983;50:399–410.
3. Brånemark P-I, Adell R, Breine U, Hansson BO, Lindström J, Ohlsson Å. Intraosseous anchorage of dental prostheses. I. Experimental studies. Scand J Plast Reconstr Surg 1969;3:81–100.
4. Brånemark P-I, Hansson BO, Adell R, Breine U, Lindström J, Hallén O, Öhman A. Osseointegrated implants in the treatment of the edentulous jaw. Experience from a 10-year period. Scand J Plast Reconstr Surg Suppl 1977;16:1–132.
5. Lekholm U, van Steenberghe D, Herrmann I, Bolender C, Folmer T, Gunne J, et al. Osseointegrated implants in the treatment of partially edentulous jaws: A prospective 5-year multicenter study. Int J Oral Maxillofac Implants 1994;9:627–635.
6. Jemt T, Chai J, Harnett J, Heath MR, Hutton JE, Johns RB, et al. A 5-year prospective multicenter follow-up report on overdentures supported by osseointegrated implants. Int J Oral Maxillofac Implants 1996;11:291–298.
7. Henry P, Laney WR, Jemt T, Harris D, Krogh P, Polizzi G, et al. Osseointegrated implants for single-tooth replacement: A prospective 5-year multicenter study. Int J Oral Maxillofac Implants 1996;11:450–455.
8. Lekholm U, Gunne J, Henry P, Higuchi K, Lindén U, Bergstrom C, van Steenberghe D. Survival of the Brånemark implant in partially edentulous jaws: A 10-year prospective multicenter study. Int J Oral Maxillofac Implants 1999;14:639–645.
9. Atwood DA. Reduction of residual ridges: A major oral disease entity. J Prosthet Dent 1971;26:266–279.
10. Tallgren A. The continuing reduction of the residual alveolar ridges in complete denture wearers: A mixed longitudinal study covering 25 years. J Prosthet Dent 1972;27:120–132.
11. Brånemark R, Lausmaa J, Ericson L, Thomsen P, Brånemark P-I, Skalak R. Anatomy of osseointegration and the transfer of load. In: Fonseca R-J, Davis WH (eds). Reconstructive Preprosthetic Oral and Maxillofacial Surgery, ed 2. Philadelphia: Saunders, 1995:165–224.
12. Brunski JB, Skalak R. Biomechanical considerations for craniofacial implants. In: Brånemark P-I, Tolman D (eds). Osseointegration in Craniofacial Reconstruction. Chicago: Quintessence, 1998.
13. Breine U, Brånemark P-I. Reconstruction of alveolar jaw bone. An experimental and clinical study of immediate and preformed autologous bone grafts in combination with osseointegrated implants. Scand J Plast Reconstr Surg 1980;14:23–48.
14. Sennerby L, Lundgren S. Histologic aspects of simultaneous implant and graft placement. In: Jensen OT (ed). The Sinus Bone Graft. Chicago: Quintessence, 1999:95–105.
15. Rasmusson L, Meredith N, Cho IH, Sennerby L. The influence of simultaneous versus delayed placement on the stability of titanium implants in onlay bone grafts. A histologic and biomechanic study in the rabbit. Int J Oral Maxillofac Surg 1999;28:224–231.
16. Lekholm U, Wannfors K, Isaksson S, Adielsson B. Oral implants in combination with bone grafts. A 3-year retrospective multicenter study using the Brånemark implant system. Int J Oral Maxillofac Surg 1999;28:181–187.
17. Sailer HF. A new method of inserting endosseous implants in totally atrophic maxillae. J Craniomaxillofac Surg 1989;17:299–305.
18. Kent JN, Block MS. Simultaneous maxillary sinus floor bone grafting and placement of hydroxyapatite-coated implants. J Oral Maxillofac Surg 1989;47:238–242.
19. Raghoebar GM, Brouwer TJ, Reintsema H, van Oort RP. Augmentation of the maxillary sinus floor with autogenous bone for the placement of endosseous implants. A preliminary report. J Oral Maxillofac Surg 1993;51:1198–1205.
20. Keller EE, Eckert SE, Tolman DE. Maxillary antral and nasal one-stage inlay composite bone grafts: Preliminary report on 30 recipient sites. J Oral Maxillofac Surg 1994;52:438–448.
21. Williamson LW, Higuchi KW. Bone graft reconstruction in conjunction with Brånemark fixture placement. Hawaii Dent J 1991;22:13–15.
22. Jensen OT (ed). The Sinus Bone Graft. Chicago: Quintessence, 1999.
23. Tulasne JF. Sinus grafting with calvarial bone. In: Jensen OT (ed). The Sinus Bone Graft. Chicago: Quintessence, 1999:107–116.
24. Tolman DE. Reconstructive procedures with endosseous implants in grafted bone: A review of the literature. Int J Oral Maxillofac Implants 1995;10:275–294.

25. Keller E, Tolman DE, Eckert SE. Maxillary antral-nasal inlay autogenous bone graft reconstruction of compromised maxillae: A 12-year retrospective study. Int J Oral Maxillofac Implants 1999;14:707–721.

26. Jensen OT, Shulman LB, Block MS, Iacono VJ. Report of the sinus consensus conference of 1996. Int J Oral Maxillofac Implants 1998;13(suppl):11–32.

27. Brånemark P-I, Gröndahl K, Nilsson P, Petrusson B, Öhrnell L-O. Osseointegration in os zygomaticum–An alternative anchorage site for oral and maxillofacial prosthetic reconstructions. Scand J Plast Reconstr Surg Hand Surg (in press).

28. Lekholm U, Zarb GA. Patient selection and preparation. In: Brånemark P-I, Zarb GA, Albrektsson T (eds).Tissue-Integrated Prostheses. Osseointegration in Clinical Dentistry. Chicago: Quintessence, 1985:199–210.

29. Brånemark P-I, Svensson B, van Steenberghe D. Ten-year survival rates of fixed prostheses on four or six implants ad modum Brånemark in full edentulism. Clin Oral Implants Res 1995;6:227–231.

30. Guedes de Azevoda R. Establishing a Protocol of Morbidity Evaluation of the Iliac Region as a Bone Graft Donor Site for Alveolar Reconstructions [thesis]. Bauru, Brazil: University of the Sacred Heart, 2000.

31. Brånemark P-I, Lindström J, Hallén O, Breine U, Jeppson PH, Öhman A. Reconstruction of the defective mandible. Scand J Plast Reconstr Surg 1975;9:116–128.

32. Kaplan EL, Meier P. Nonparametric estimation from incomplete observations. J Am Stat Assoc 1958;53: 457–462.

33. Peto R, Pike MC, Armitage P, Breslow NE, Cox DR, Howard SV, et al. Design and analysis of randomized clinical trials requiring prolonged observation of each patient. II. Analysis and examples. Br J Cancer 1977;35:1–39.

34. Cox DR. Regression models and life tables (with discussion). J Royal Stat Soc B 1972;34:187–220.

35. Bradley JV. Distribution-Free Statistical Test. London: Prentice-Hall, 1968:73–76.

36. Bradley JV. Distribution-Free Statistical Test. London: Prentice-Hall, 1968:78–80.

37. Bradley JV. Distribution-Free Statistical Test. London: Prentice-Hall, 1968:76–78.

38. Hirsch JM, Brånemark P-I. Fixture stability and nerve function after transposition and lateralization of the inferior alveolar nerve and fixture installation. Br J Oral Maxillofac Surg 1995;33(5):276–281.

39. Sullivan DY, Sherwood RL, Collins TA, Krogh PH. The reverse-torque test: A clinical report. Int J Oral Maxillofac Implants 1996;11:179–185.

40. Ahlqvist J, Borg K, Gunne J, Nilson H, Olsson M, Åstrand P. Osseointegrated implants in edentulous jaws: A 2-year longitudinal study. Int J Oral Maxillofac Implants 1990;5:155–163.

41. Öhrnell L-O, Engstrand P, Palmkvist J, Gröndahl K, Svensson B, Brånemark P-I. Osseointegration in single tooth rehabilitation. A long-term multicenter study. In: Francischone CE, Vasconcelos LW, Brånemark P-I (eds). Osseointegration and Esthetics in Single Tooth Rehabilitation. São Paulo: Quintessence, 2000.

42. Williams E, Rydevik B, Johns R, Brånemark P-I. Osseoperception and musculoskeletal function. [Report on the Workshop on Osseoperception and Musculoskeletal Function, 16 Sept 1998, London]. Göteborg, Sweden: Brånemark Osseointegration Center, 1999.

43. Adell R, Eriksson B, Lekholm U, Brånemark P-I, Jemt T. A long-term follow-up study of osseointegrated implants in the treatment of the totally edentulous jaws. Int J Oral Maxillofac Implants 1990;5: 347–359.

44. Åstrand P, Nord PG, Brånemark P-I. Titanium implants and onlay bone graft to the atrophic edentulous maxilla: A 3-year longitudinal study. Int J Oral Maxillofac Surg 1996;25:25–29.

45. van Steenberghe D, Naert I, Bossuyt M, deMars G, Calberson L, Ghyselen J, Brånemark P-I. The rehabilitation of the severely resorbed maxilla by simultaneous placement of autogenous bone grafts and implants: A 10-year evaluation. Clin Oral Investig 1997;1:102–108.

46. Widmark G, Andersson B, Andrup B, Carlsson GE, Ivanoff CJ, Lindvall AM. Rehabilitation of patients with severely resorbed maxillae by means of implants with or without bone grafts. A 1-year follow-up study. Int J Oral Maxillofac Implants 1998;13: 474–482.

47. Schliephake H, Neukam FW, Wichmann M. Survival analysis of endosseous implants in bone grafts used for the treatment of severe alveolar ridge atrophy. J Oral Maxillofac Surg 1997;55:1227–1234.

48. Johansson B. Bone Grafts and Dental Implants in the Reconstruction of the Severely Atrophied, Edentulous Maxilla [thesis]. Uppsala, Sweden: Uppsala University, 2001.

49. Brånemark P-I, Higuchi KW, Ferraz de Oliveira M (eds). Rehabilitation of Complex Cleft Palate and Craniomaxillofacial Defects: The Challenge of Bauru. Chicago: Quintessence, 1999.

50. Granström G, Tjellström A, Brånemark P-I, Fornander J. Bone-anchored reconstruction of the irradiated head and neck cancer patient. Otolaryngol Head Neck Surg 1993;108:334–343.

51. Granström G, Tjellström A, Brånemark P-I. Osseointegrated implants in irradiated bone: A case-controlled study using adjunctive hyperbaric oxygen therapy. J Oral Maxillofac Surg 1999;57:493–499.